CONTENTS

Berjinia Lopez   *619-471-4574*

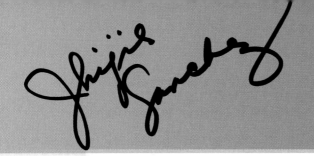

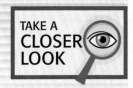

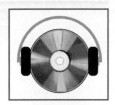

Medical Terminology: A Programmed Systems Approach, Ninth Edition, is a medical terminology textbook that teaches a word-building system using a programmed learning format. Thousands of medical words may be built by learning the Latin and Greek prefixes, suffixes, and word roots from which our English medical terms originate. Genevieve Smith and Phyllis Davis were the first to apply programmed learning to the teaching of medical terminology when they designed this textbook over 38 years ago. This system continues with the ninth edition to refine the process as well as to enhance this system using current educational technology.

Medical Terminology: A Programmed Systems Approach, Ninth Edition, is designed to provide a comprehensive entry-level study of medical language for health career learners with little or no previous experience. During 26 years of teaching medical terminology, I have been amazed by course assessment statistics showing positive results using this textbook. Instructor and student reviews also express their satisfaction and enthusiasm for using the materials in this textbook and its supplemental package.

ORGANIZATION

This book contains fifteen units progressively organized by word-building subject matter and body systems that may be easily organized for semester assignments.

The programmed learning, word-building system format presents and reinforces word parts and word building with over 2,000 frames—more than any other programmed medical terminology textbook. This format requires active participation through reading, writing, answering questions, labeling, repetition, and providing immediate feedback.

Various types of tables offer word part summaries, medical report data, and additional information about subjects that may not be included in the frames. Abbreviation tables appear at the end of each unit that include correct medical abbreviations. Abbreviation lists are included in Appendix B and organized by subjects including weights and measures, chemical symbols, diagnoses, procedures, health professions and organizations, and charting.

Several special features in each unit enhance the learning of medical terminology. See "About this Programmed System" on pages xiii–xv for a detailed description of each feature.

Practice software with review exercises, activities, and games with valuable feedback make learning fun. See "How to Use the Practice Software" on pages xvi–xviii.

CHANGES TO THE NINTH EDITION

- *New Unit 1.* We listened! Based on feedback from instructors, this unit was created by combining the previous Section B that contained material on the word-building system with portions of former Unit 1. This new unit places more emphasis on the importance of this beginning material. Review activities are revised, and a glossary is also added.
- *New Unit 2.* Formerly Unit 1, this new unit now focuses more clearly on surgical suffixes, dermatology, hematology, and diagnostic imaging. The rationale for this change is that former Unit 1 included too much content for an introductory chapter.
- *New Unit 3.* This unit includes all material from former Unit 2 and histology terms from former Unit 6.
- *New Unit 4.* This unit contains all material from former Unit 3, and includes new illustrations and an art labeling review activity.
- *New Unit 5.* This unit contains all material from former Unit 4. New vocabulary is also added to the glossary.
- *New Unit 6.* This unit contains all material from former Unit 5. A new table on urinalysis is added. New vocabulary is also added to the glossary.
- *New Unit 7.* This unit contains all material from former Unit 6.
- *New Unit 8.* This unit combines material from former Units 7 and 8 so that neurology and psychology terms are now in one unit instead of spread across two units.
- *New Unit 9.* Material on anatomic terminology from former Unit 8 and former Unit 9 is combined to form this new unit that focuses on location prefixes related to anatomic terms.
- *New Unit 10.* Material on surgical terms, diabetes terms, immunology, and number prefixes from former Unit 9 and all material from former Unit 10 are combined to create this new unit.

COMPREHENSIVE TEACHING AND LEARNING RESOURCES

Audio CDs ISBN: 1-4018-3224-5

Audio CDs to accompany *Medical Terminology: A Programmed Systems Approach,* Ninth Edition, include specific frame references and pronunciation of most terms, presented in unit order. The audio CDs are designed to allow learners to listen to the term, pronounce it aloud, and in many cases hear the term used in context or defined. The audio CDs may also be used as dictation by listening to the term, writing the word, and then checking the spelling of the terms in the textbook.

Also Available: Text/Audio CDs Value Package ISBN: 1-4018-5471-0

Instructor's Manual ISBN: 1-4018-3219-9

The *Instructor's Manual* features a correlation guide from the eighth to ninth edition, sample syllabi for 10-week and 16-week courses, quizzes for each unit, midterm exam, and comprehensive final exam. In addition, suggestions for course design, class activities, games, and unit word part lists are also included.

Computerized Test Bank ISBN: 1-4018-3218-0

The *Computerized Test Bank* includes over 1,400 questions with answers organized according to the fifteen units in the textbook. This CD-ROM test book assists you in creating personalized unit, midterm, and final examinations.

Features include:

- An interview mode or wizard, to guide you through the steps of creating a test in less than 5 minutes
- The capability to edit questions or to add an unlimited number of questions
- Online (Internet-based) testing capability
- Online (computer-based) testing capability
- A sophisticated word processor
- Numerous test layout and printing options
- Link groups of questions to common narratives

WebTUTOR™ Advantage

Designed to compliment the text, WebTUTOR™ is a content-rich, web-based teaching and learning aid that reinforces and clarifies complex concepts. Animations enhance learning and retention of material. The WebCT™ and Blackboard™ platforms also provide rich communication tools to instructors and learners, including a course calendar, chat, email, and threaded discussions.

> WebTUTOR™ Advantage on WebCT™ (ISBN: 1-4018-3220-2)
> Text Bundled with WebTUTOR™ Advantage on WebCT™
>   (ISBN: 1-4018-5382-X)
> Text Bundled with WebTUTOR™ Advantage on WebCT™ and Audio CDs
>   (ISBN: 1-4018-5473-7)
> WebTUTOR™ Advantage on Blackboard™ (ISBN: 0-7668-3221-0)
> Text Bundled with WebTUTOR™ Advantage on Blackboard™
>   (ISBN: 1-4018-5384-6)
> Text Bundled with WebTUTOR™ Advantage on Blackboard™ and Audio CDs
>   (ISBN: 1-4018-5472-9)

Delmar Learning's Medical Terminology Audio Library

This extensive audio library of medical terminology includes four audio CDs with over 3,600 terms pronounced, and a software CD-ROM. The CD-ROM presents terms organized by body system, medical specialty, and general medical term categories. The user can search for a specific term by typing in the term or key words, or clicking on a category to view an alphabetical list of all terms within the category. Hear the correct pronunciation of one term or listen to each term on the list pronounced automatically. Definitions can be viewed after hearing the pronunciation of terms.

> Institutional Version ISBN: 1-4018-3223-7
> Individual Version ISBN: 1-4018-3222-9

Medical Terminology: A Programmed Systems Approach, Eighth Edition, Complete On-Line Course

Designed as a stand-alone course, there is no need for a separate book. Everything is online! Content is presented in four major sections: study, practice, tests, and reports.

Study includes the content from the text, along with graphics and audio links. Practice includes exercises and games to reinforce learning. The test section includes tests with a variety of question types for each unit. A midterm and final exam are also available. The report section features student and instructor reports.

Individual Course ISBN: 0-7668-2754-2
Educational Course ISBN: 0-7668-2753-4

Delmar's Medical Terminology Image Library CD-ROM, Second Edition
ISBN: 1-4018-1009-8

This CD-ROM includes over 600 graphic files. These files can be incorporated into a PowerPoint, Microsoft Word, or WordPerfect presentation, used directly off the CD-ROM in a classroom presentation, or used to make color transparencies. The Image Library is organized around body systems and medical specialties. The library will include various anatomy, physiology, and pathology graphics of different levels of complexity. Instructors will be able to search and select the graphics that best apply to their teaching situation. This is an ideal resource to enhance your teaching presentation of medical terminology or anatomy and physiology.

Delmar's Medical Terminology CD-ROM Institutional Version
ISBN: 0-7668-0979-X

This exciting interactive reference, practice, and assessment tool is designed to compliment any medical terminology program. Features include the extensive use of multimedia—animations, video, graphics, and activities—to present terms and word-building features. The difficult functions, processes, and procedures help learners to more effectively learn from a textbook.

Delmar's Medical Terminology Video Series

This series of fourteen medical terminology videotapes is designed for allied health and nursing students who are enrolled in medical terminology courses. The videos may be used in class to supplement a lecture or in a resource lab by users who want additional reinforcement. The series can also be used in distance learning programs as a telecourse. The videos simulate a typical medical terminology class, and are organized by body system. The on-camera "instructor" leads students through the various concepts, interspersing lectures with graphics, video clips, and illustrations to emphasize points. This comprehensive series is invaluable to students trying to master the complex world of medical terminology.

Complete Set of Videos ISBN 0-7668-0976-5 (Videos can also be purchased individually.)

Delmar's Medical Terminology Flash!: Computerized Flashcards
ISBN: 0-7668-4320-3

Learn and review over 1,500 medical terms using this unique electronic flashcard program. Flash! is a computerized flashcard-type question and answer association program designed to provide learners with correct spellings, definitions, and pronunciations. The use of graphics and audio clips make it a fun and easy way for users to learn and test their knowledge of medical terminology.

It is our intent that *Medical Terminology: A Programmed Systems Approach,* Ninth Edition, Delmar Learning, be the best edition yet and continues to serve the needs of the learners and teachers who use it. We maintain our commitment to the original philosophy and integrity of this classic textbook.

ACKNOWLEDGMENTS

Medical Terminology: A Programmed Systems Approach, Ninth Edition, would not have been possible without many people contributing their expert observations, testing, evaluation, and skills. I would like to first thank the following team members from Delmar Learning whose dedicated professional publishing skills maintain the quality and integrity of this work.

Marah Bellegarde, Acquisitions Editor
Deb Flis, Developmental Editor
Daniel Branagh, Project Editor
Robert Plante, Art and Design Specialist
Bridget Lulay, Production Coordinator
Victoria Moore, Technology Project Manager

For many years I have been able to count on a number of healthcare practitioners and experienced medical terminology instructors in the community of Jackson, Michigan, who have made content contributions to this and previous editions. I extend my continued thanks to:

Billie Jean Buda, CMA, Medical Assistant Instructor
Lynne Schreiber MA, RT(R), RDMS, Diagnostic Medical Sonography Director
Ann Wentworth, BS, RT(R), RDMS, Medical Terminology Instructor
Marina Martinez-Kratz, MSN, Nursing Instructor
Grant Brown, Pharm D, Brown's Option Care
Andrew J. Krapohl, MD, Retired Obstetrician and Gynecologist
Patricia Krapohl, RN, MPH
Chip Smith, EMT-P
Denise Brzozowski, AAS, COT
Ann Blaxton, CCC-A, Professional Hearing Services
Sharon Rooney-Gandy, DO, General Surgery Board Certified
Paul H. Ernest, MD, TLC Eye Care PC
Shawn McKinney, COMT, American College of Ophthalmic Technology
Noreen Calus, MS, RHIA (posthumous)

W.A. Foote Memorial Hospital employees:

Shannon Griggs, RHIA, Assistant Director Health Information Department
Sally Mulnix, OT(R) and Maris Kalmbach OT(R), Occupational Therapists
Eva Maga, ASCP (MT), Medical Technologist
Cathy Rayl, RT(R), Diagnostic Imaging Clinical Education Supervisor
Mary Beth Reilly, Promotion Coordinator
Diane Jonas, CMT, Medical Transcription Supervisor

I also thank the following reviewers:

Lisa M. Carrigan, RN
Instructor
Applied Technology Center
Rock Hill, South Carolina

Barbara Hogg, MLT, RN, BSN
Nursing Faculty
South Arkansas Community College
El Dorado, Arkansas

Patricia A. Ireland, CMT, FAAMT
Freelance Medical/Technical Editor
Facilitator, Gatlin Education Services Medical Terminology/Medical
    Transcription course (medical transcriptionist since 1968)

Marina Martinez-Kratz, RNC, MS
Assistant Professor of Nursing
Jackson Community College
Jackson, Michigan

Donald C. Rizzo, PhD
Head: Science and Mathematics Academic Unit
Professor of Biology
Marygrove College
Detroit, Michigan

Victoria Wetle, RN, EdD
Chair, Health Services Management
Chemeketa Community College
Oregon

I would also like to acknowledge the contribution that 26 years of medical terminology students have made at Jackson Community College in Jackson, Michigan, and other students from around the world. Through direct comments, letters, and emails, they remind me what it is like to be a beginning medical terminology student, what improvements are needed in the textbook to enhance learning, and what details must be addressed.

Finally, I am grateful for the continued support and understanding of my husband and computer technician, Timothy J. Dennerll, PhD; my daughter, Diane; my son, Raymond; and my mother, Helen Stamcos Tannis. You are my inspiration.

Sincerely,
Jean M. Tannis Dennerll BS CMA

LIST OF ILLUSTRATIONS

ABOUT THIS PROGRAMMED SYSTEM

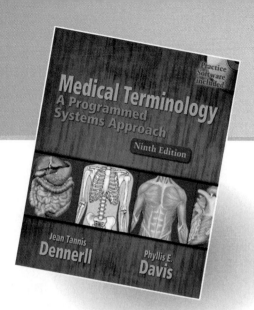

Medical Terminology: A Programmed Systems Approach, Ninth Edition, is carefully designed to help you learn medical terminology.

OBJECTIVES OF THE LEARNING SYSTEM

Upon completion of this system, the learner should be able to:

1. Build literally thousands of medical words from Greek and Latin prefixes, suffixes, word roots, and combining forms.
2. Define medical words by analyzing their Greek and Latin parts.
3. Spell medical words correctly.
4. Use a medical dictionary.
5. Pronounce medical words correctly.
6. Recall acceptable medical abbreviations that represent phrases and terms.

To maximize the benefits of this learning system, familiarize yourself with the following features.

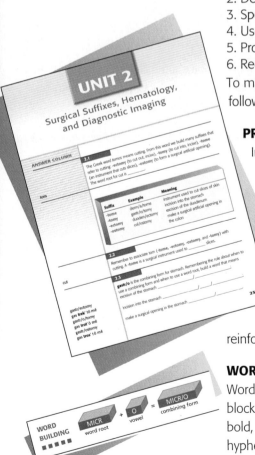

PROGRAMMED LEARNING FORMAT

Information is presented and learned in small numbered sections called frames. You will have an active part in learning medical terminology using this successful programmed approach. The right column contains a statement and an answer blank; the left column provides the answer. Cover the answer column with a bookmark (two are provided as part of the back cover). Read the right column of the frame and write your answer in the blank. Pull down the bookmark to reveal the answer and confirm your response. Then move on to the next frame. Learning one bit of information at a time is part of programmed learning. Another part is continual reinforcement of word parts and terms throughout the book.

WORD-BUILDING SYSTEM AND WORD PARTS

Word roots, combining forms, prefixes, and suffixes are important building blocks in the word-building system. **Combining forms** are highlighted in bold, **prefixes** in blue with a hyphen after each, and **suffixes** in red with a hyphen preceding each.

FEATURES FRAMES

Information—present interesting facts to help retention

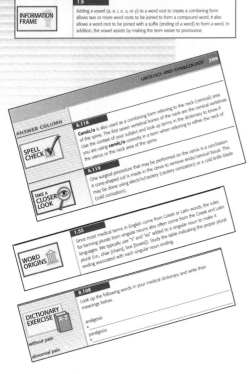

Spell Check—clues and special notes on troublesome spelling

Take a Closer Look—analyzes similar terms

Word Origins—encourages memory retention through fascinating references using Greek and Roman mythology, legends, and etymology

Dictionary Exercise—provides learners with practice using a medical dictionary

FULL-COLOR ART

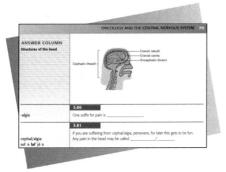

Even more full-color illustrations and photos are included in this edition. Art and photos are placed near their reference—not in a separate color section. A complete list of all art is on pages xi and xii.

PROFESSIONAL PROFILES

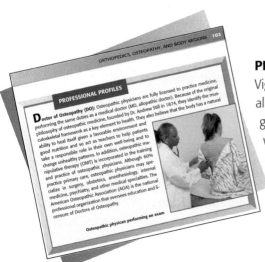

Vignettes and photos describing the function and credentials of many allied health professions are placed throughout the text. These profiles give information about various professions and possible career paths as well as reinforce the importance of medical terminology for all health professionals.

ABBREVIATIONS

Abbreviations are covered many ways. Several frames work abbreviations, a list of abbreviations and meanings is included in each unit, and activities specifically identify and test abbreviations. Appendix B includes a comprehensive list of abbreviations.

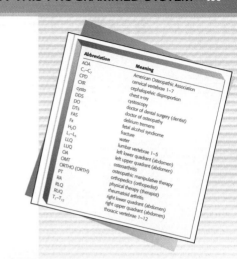

AUDIO CDS

After completing each unit, you may want to listen to the audio CDs that accompany the text. You can use the audio CDs to listen to each term and repeat the term aloud for pronunciation practice. You may also write the term and its definition to check spelling and meaning comprehension.

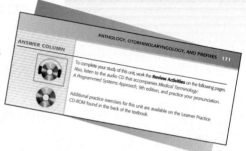

GLOSSARY

Unit end glossaries summarize terms and definitions in a frame-type format for easy study and review.

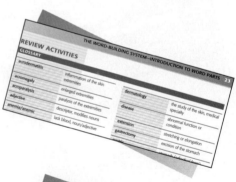

REVIEW ACTIVITIES

Activities include a variety of exercises to reinforce terms learned within the frames. Also included are *case study* excerpts from actual medical records featuring medical terms in context along with questions to test and reinforce spelling and definitions. *Crossword puzzles* provide definition to term review in an easy, fun format.

HOW TO USE THE PRACTICE SOFTWARE

The Practice Software is designed to accompany *Medical Terminology: A Programmed Systems Approach*, Ninth Edition, so you can learn even the toughest medical terms. By using these exercises and games, you'll challenge yourself to make your study of medical terms more effective, and have fun!

GETTING STARTED

Getting started is easy. Follow these simple steps to install the program on your computer:

1. Double click on My Computer.
2. Double click the Control Panel icon.
3. Double click Add/Remove Programs.
4. Click the Install button and follow the on-screen prompts from there.

Now you can take advantage of the following features.

MAIN MENU

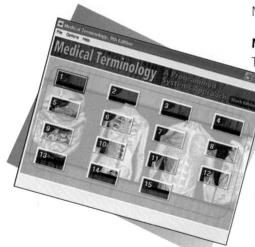

The main menu follows the unit organization of the text exactly—which makes it easy for you to find your way around. Just click on the button for the unit opening screen to select the exercises and games for that unit.

As you navigate through the software, check the toolbar for other exercises, games, and resetting and printing features. The button bar allows you to retrace your steps, while the Exit button lets you end your practice session quickly and easily.

ONLINE HELP

If you get stuck, just press F1 or click Help on the toolbar for assistance. The online help includes instructions for all parts of the Practice Software.

Basic System Requirements:

- Microsoft ®Windows® 95 or better
- Pentium or faster processor
- 24 MB or more RAM
- Double-spin CD-ROM drive
- 10 MB or more free hard drive space

UNIT SCREEN

The program lets you choose how you want to learn the material. Select one of the exercises for practice, review, or self-testing or click on a game to practice unit terms in a fun format.

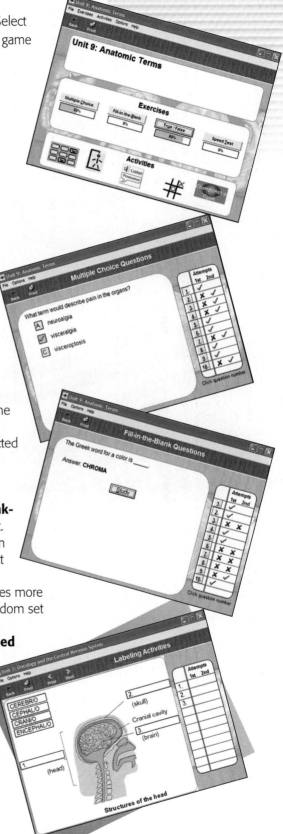

EXERCISES

The software acts as your own private tutor. For each exercise, it chooses from a bank of over questions covering all fifteen units. To start, simply:

- Choose an exercise from those displayed such as **multiple choice**, **fill-in**, **true/false**, or **labeling** exercise, whichever appeals to you. Highlighted terms throughout the exercises are directly hyperlinked to the audio pronunciation of that term. Click the term to hear it pronounced.
- Each exercise offers you a series of ten questions randomly selected from that unit's bank of questions. Each question gives you two chances to answer correctly.
- Instant **feedback** tells you whether you are right or wrong. **Rationales** explain why an answer was correct and **critical thinking hints** are provided when your first-choice answer is incorrect.
- The percentage of correct answers displays on the unit screen. An on-screen score sheet (which you can print) lets you track correct and incorrect answers.
- Review of previous questions and answers for an exercise provides more in-depth understanding. Or start an exercise over with a new, random set of questions.
- When you're ready for an additional challenge, try the timed **Speed Test**. Once you've finished, it displays your score and the time you took to complete the test, so you can see how much you've learned.

GAMES

To further reinforce your skill and knowledge, play one of the five games that you can enjoy alone, with a partner, or on teams.

- **Concentration:** Match terms or abbreviations to their corresponding definitions under the cards as the seconds tick by.
- **Hangman:** Review your spelling and vocabulary by choosing the correct letters to spell medical terms before you're "hanged."
- **Crossword Puzzles:** Using the definition clues provided, fill in the medical terms to complete each puzzle. A click of the Check button highlights incorrect answers in blue.
- **Board Game:** Challenge your classmates and increase your knowledge by playing this question-and-answer game.
- **Tic-Tac-Toe:** You or your team must correctly answer a medical question before placing an X or an O.

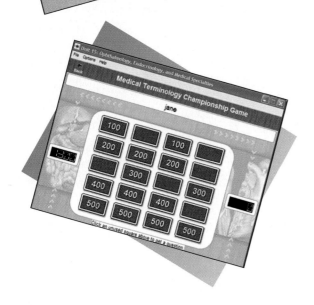

How to Work the Program—
Directions for Use
of Programmed Learning

SECTION A

ANSWER COLUMN

A.1

Directions: Tear off the bookmark from the back cover and use it to cover the answer column.

frame
Now go on to Frame A.2

A frame is a piece of information, plus a blank (_____) in which you write. All this material following the number A.1 is a _____.
Check your answer by sliding down your bookmark.

A.2

By checking your answer immediately, you know if you are correct. This immediate knowledge helps you to learn only what is (choose one)

correct
Now go on to Frame A.3

_____ (correct/incorrect).
Check your answer by sliding down your bookmark.

A.3

Programmed learning is a way of learning that gives you immediate feedback and allows you to work at your own speed. When you work a series of frames and are

program

certain that you know the terms, you are learning from a _____.
Check your answer by sliding down your bookmark.

A.4

check
Write

Always _____ your answers immediately. _____ your answers in the blank or on a separate paper.

The first time you read the frames you may want to just think of the answer. Then read the frames a second time and write the answer on the blank provided or on a separate sheet of paper and check your answer again.

ANSWER COLUMN

INFORMATION FRAME

A.5

When you write a new word and check your answer, you will usually find the pronunciation given. Pronounce the word aloud and listen to what you are saying. Practice proper pronunciation by listening to the audio CDs prepared to accompany *Medical Terminology: A Programmed Systems Approach* Ninth Edition. Pronouncing words correctly assists in spelling correctly, speaking medical phrases correctly and understanding medical terms when you hear them pronounced (as in dictation).

A.6

prō′nun sē ā′shun

The front inside cover presents a pronunciation key to vowel and consonant sounds and the phonetic system used in this text. The syllable with the major accent is highlighted in bold print.

A.7

aloud

Practice saying each new medical word _____ several times. Practicing pronunciation helps you to focus on each syllable so you do not miss any part of the word as you read. Pronunciation will also help you see each letter of the word and improve your spelling.

A.8

medical
one

When you see a blank space (_____) your answer will need only one word. In the sentence, "This is a program in _____ terminology," you know to use _____ word.

A.9

long

A single blank (_____) contains a clue. It is proportional to the length of the word needed. A short blank (_____) means one short word. A long blank (_____) means one _____ word.

A.10

medical terminology
more than one word

When you see an asterisk and a blank (*_____), your answer will require more than one word. In the sentence, "This is a programmed course in
*_____,"
your answer requires *_____.

A.11

more than one word

In (*_____) there is no clue to the length of the words. The important thing to remember is that an asterisk and a blank means
*_____.

ANSWER COLUMN

	A.12
aloud	Use the pronunciation key on the inside front cover to aid in proper practice when saying words _____.
	A.12
spelling	Saying each term aloud will also improve your _____.
	A.13
anything from interesting to dull (if you did not answer this one, it doesn't matter) use your own words	When you see a double asterisk and a blank (**_____), use your own words. In the sentence, "I think a programmed course in medical terminology will be **_____," you are expected to **_____.
	A.14
never look ahead	When working a program, *never look ahead.* The information presented in the frames is in a special order, so do not skip around and *_____.
	A.15
one length more than one use your own aloud never look ahead	Now summarize what you have learned so far. A single blank means _____ word. A single blank gives a clue about the _____ of the word. A single asterisk means *_____ word. A double asterisk means *_____ words. Practice saying each term _____. The frames are in a special order so *_____.
	A.16
	Saying, listening, seeing, writing, and *thinking* will do much for your learning. On the following drawing, find the parts of the brain used when saying, listening, seeing, writing, and thinking.

1. thinking area
2. hearing area
3. saying area
4. seeing area
5. writing area

INFORMATION FRAME

A.17

If you have five parts of the brain working for you at the same time, you will learn much faster. This is efficient learning. It makes sense to say a word, listen to it, look at it, write it, and think about it in one operation.

A.18

This programmed learning, word-building system encourages you to *read* (look and understand) about medical terms, *say* them aloud correctly, *listen* to them on audio CDs, *write* the terms as answers in the blanks and review activities, and *think* about the terms as you use them to complete statements. Doing this uses at least _____ areas of your brain and helps you learn more efficiently.

five

See how efficiently you are learning!

You are now ready to move on to an introduction of the word-building system and learning your first medical terms.

UNIT 1

The Word-Building System—Introduction to Word Parts Including Word Roots, Suffixes, Prefixes, Parts of Speech, and Plural Formation

ANSWER COLUMN

1.1

This word-building system is used throughout the textbook to help you learn medical terminology. By combining programmed learning and the word-building system, you

medical

will soon be learning hundreds, even thousands, of _____ terms.

1.2

It would be impossible to simply memorize thousands of medical terms and remember them for very long. The word-building system teaches word parts including word roots, combining forms, prefixes, and suffixes as well as rules about grammar usage and spelling. In a short time you will be easily using the

word-building system

*_____.

1.3

All words have a word root. Even ordinary, everyday words have a

word root

*_____.

1.4

The word root is the foundation of a word. Trans/port, ex/port, im/port, and

word root

sup/port have port as their *_____.

1.5

word root

Suf/fix, pre/fix, af/fix, and fix/ation have fix as their *_____.

1.6

The word root for stomach in gastr/itis, gastr/ectomy, and gastr/ic is

gastr

_____.

NOTE: Notice that when a combining form is presented by itself it is printed in bold text.

1.7

word root

The foundation of the word is the *_____.
NOTE: A slash mark (diagonal) "/" is used to divide words into their word parts.
EXAMPLE:

gastr/	**o/**	duoden/	**-ostomy**
word root	combining vowel	word root	suffix

1.8

combining form

A *combining form* is a word root plus a vowel. In the word therm/o/meter, **therm/o** is the *_____.

WORD BUILDING ▪▪▪▪▪	MICR + O = MICR/O
	word root vowel combining form

1.9

INFORMATION FRAME 💡

Adding a vowel (a, e, i, o, u, or y) to a word root to create a combining form allows two or more word roots to be joined to form a compound word. It also allows a word root to be joined with a suffix (ending of a word) to form a word. In addition, the vowel assists by making the term easier to pronounce.

1.10

vowel or letter o

In the word cyt/o/meter (instrument used to measure [count] cells), the *_____ allows cyt to be joined to meter.

1.11

combining form

In the words micr/o/scope, micr/o/film, and micr/o/be, **micr/o** is the *_____.

1.12

INFORMATION FRAME 💡

Usually a combining form is used when joining a word root to a suffix or other word root that begins with a *consonant* (for example, b, d, p, s, t, v).

WORD BUILDING ▪▪▪▪▪	GASTR/O + DUODEN/O + SCOPY = GASTRODUODENOSCOPY
	combining form combining form suffix compound word

Compound microscope

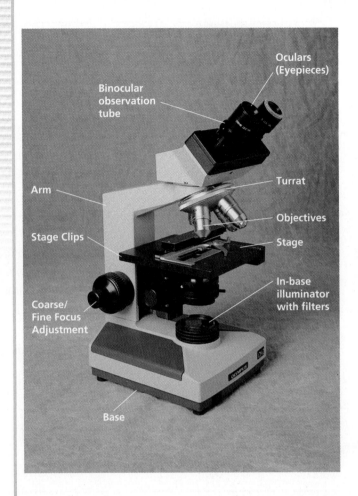

Binocular observation tube

Oculars (Eyepieces)

Arm

Turrat

Objectives

Stage Clips

Stage

In-base illuminator with filters

Coarse/ Fine Focus Adjustment

Base

1.13

would
neur/o/spasm

You (choose one) _____ (would/would not) use a combining form to join the word roots neur and spasm to form _____/____/_____.

1.14

> INFORMATION FRAME

Use a word root, not a combining form, when joining a word root with a suffix or another word root that begins with a vowel (a, e, i, o, u, y).

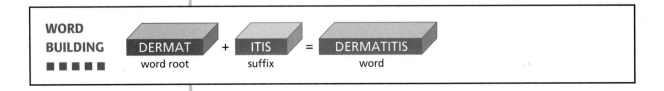

WORD BUILDING
■ ■ ■ ■ ■

DERMAT + ITIS = DERMATITIS
word root   suffix   word

ANSWER COLUMN

1.15

would not

lymph/adenopathy

You (choose one) _____ (would/would not) use a combining form to join the word parts lymph and adenopathy to form

_____/_____.

NOTE: Combining forms are never used as a suffix. They require an ending to complete a word. There are many exceptions to the rules about combining form usage stated above. Always consult your medical dictionary for correct spelling of new terms. That way you will know if the new word you created is actually a medical word.

1.16

compound words

Compound words can be formed when two or more word roots are used to build the word. Even in ordinary English, two or more word roots are used to form

*_____ (for example, shorthand or download).

1.17

compound word

Sometimes word roots are words. Two or more word roots still form a compound word. Chickenpox is a *_____.

WORD BUILDING
■ ■ ■ ■ ■

CHICKEN + POX = CHICKENPOX
word root   word root   compound word
(word)   (word)

1.18

underage

Form a compound word using the word roots under and age.

_____

Varicella—chickenpox
(Courtesy of Robert A. Silverman, MD, Clinical Associate Professor, Department of Pediatrics, Georgetown University)

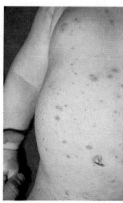

ANSWER COLUMN

1.19

Form a compound word from the word roots brain and stem.

brainstem

_____

1.20

Because they are formed by joining two or more word roots, therm/o/meter, cyt/o/meter, micr/o/scope, and micr/o/surgery are all

compound words

*_____.

1.21

Compound words can also be formed from a combining form and a whole word. Thermometer is a compound word built from a combining form and a word. In

combining form
whole word (suffix)

the word therm/o/meter, **therm/o** is the *_____,

meter is the *_____.

1.22

Build a compound word using the combining form **micr/o** plus

-scope

micr/o/scope
mī′ krō skōp
micr/o/surgery
mī krō **ser**′ jer ē
micr/o/meter
mī **kro**′ me ter

micr/o/_____ (instrument used to see small things);

-surgery

micr/o/_____ (surgery using a microscope);

-meter

micr/o_____ (device used to measure small things).

Remember practice pronouncing the terms aloud as well.

1.23

Build a compound word using the combining form **hydr/o** plus

-phobia

hydr/o/phobia
hī drō **fō**′ bē ə
hydr/o/cele
hī′ drō sēl
hydr/o/therapy
hī drō **thair**′ ə pē

hydr/o/_____(fear of water);

-cele

hydr/o/_____(fluid in a saclike cavity);

-therapy

hydr/o/_____(treatment using water).

1.24

-**ic** is an adjective suffix. In medical terminology, compound words are usually built from a combining form, a word root, and a suffix. In the word micr/o/scop/ic,

micr/o is the combining form;

scop is the word root;

suffix

-**ic** is the _Suffix_ .

ANSWER COLUMN

1.25

In medical terminology, compound words are usually built in the following order: combining form + word root + suffix. The word part coming first is usually a

combining form   *_____. The word part that comes last is the

suffix   _____.

NOTE: The suffixes are highlighted in **[red]** print throughout this textbook for easy identification.

1.26

In the word therm/o/metr/ic,
therm/o is the combining form;

word root   metr is the *_____;

suffix   **-ic** is the _____.

1.27

radi/o/grapher   Build a word from the combining form **radi/o**;
rā dē **og**′ raf er   the suffix **-grapher**.

1.28

Build a word from the combining form **acr/o**; the word root dermat;

acr/o/dermat/itis   and the suffix **-itis**. ACR / O / DERMAT / iTiS
a′ krō der′ ma **ti**′ tis

1.29

INFORMATION
FRAME

If you had difficulty with either of the last two frames, rework the program starting with Frame 1.24.
NOTE: The suffix is usually described first in the definition; for example,
(1) pertaining to (**-ic**), (2) electricity—electric; or
(1) inflammation (**-itis**) of the (2) bladder (cyst)—cystitis.

1.30

The ending that follows a word root is called a **suffix**. You can change the meaning of a word by putting another part after it. This other part is also called a

suffix   _____ (highlighted in **red**).
NOTE: Notice in this textbook the suffixes are highlighted in **red** and proceded by a hyphen (-).

1.31

The suffix **-er** means either one who or one which. The word root port (to carry) is changed by putting **-er** after it. In the word port/er (one who carries), **-er** is a

suffix   _____.

1.32

one who

A medical practitioner is *_____ practices medicine.

1.33

suffix

In the word read/able, **-able** changes the meaning of read.
-able is a _____.

WORD BUILDING
■ ■ ■ ■ ■

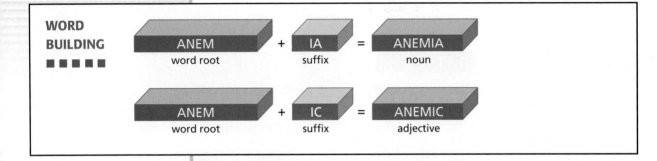

1.34

INFORMATION FRAME

Suffixes also may change a word's part of speech. For example, nouns (naming persons, places, or things) may be changed to adjectives (descriptors) such as the following.

Noun	Suffix	Adjective	Suffix
cyanosis	**-osis**	cyanotic	**-otic**
anemia	**-ia**	anemic	**-ic**
mucus	**-us**	mucous	**-ous**
ilium	**-um**	iliac	**-ac**
condyle	**-e**	condylar	**-ar**
carpus	**-us**	carpal	**-al**

1.35

-osis
-ia
-um

In the words cyan/osis, anem/ia, and ili/um, the noun suffixes are
oasis ,
_ia_ ,
and _um_ .

1.36

By now you may be curious about the meanings of several of these medical terms. Look up the following words in your medical dictionary, then write the meaning below.

Word   Meaning

cyanosis = *abnormal bluish discoloration of the lips, skin and mucous membranes, due to lack of oxygen in the blood*

condyle = *a bony projection that fits into a joint*

anemia = *lack of blood*

emetic = *an agent that induces vomiting*

Good work.

1.37

List the suffixes that make the following nouns adjectives.

<table>
<tr><td>**Adjective**</td><td>**Nouns**</td></tr>
<tr><td>ili/ac</td><td>ilium</td></tr>
<tr><td>cyan/otic</td><td>cyanosis</td></tr>
<tr><td>anem/ic</td><td>anemia</td></tr>
<tr><td>duoden/al</td><td>duodenum</td></tr>
<tr><td>vomit/ous</td><td>vomit</td></tr>
<tr><td>condyl/ar</td><td>condyle</td></tr>
<tr><td>man/iac</td><td>mania</td></tr>
<tr><td>arthr/itic</td><td>arthritis</td></tr>
<tr><td>eme/tic</td><td>emesis</td></tr>
</table>

Answer column:
-ac
-otic
-ic
-al
-ous
-ar
-iac
-itic
-tic

INFORMATION FRAME

1.38

Verbs are words that represent action or a state of being.
EXAMPLE: incise, ambulate, love.

1.39

The suffixes **-ed** or **-ing** added to the word vomit alter the tense of this verb (when the action takes place). Create the past tense by adding **-ed** to
vomit: _____, and the present participle by adding **-ing** to
vomit: _____.

Answer column:
vomited
vomiting

1.40

Use the suffixes **-ed** and **-ing** with the word inject.
_____ past tense;
_____ present participle.

Answer column:
injected
injecting

ANSWER COLUMN

Injectable forms of medication: (A) ampule, (B) cartridge, (C) multidose vial

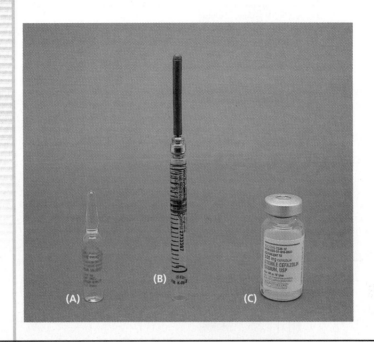

Read and study this table. Then move on to the next frame.

Noun Suffixes	Examples
-ism—condition, state, or theory	hyperthyroidism
-tion—condition	contraction, relaxation
-ist—specialist	psychiatrist
-er—one who	radiographer
-ity—quality	sensitivity
Adjectival Suffixes	**Examples**
-ous—possessing, having, full of	nervous, mucous
-able ⎱ —ability	injectable
-ible ⎰	edible

1.41

condition or state

Hyper/thyroid/ism is a _____*condition*_____ of too much secretion by the thyroid gland.

1.42

theory

Darwin/ism presents a theory of evolution. Mendel/ism presents a _____*theory*_____ of heredity.

ANSWER COLUMN

1.43

condition
condition

Contrac/tion is a _____ of muscle shortening. Relaxa/tion is the _____ of diminished tension.

1.44

nouns

Contraction and relaxation are (choose one) _____ (nouns/adjectives) because they name a condition.

1.45

a specialist
one who

A psychiatr/ist is *_____ who practices psychiatry. A medical practition/er is *_____ practices medicine.

1.46

noun

The word practitioner is a (choose one) _____ (noun/adjective).

1.47

quality

quality

-ity indicates a quality. Conductiv/ity expresses the _____ of conducting nerve and muscle impulses. Sensitiv/ity expresses the _____ of nervous tissue excitability related to receiving stimuli.

1.48

noun

Irritabil/ity is a (choose one) _____ (noun/adjective).

1.49

having a material
(substance)
having, possessing

Mucus, a noun, is a watery secretion. Muc/ous, an adjective, refers to the nature of *_____ secreted by the mucous membrane.
Ser/ous refers to the nature of _____ material lining closed body cavities such as the abdomen.

1.50

having, possessing
nerve

Nerv/ous refers to _____ too much stress, or having a type of tissue made of _____ cells.

1.51

adjectives

Words ending in **-ous** are (choose one) _____ (nouns/adjectives).

ANSWER COLUMN

	1.52
ability	**-ible** and **-able** indicate ability. To say a food is digestible is to say it has the
ability	_____ to be digested. To say a fracture is reducible is to say that it has the _____ to be reduced.

	1.53
ability	To say that lungs are inflatable is to say that they have the _____ to inflate.

	1.54
adjectives	Words ending in **-ible** or **-able** are (choose one) _____ (nouns/adjectives).

1.55

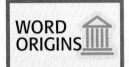

WORD ORIGINS

Since most medical terms in English come from Greek or Latin words, the rules for forming plurals from singular nouns also often come from the Greek and Latin languages. We typically use "s" and "es" added to a singular noun to make it plural (i.e., chair [chairs], box [boxes]). Study the table indicating the proper plural ending associated with each singular noun ending.

Singular Suffixes	Plural Suffixes
Greek	
-on	**-a**
-ma	**-mata**
-sis	**-ses**
-nx	**-ges**
Latin	
-a	**-ae**
-us	**-i**
-um	**-a**
-is	**-es**
-ex	**-ices**
-ix	**-ices**
-ax	**-aces**

ANSWER COLUMN

1.56

Now see if you are able to recognize the suffix patterns and write them in the blanks provided. Check your answers. Then look up each word in the medical dictionary.

Greek Singular Noun	Greek Plural Form
spermatozoon	spematozoa
ganglion	ganglia

-on, -a

suffix _____on_____   suffix _____a_____

carcinoma   carcinomata
lipoma   lipomata

-ma, -mata

suffix _____ma_____   suffix _____mata_____

crisis   crises
prognosis   prognoses

-is, -es

suffix _____is_____   suffix _____es_____

larynx (**laryng/o**)   larynges
pharynx (**pharyng/o**)   pharynges

-nx, -ges

suffix _____nx_____   suffix _____ges_____

Use what you just learned about Greek to form the plurals for the following terms.

protozoa   protozoan (protozoon)   _____
sarcomata   sarcoma   _____
diagnoses   diagnosis   _____
phalanges   phalanx (**phalang/o**)   _____

Great! Now go on to the Latin forms.

1.57

Latin Singular Noun	Latin Plural Form
vertebra	vertebrae
conjunctiva	conjunctivae

-a, -ae

suffix _____a_____   suffix _____ae_____

bacillus   bacilli
bronchus   bronchi

-us, -i

suffix _____us_____   suffix _____i_____

testis   testes

-is, -es

suffix _____is_____   suffix _____es_____

ilium   ilia
bacterium   bacteria

-um, -a

suffix _____um_____   suffix _____a_____

cortex (**cortic/o**)   cortices

-ex, -ices

suffix _____ex_____   suffix _____ices_____

appendix (**appendic/o**)   appendices

-ix, -ices

suffix _____ix_____   suffix _____ices_____

thorax (**thorac/o**)   thoraces

-ax, -aces

suffix _____ax_____   suffix _____aces_____

ANSWER COLUMN

1.58

Use what you just learned about Latin to form the plurals for the following terms.

cocci

calcanea

vertices

cervices

thoraces

coccus   _occci_

calcaneum   _calcarea_

vertex (**vertic/o**) _Vertices_

cervix (**cervic/o**) _Cervices_

thorax (**thorac/o**) _thoraces_

Great work! As you continue through the text, you may wish to refer back to this section to review the rules for plural formation. Plural forms will be included with many of the frames as you learn the singular noun form. When in doubt, consult your dictionary.

1.59

prefix

A **prefix** is a word part that goes in front of a word root. You can change the meaning of the word by putting another word part in front of it. This other part is a _prefix_.

NOTE: Notice in this book the prefixes are highlighted in **blue** and are followed by a hyphen.

Prefix	Word	New Word
ex-	tension	extension
ex-	press	express
dis-	please	displease
dis-	ease	disease

1.60

prefix

The prefix **ex-** means either from or out from. The word press means to squeeze or push on. Placing **ex-** in front of press changes its meaning to "squeeze out." In the word ex/press, **ex-** is a _____.

1.61

prefix

In the word dis/ease, **dis-** changes the meaning of ease. **dis-** is a _____.

1.62

im-

sup-, trans-

In the words im/plant, sup/plant, and trans/plant, the prefixes are _____, _____, and _____.

1.63

word root

Before learning more, review what you have learned. The foundation of a word is a *_____.

ANSWER COLUMN

	1.64
prefix	The word part that is placed in front of a word root to change its meaning is a _____. In a later unit, you will learn many prefixes.
	1.65
suffix	The word part that follows a word root is a _____.
	1.66
adjective verb	A suffix may change a noun to an _____ or change the tense of a _____. Good!
	1.67
combining form	When a vowel is added to a word root, the word part that results is a *_____.
	1.68
compound word	When two or more word roots are used to form a word, the word formed is called a *_____.

Notice the diagrammed sentence below, which illustrates the use of adjectives, nouns, and verbs.

```
        adj    noun    verb      adj    noun     adj    noun
The medical assistant charted the patient's history of duodenal ulcer.
      |_____|                |_____|
           |                                      |
        subject                               predicate
```

Notice the diagrammed words below indicating their word parts.

dysmenorrhea

dys-	men	o	-rrhea
prefix	word root		suffix
	combining form (vowel)		

acrodermatitis

acr	o	dermat	-itis
word root		word root	suffix
combining form (vowel)			

PRONUNCIATION NOTE

Pronunciation symbols, descriptions, and rules are described on the inside front cover. They will also appear through the text below new terms and at other

ANSWER COLUMN

appropriate times. Refer to this Pronunciation Key or your medical dictionary when in doubt about how to say a word. Also, listen to the audio CDs that accompany *Medical Terminology: A Programmed Systems Approach,* 9th edition.

INFORMATION FRAME

1.69

How do you know what to put where? The following material will assist you with word building. This is a system that you may have already figured out. If not, study these rules.

RULE I: Most of the time the definitions indicate the last part of the word first. The descriptive phrases usually start with the suffix and then indicate the body part.

EXAMPLES

1. Inflammation (1) of the bladder (2)
   inflammation
   (of the) bladder

   cystitis

   cyst/**itis**
   cyst/*itis*
   cyst/itis
   (2) (1)

2. One who specializes (1) in skin disorders (2)
   one who specializes (studies)
   (in) skin (disorders)

   dermatologist

   dermat/o/**logist**
   dermat/o/*logist*
   dermat/o/logist
   (2)   (1)

3. Pertaining to the abdomen (1) and
   bladder (2) pertaining to
   (the) abdomen
   (and) bladder

   abdominocystic

   abdomin/o/cyst/**ic**
   abdomin/o/cyst/*ic*
   abdomin/o/cyst/*ic*
   abdomin/o/cyst/ic
   (2)   (1)

RULE II: Where body systems are involved, words are usually built in the order that organs are studied in the system.

EXAMPLES

1. Inflammation of the stomach and small intestine
   inflammation
   (of the) stomach
   (and) small intestine

   gastroenteritis

   ___/ /___ /**itis**
   gastr/o/ /
   ___/ /enter/
   gastr/o/enter/itis

2. Removal of the uterus, fallopian tubes, and ovaries
   removal of
   (the) uterus
   fallopian tubes
   (and) ovaries

   hysterosalpingooophorectomy

   hyster/o/salping/o/oophor/**ectomy**
   hyster/o/salping/o/oophor/ectomy
   hyster/o/**salping/o/**oophor/ectomy
   hyster/o/salping/o/-oophor/ectomy
   hyster/o/salping/o/-oophor/ectomy

ANSWER COLUMN

RULE III: The body part usually comes first and the condition or procedure is the ending.

EXAMPLES
1. dermat/o/mycosis
   (skin) (fungal condition)
2. cyst/o/scopy
   (bladder) (process of examining the urinary bladder with a scope)

1.70

word root	In this learning program, the word root is followed by a slash and a vowel to make a combining form. In **acr/o**, acr is the *_____;
vowel	**o** is the _____;
combining form	and **acr/o** is the *_____.

1.71

acr/o or acr	**acr/o** is used to build words that refer to the *extremities.* To refer to extremities, physicians use these word parts _____.

1.72

acr/o	**acr/o** is found in words concerning the extremities, which in the human body are the arms and legs. To build words about the arms use _____/_____. NOTE: Think of an acrobat.

1.73

acr/o	To build words about the legs, use _____/_____.

1.74

extremities	**acr/o** any place in a word should make you think of the extremities. When you read a word containing acr or **acr/o**, you think of _____.

1.75

extremities	In the word acr/o/paralysis (acroparalysis), **acr/o** refers to _____.

1.76

word root	In **megal/o** (enlarged, large), megal is the *_____;
vowel	**o** is the _____;
combining form	and **megal/o** is the *_____.

1.77

extremities	**-megaly** is used as a suffix for enlarged. The words acr/o/megaly (acromegaly), acr/o/cyan/osis (acrocyanosis), and acr/o/dermat/itis (acrodermatitis) refer to the ___EXTREMITIES___.

ANSWER COLUMN

Acromegaly

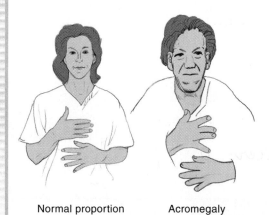

Normal proportion   Acromegaly

	1.78
enlarged	A word containing **megal/o** or **-megaly** will mean something is _enlarged_.
	1.79
acr/o/megaly ak ró **meg′** ə lē	Acr/o/megaly means enlargement of the extremities. The word that means a person has either enlarged arms and legs or hands and feet is _acr_ / _o_ / _megaly_.
	1.80
acromegaly	Acr/o/megal/ic gigantism is a specific disorder of the body. The signs are enlargement of the bones of the hands and feet as well as some of the bones of the head. The term describing these signs is _acromegaly_.
	1.81
noun	**-y** is a suffix meaning the process or condition that makes a word a noun. Acromegaly is a _noun_.
	1.82
skin	**dermat/o** refers to the skin. When you see dermat or **dermat/o**, think immediately of _Skin_.
	1.83
	-logy and **-logist** are suffixes. **-logos** is Greek for study **-logy**—noun, study of **-logist**—noun, one who studies

ANSWER COLUMN

skin
dermat/o/logy
dûr mə **tol′** ō gē

A dermat/o/logist (dermatologist) is a specialist studying diseases of the ___SKIN___ . The study of skin is ___dermat___ / ___O___ / ___logy___ .

1.84

acr/o/dermat/itis
ak′ rō dûr mə **tī′** tis

Acr/o/dermat/itis (acrodermatitis) is a word that means inflammation of the skin of the extremities. A person with red, inflamed hands has ___acr___ / ___O___ / ___dermat___ / ___itis___ .

1.85

inflammation

Remembering the word acrodermatitis, which means inflammation of the skin of the extremities, draw a conclusion. **-itis** is a suffix that means ___inflammation___ .

1.86

acr/o/paralysis
ak′ rō pə **ral′** ə sis

Paralysis is a word that means loss of movement. Form a compound word meaning paralysis of the extremities: ___acr___ / ___O___ / ___paralysis___ .

1.87

word root
vowel
combining form

In **dermat/o**, dermat (skin) is the *_____ ;
o is the _____ ;
and **dermat/o** is the *_____ .

Contact dermatitis—poison oak (Courtesy of Timothy Berger, MD, Associate Clinical Professor, University of California, San Francisco)

1.88

skin

Analyze the word dermat/itis. **-itis** means inflammation; dermat means of the ___skin___ .

1.89

-osis

Dermat/osis means any skin condition. This word denotes an abnormal skin condition. The suffix that means condition, status, or process is ___osis___ .

ANSWER COLUMN

1.90

Signs of inflammation include redness, swelling, pain, and heat. Acrodermatitis could result from stepping in a patch of poison ivy. A person with red, inflamed skin on his or her feet has ___*acrodermatitis*___.

acrodermatitis

1.91

Dermat/itis means inflammation of the skin. There are many causes of inflammation, including infection, allergic reaction, and trauma. The suffix that means inflammation is ___*itis*___.

-itis

1.92

Bacterial, fungal, or parasitic infections may cause red, inflamed skin called ___*dermat*___ / ___*itis*___.

dermat/itis
dûr m ə **tĭ′** tis

To complete your study of this unit, work the **Review Activities** on the following pages. Also, listen to the Audio CD that accompanies *Medical Terminology: A Programmed Systems Approach*, 9th edition, and practice your pronunciation.

Additional practice exercises for this unit are available on the Learner Practice CD-ROM found in the back of the textbook..

REVIEW ACTIVITIES

CIRCLE AND CORRECT

Circle the correct answer for each question. Then check your answers in Appendix A.

1. The base of the word is the
   - a. prefix
   - b. combining form
   - c. ending
   - d. word root

2. The _____ comes in front of a word root to change its meaning.
   - a. prefix
   - b. combining form
   - c. suffix
   - d. pronoun

3. The suffix may change the
   - a. part of speech
   - b. meaning
   - c. plural/singular form
   - d. all of these

4. If two or more word roots are combined to build a word, this is a _____ word.
   - a. combining form
   - b. complex
   - c. compound
   - d. plural

5. When joining two word roots together you may need to use a(n)
   - a. combining form
   - b. consonant
   - c. adjective
   - d. prefix

REVIEW ACTIVITIES

6. Which word part would indicate inflammation when building a word meaning inflammation of the stomach"?
   a. prefix
   b. word root
   c. compound word
   d. suffix

7. When building words about conditions of body parts, the word root for the body part usually comes
   a. first
   b. last
   c. the suffix comes first
   d. the condition comes first

8. –y is a suffix that usually makes a word a(n) _____.
   a. adjective
   b. verb
   c. noun
   d. plural

9. When building words with a suffix that begins with a vowel, for example, -itis, you would
   a. put the suffix first
   b. use a combining form in front
   c. use a word root in front
   d. all of these

10. The correct plural form for thorax is
   a. thoraces
   b. thoraxes
   c. thora
   d. thoranges

11. The part of speech that indicates action or state of being is a(n)
   a. noun
   b. adjective
   c. verb
   d. plural

12. –ity is a suffix that indicates
   a. a condition
   b. quantity
   c. lack of
   d. quality

13. –ism is a suffix that indicates
   a. condition or theory
   b. inflammation
   c. adjective
   d. lack of

14. –ed and –ing are usually suffixes used to make a word a
   a. noun
   b. adjective
   c. verb
   d. plural

15. The suffix indicating a condition is
   a. –tic
   b. –itis
   c. –tion
   d. –er

16. The suffix indicating being full (i.e., full of a substance) is
   a. –ist
   b. –ous
   c. –er
   d. –tion

SELECT AND CONSTRUCT

Select the correct word parts (some may be used more than once) from the following list and construct medical terms that represent the given meaning.

acr/o	an-	cyt/o	dermat/o	duoden/o	em/ia/ic
-er	gastr/o	-graph	hydr/o	-ic	-itis
-megal/y	-meter	micr/o	-phobia	radi/o	-scope
-scopy	surgery	therm/o			

1. enlargement of the extremities ___acromegaly___
2. instrument used to look at small things ___microscope___
3. pertaining to lack of blood ___anemic___
4. one who makes x-ray images ___radiographer___
5. inflammation of the skin on the extremities ___acro dermatitis___
6. fear of water ___hydrophobia___
7. instrument used to measure heat ___thermometer___
8. surgery using a microscope ___micro surgery___
9. looking into the stomach and duodenum with a scope ___gastroduodenoscopy___
10. instrument used to measure (count) cells ___cytometer___

REVIEW ACTIVITIES

PLURAL/SINGULAR FORMS

Using the rules you have learned, form the plural for each of these singular terms.

1. bursa _____bursae_____
2. coccus _____cocci_____
3. carcinoma _____carcinomata_____
4. protozoan _____protozoa_____
5. crisis _____crises_____
6. appendix _____appendices_____
7. ovum _____ova_____

DEFINE AND DISSECT

Give a brief definition and dissect each listed term into its word parts in the space provided. Check your answers by referring to the frame listed in parentheses and to your medical dictionary. Then listen to the CD to practice pronunciation.

Key: rt (word root), v (vowel)

1. gastritis (1.6)

   meaning _inflammation of the stomach_   gastr / itis
                                                       rt   suffix

2. practitioner (1.32)

   meaning _the one who practice med._   ___/___/_____/_____
                                                        rt   v   suffix   suffix

3. cytometer (1.20)

   meaning _instrument use to count cell_   ___/___/_____
                                                        rt   v   suffix (word)

4. micrometer (1.22)

   meaning _device use to measure. small thg_   ___/___/_____
                                                        rt   v   suffix (word)

5. gastroduodenoscopy (1.12)

   meaning _looking into the stomach & deodenum o/scope_   ___/___/___/___/_____
                                                        rt   v   rt   v   suffix

6. lymphadenopathy (1.15)

   meaning _disease of the lymph nodes Particularly enlargement of the lymph notes_   ___/___/___/_____
                                                        rt   rt   v   suffix

7. chickenpox (1.17)

   meaning _varicella_   ___/_____
                                                        rt (word)   rt (word)

8. hydrocele (1.23)

   meaning _accumulation of fluid around the testicle_   ___/___/_____
                                                        rt   v   suffix

9. hyperthyroidism (1.41)

   meaning _is a condition of too much secretion by the thyroid gland_   ___/_____/_____
                                                        pre   rt   suffix

10. psychiatrist (1.45)

    meaning _is a specialist who practices psychiatry_   ___/_____
                                                         rt   suffix

REVIEW ACTIVITIES

ADJECTIVE FORMS

Write the adjective for each of the following nouns.

1. cyanosis ___CYANOTIC___
2. anemia ___ANEMIC___
3. duodenum ___duodenal___
4. mucus ___mucous___
5. arthritis ___arthritic___

CROSSWORD PUZZLE

Check your answers by going back through the frames or checking the solution in Appendix C.

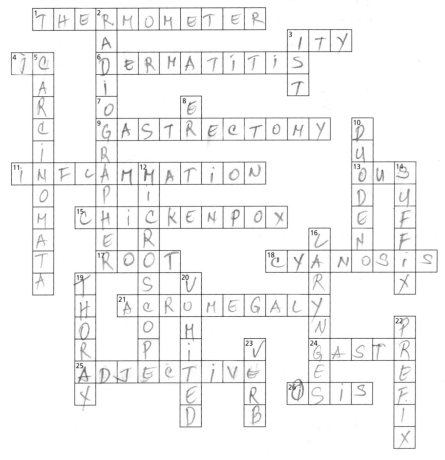

Across
1. instrument: used to measure temperature
3. suffix; quality
4. adjective suffix: pertaining to
6. inflammation of the skin
7. combining vowel
9. excision of the stomach
11. redness, swelling, pain, warmth
13. adjective suffix: full of, possessing
15. compound word for Varicella infection
17. The word _____ is the base of a word.
18. condition of blueness
21. enlarged extremities
24. word root for stomach
25. part of speech: describes a noun
26. suffix: condition

Down
2. one who makes radiographic images
3. suffix: specialist
5. plural of carcinoma
8. suffix: one who
10. combining form for duodenum
12. instrument: looks at very small things
14. placed at the end of a word
16. plural of larynx
19. singular of thoraces
20. past tense verb: vomit
22. placed in front of the word root
23. part of speech: shows action or a state of being

REVIEW ACTIVITIES

GLOSSARY

acrodermatitis	inflammation of the skin extremities	dermatology	the study of the skin, medical specialty
acromegaly	enlarged extremities	disease	abnormal function or condition
acroparalysis	paralysis of the extremities	extension	stretching or elongation
adjective	descriptor, modifies nouns	gastrectomy	excision of the stomach
anemia/anemic	lack blood, noun/adjective	gastric	stomach (adjectival form)
appendix/appendices	glandular tissue below the cecum, singular/plural	gastritis	inflammation of the stomach
bacillus/bacilli	rod-shaped bacteria, singular/plural	gastroduodenoscopy	examination by looking into the stomach and the duodenum with a scope
bacterium/bacteria	microorganism group, singular/plural	gastroduodenostomy	make a surgical opening between the stomach and duodenum
brainstem	midbrain, pons, medulla oblongata	hydrocele	herniation or sac containing fluid
carcinoma/carcinomata	cancer (epithelial origin), singular/plural	hydrophobia	abnormal fear of water
carpus, carpal	wrist bone, (noun/adjective)	hydrotherapy	therapy using water
chickenpox	viral infection with Varicella zoster	hyperthyroidism	overactive thyroid condition
combining form	word root plus a vowel	ilium/iliac	upper pelvic bone, noun/adjective
compound word	word made of two or more word roots	inflammation	condition defined by redness, swelling, pain, and warmth
condyle/condylar	rounded bony process (noun/adjective)	inject, injected, injecting	put in using a needle, verbs
contraction	condition of shortening a body part (tensing)	injectable	able to be injected
crisis/crises	acute (severe) situation (singular/plural)	larynx/larynges	voice box (singular/plural)
		lymphadenopathy	disease of a lymph gland
cyanosis/cyanotic	condition of blueness (noun/adjective)	microbe	very small organism
cytometer	instrument that measures (counts) cells	microfilm	image reduced to small size on film
		micrometer	one millionth of a meter
dermatitis	inflammation of the skin	microscope	instrument used to look at small structures

(handwritten annotation near "appendix/appendices": LARGE INTESTINE)

REVIEW ACTIVITIES

microsurgery	surgery using a microscope	**spermatozoon**	sperm (pl. spermatozoa)
mucus/mucous	watery substance produced by a membrane, (noun/adjective)	**suffix**	follows a word root to change its meaning or part of speech
neurospasm	nerve spasm (twitching)	**thermometer**	instrument that measures temperature
noun	name of a person, place, or thing	**transport**	carry across
practitioner	one who practices	**verb**	action or state of being word
prefix	placed before a word root to change its meaning	**vertebra/vertebrae**	spinal bones (singular/plural)
psychiatrist	specialist in treating mental disorders	**vomit, vomited, vomiting**	evacuate stomach contents (verbs)
radiographer	one who makes x-ray images	**word root**	base of a word
sensitivity	quality of being sensitive		

Surgical Suffixes, Hematology, and Diagnostic Imaging

ANSWER COLUMN	

2.1

The Greek word *tomos* means cutting. From this word we build many suffixes that refer to cutting: **-ectomy** (to cut out, incise), **-tomy** (to cut into, incise), **-tome** (an instrument that cuts slices), **-ostomy** (to form a surgical artificial opening). The word root for cut is _____.

tom

Suffix	Example	Meaning
-tome	derm/a/tome	instrument used to cut slices of skin
-tomy	gastr/o/tomy	incision into the stomach
-ectomy	duoden/ectomy	excision of the duodenum
-ostomy	col/ostomy	make a surgical artificial opening in the colon

2.2

INSTRUMENT   EX-   SURGICAL OPENING   IN-

Remember to associate tom (**-tome, -ectomy, -ostomy,** and **-tomy**) with cutting. A **-tome** is a surgical instrument used to ___cut___ slices.

cut

2.3

gastr/o is the combining form for stomach. Remembering the rule about when to use a combining form and when to use a word root, build a word that means

excision of the stomach ___gastr (ø) / ectomy___;

incision into the stomach ___gastr / o / tomy___;

make a surgical opening in the stomach ___gastr / ostomy___.

gastr/ectomy
gas trek′ tō mē
gastr/o/tomy
gas trot′ ō mē
gastr/ostomy
gas tros′ tō mē

ANSWER COLUMN

2.4

derm/a/tome
dûr′ mə tōm

A derm/a/tome is an instrument that cuts skin. When a surgeon needs to excise a thin slice of skin for examination, she or he may use a __DERM/ A / toME__.

2.5

tom/o is used as a combining form meaning to cut in slices. Tom/o/graphy is a process that makes images of slices (planes) of the body. The body is not actually cut to make these images. The tom/o/graph, (x-ray machine) makes picture-like images that look like a cross-sectional slice. When you see **tom/o** in a word, think

slices or planes

of __SLICES__.

2.6

excision or removal

Recall that **-tome** referred to cutting or a cutting instrument. Gastr/ectomy means excision (removal) of all or part of the stomach. **-ectomy** is a suffix meaning

__EXCISION__. (Refer to Frame 2.7.)

2.7

INFORMATION FRAME

This is a free frame for those who are interested. Others may go on.

		meaning
ect/o	combining form	outside
tom/e	combining form	cut
-y	noun suffix	

Add **ect** + **om** + **y** = ectomy means excision
NOTE: One "t" is dropped when **-tome** is preceded by "ect."

2.8

INFORMATION FRAME

Here's another free frame for those interested in **-ostomy**.

		meaning
os	combining form	mouth, opening
tom/e	combining form	cut
-y	noun suffix	

Add **os** + **tom** + **y** = ostomy means opening by cutting

2.9

gastr/ostomy
gas **tros′** tō mē

gastr/o means stomach.
If a person is unable to swallow and a tube feeding directly into the stomach is necessary, a new opening may be made through the stomach, called a
__gastr / ostomy__.

2.10

duoden/o means duodenum.

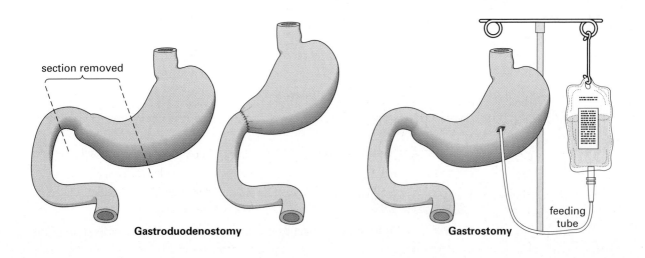

section removed

Gastroduodenostomy

feeding tube

Gastrostomy

ANSWER COLUMN

gastr/o/duoden/ostomy
gas′ trō dōō ō′ də
nos′ tə mē

Gastr/o/duoden/o/stomy means forming a new opening between the stomach and duodenum. A surgeon who removes the natural connection between the duodenum and stomach and then forms a new connection is doing a _gastr / o / duoden / ostomy_.

2.11

gastroduodenostomy

A gastroduodenostomy is a surgical procedure. When the pyloric sphincter (a valve that controls the amount of food going from the stomach to the duodenum) no longer functions, a _gastroduodenostomy_ may be necessary.

2.12

gastroduodenostomy

When a portion of the first part of the small intestine is removed because of cancer, a new artificial surgical opening is created by performing a _gastroduodenostomy_.

2.13

duoden/um
dōō ō **dē**′ nəm
dōō **od**′ ə nəm

-tomy is a suffix meaning incision into. A duoden/o/tomy is an incision into the _duoden / um_.

2.14

duoden/o/tomy
dōō ō də **not**′ ə mē

An incision into the duodenum is a _duoden / o / tomy_

ANSWER COLUMN

2.15

A gastr/ectomy is a surgical procedure. When a gastr/ic ulcer has perforated, a partial _____/_____ may be indicated to remove part of the stomach. NOTE: The combining form is not used when the suffix begins with a vowel.

gastr/ectomy
gas **trek**′ tə mē

2.16

Cancer of the stomach may also be treated by removal of the stomach, called _____.

gastrectomy

2.17

-itis is the suffix used for inflammation. A word that means inflammation of the stomach is _____/_____.

gastr/itis
gas **trī**′ tis

2.18

-megaly is a suffix meaning *enlarged*. Gastromegaly is one word for enlarged stomach. **gastr/o** is the combining form for _____.

stomach

2.19

Two words that mean enlargement of the stomach
are _____/_____/_____
and _____/_____/_____.

gastr/o/megaly
megal/o/gastria

2.20

duoden/o is used in words that refer to the first part of the small intestine, the duoden/um. To build words about the duodenum, use _____/____. An outline of terms and illustration showing the digestive system may be found in Unit 7.

duoden/o

2.21

The duoden/um is the first part of the small intestine that connects with the stomach. **duoden/o** is a combining form that refers to the _____/_____.

duoden/um

2.22

A surgeon who incises the duodenum is performing a _____.

duodenotomy

2.23

Inflammation is characterized in part by redness and swelling of a body part. **-itis** is a suffix for inflammation. When physicians are listing conditions of the duodenum and they want to say it is inflamed, they use the word _____.

duodenitis

ANSWER COLUMN

2.24

-itis
duoden/itis
dōō ō də **nī**′ tis
dōō od′ e **nī**′ tis

The suffix for inflammation is _____. The word for inflammation of the duodenum is _____/_____.

2.25

-al or -ic

Gastric and duoden/al are adjectives. **-al** and **-ic** are adjectival suffixes meaning pertaining to (whatever the adjective modifies). One adjectival suffix is _____.

2.26

duoden/al
dōō ō **dē**′ nəl
dōō **od**′ ə nəl
ulcer
lesion

In duoden/al ulcer and duoden/al lesion, the adjective is _____/_____, and the nouns modified are _____.

WORD BUILDING
■ ■ ■ ■ ■

GASTR (word root) + O (vowel) + DUODEN (word root) + OSTOMY (suffix)

2.27

duodenal

In the phrase, "Duodenal carcinoma was present," the adjective meaning that pertains to the duodenum is _____.

2.28

duoden/ostomy
dōō ō də **nos**′ tə mē

Recall that **-ostomy** means making a new artificial surgical opening. The word to form a new opening into the duodenum is _____/_____.

2.29

gastr/o/duoden/ostomy
gas′ trō dōō ō dēn **os**′ tō mē

A duodenostomy can be formed in more than one manner. If it is formed with the stomach, it is called a _____/_____/_____/_____.

2.30

-ectomy
-tomy
-ostomy

The suffix for excision is ___ECTOMY___.
The suffix for incision is ___toMY___.
The suffix for forming a new opening is ___OSTOMY___.

(A) Computed tomography and (B) conventional x-ray procedure

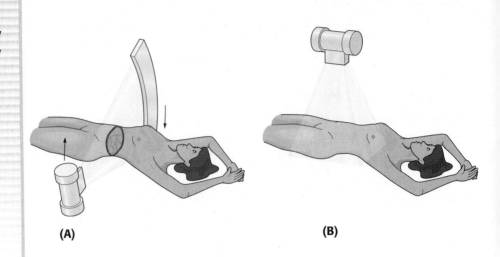

(A) (B)

2.31

Diagnostic imaging has emerged as an important assessment tool in medicine today. It includes any modality that creates a graph, picture, or other visual representation of body structures and/or their function. The cardi/o/pulmon/ary, radi/o/logy, neur/o/logy, and information processing departments have been responsible for the development and study of most imaging systems used today.

2.32

-graph is a suffix taken from the Greek verb *graphein*, meaning to write or record. In medical words, **-graph** refers to an instrument used to record data. A tom/o/graph is an x-ray instrument used to show tissue or organs in one plane (slice, so to speak). To obtain an x-ray of a slice of an organ, the radiographer would use a _____/____/_____.

NOTE: The word root for to cut is tom; the combining form is **tom/o**.

tom/o/graph
tō′ mō graf

2.33

-gram indicates a picture or record.

Adding a **-y** to **-graph** (as in biography) creates a suffix indicating the process of making a recording of data. The process of using a tomograph is called _____/____/_____.

tom/o/graphy
tō **mog**′ raf ē

Computed tomography (CT) allows the radiologist to obtain a three-dimensional view of internal structures. A CT (or CAT) scanner is a type of _____.

tomograph

The CT image is a _____/_____/_____.

tom/o/gram
tō mō gram

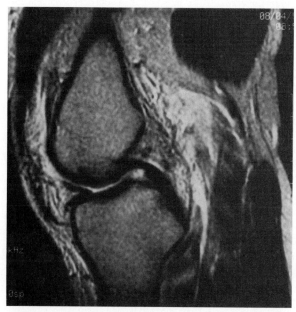

(A) MRI (magnetic resonance imaging) of the knee acquired in the sagittal plane

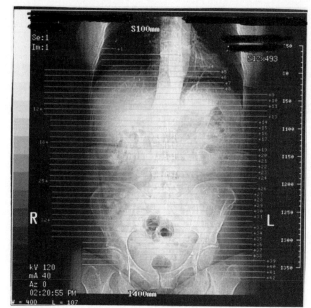

(B) This scout view of the abdomen helps localize the scan parameters of a CT (computed tomography) scan. Each horizontal line indicates the level of one slice.

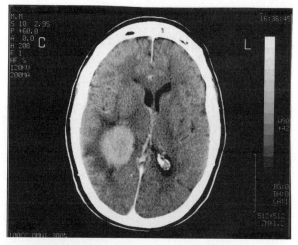

(C) CAT (computed axial tomography) scan demonstrates a meningioma surrounded by edema.

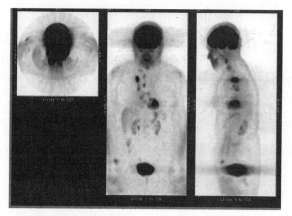

(D) PET (positron emission tomography) scan demonstrating tumor in right lung

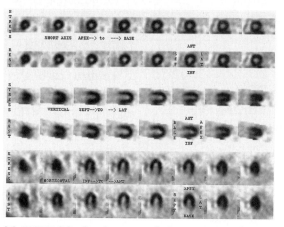

(E) SPECT (single photon emission computed tomography)

ANSWER COLUMN

2.34

INFORMATION FRAME

Tomography is a radiographic procedure that uses x-rays to produce images of a slice or plane of the body. Each of the following imaging procedures is a type of tomography.

MRI	magnetic resonance imaging
CT	computed tomography (CAT scan)
PET	positron emission tomography
SPECT	single photon emission computed tomography

For more information use your medical dictionary or perform a library or Internet search of these topics.

2.35

tomography

MRI, CT, PET, and SPECT are all types of _____.

2.36

cardi/algia
kär′ de **al**′ jē ə

-algia is one suffix that means pain. Form a word that means heart pain.
(Clue: **-algia** is a suffix that begins with a vowel, you will use the word root rather than the combining form.) _____/_____

2.37

cardialgia

Gastr/algia means pain in the stomach. When a patient complains of pain in the heart, this symptom is known medically as _____.

2.38

algia
gastr/algia
gas **tral**′ jē ə

One suffix for pain is _____. Stomach pain is
_____/_____.

2.39

SPELL CHECK ✓

cardi/o (**card/o**) is used in building words that refer to the heart. Card/itis is inflammation of the heart.
When using a suffix that begins with a vowel (i.e., **-itis, -ectomy**), use the word root. When using a suffix that begins with a consonant (i.e., **-dynia, -logy**), you will need a combining form. Examples are card/itis, cardi/ectomy, cardi/o/dynia, and cardi/o/logy.

2.40

cardiologist

A cardi/o/logist discovers irregularities in the flow of the blood in the heart. The physician catheterizes the heart to view blood flow through the vessels of the heart. This heart specialist is a _____.

Computed tomography (CT) planes

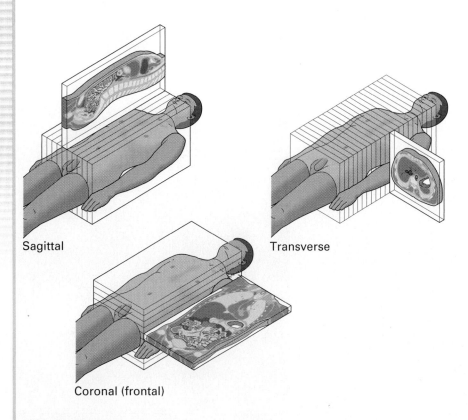

Sagittal

Transverse

Coronal (frontal)

2.41

cardiologist
kär dē **ol′** ō jist

A person who reads electr/o/cardi/o/grams (records of electrical impulses given off by the heart) is also a _____.

2.42

INFORMATION FRAME

When hospitalized, a patient with a severe heart condition is usually treated in a cardiac care unit (CCU). An electr/o/cardi/o/gram (EKG or ECG) may be performed to assess heart function.

2.43

a picture or record
of electrical activity
of the heart

-gram is the suffix meaning record or a picture. **electr/o** is the combining form for *electrical*. Give the meaning of electr/o/cardi/o/gram. ** _____

_____.

2.44

electr/o/cardi/o/gram
e lek′ trō **kär′** dē ō gram

-graph is a suffix indicating an instrument used to make a recording or any pictorial device. An electr/o/cardi/o/gram is the record produced. The electr/o/cardi/o/graph is the instrument used to record the picture, or

_____/____/_____/____/_____.

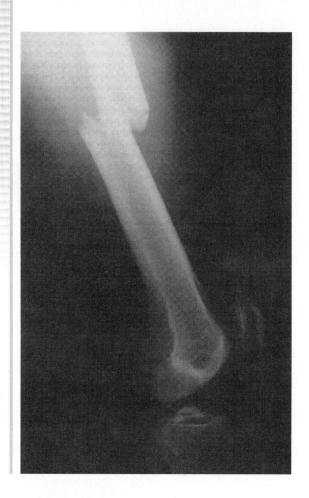

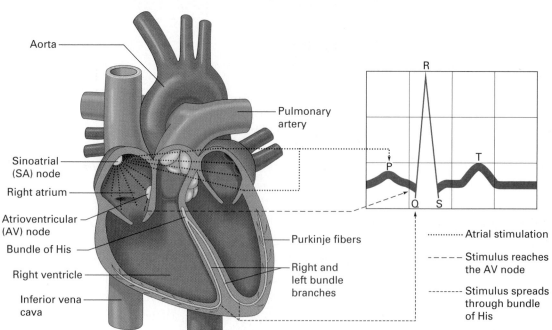

Conduction system of the heart showing the source of electrical impulses produced on an ECG (EKG)

ANSWER COLUMN

2.45

-graphy is a suffix for the *process* of making a recording or image (EKG or ECG). The electr/o/cardi/o/gram is a record obtained by the process of electr/o/cardi/o/graphy. A technologist can learn electrocardiography, but it takes a cardiologist to read the _____.

electrocardiogram

NOTE: The suffix **-gram** refers to the actual paper readout or picture on a computer screen. Think of obtaining a telegram from a telegraph.

2.46

A physician can read a tracing that looks like this,

Ventricular fibrillation

atrial tachycardia (atrial rate, 107; ventricular rate, 43)

and learn something about a person's heart. The physician is a _____ and is reading an _____.

cardiologist
electrocardiogram

2.47

son/o is a combining form taken from the Latin word *sonus,* meaning sound. A supersonic transport travels above the speed of sound. A son/o/gram is a picture made by a sonograph. The process of obtaining the sonogram is called _____/_____/_____ (ultrasonography).

son/o/graphy
son **og**′ ra fē

2.48

Recall that the suffix **-er** means one who. The person who (one who) performs sonography is called a ____/____/_____/____.

son/o/graph/er
son **og**′ ra fer

2.49

ech/o is a combining form meaning sound made by *reflected sound* waves. A record of sound waves reflected through the heart is an ____/____/_____/____/_____.

ech/o/cardi/o/gram
ek′ō **kär**′ dē ō gram

ANSWER COLUMN

ech/o/cardi/o/graphy
ek′ ō kär dē **og**′ ra fē

2.50

The process of making the ech/o/cardi/o/gram is called
_____/_____/_____/_____/_____.

NOTE: *Echo*cardiography uses sound waves; *electro*cardiography uses electricity.

radi/o/gram
rād′ ē ō gram

2.51

radi/o is a combining form from the Latin word *radius*, meaning a ray coming from a central point. **radi/o** is used to refer to radiation such as that used in x-rays. A picture made by using x-rays (XR) is called a _____/_____/_____.

NOTE: In practice, this is usually called a radiograph.

Electrocardiogram ECG tracing or recording

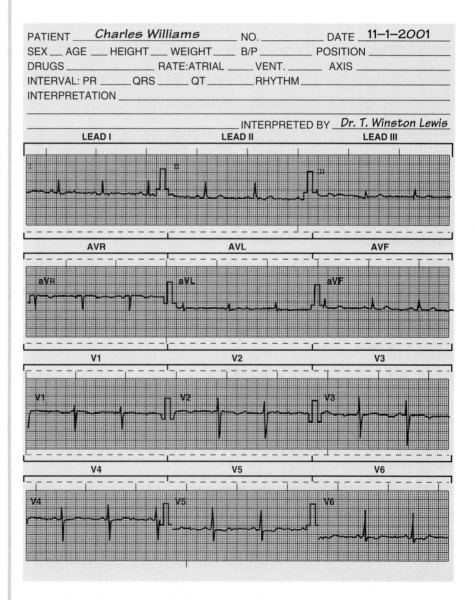

PATIENT ____*Charles Williams*____ NO. _____ DATE __11–1–2001__
SEX ___ AGE ___ HEIGHT ___ WEIGHT _____ B/P _____ POSITION _____
DRUGS _____ RATE:ATRIAL _____ VENT. _____ AXIS _____
INTERVAL: PR _____ QRS _____ QT _____ RHYTHM_____
INTERPRETATION _____
_____
_____ INTERPRETED BY __Dr. T. Winston Lewis__
LEAD I   LEAD II   LEAD III

AVR   AVL   AVF

V1   V2   V3

V4   V5   V6

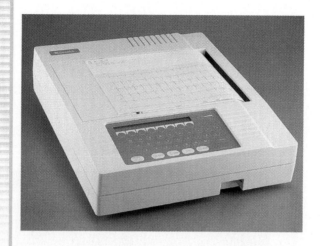

2.52

radi/o/grapher
rād′ ē **og′** ra fer
radi/o/logist
rād ē **ol′** ō jist

Build words for the following meanings:
one who takes x-rays _____/____/_____;
a physician specialist who studies (interprets) x-rays
_____/____/_____.

2.53

radiologist

Radiation therapists (RATx) use x-rays to irradiate a cancerous area.
These treatments would be supervised by a physician specialist called a

_____.

2.54

skin

-pathy is a suffix meaning disease. Dermat/o/pathy means a disease condition
of the ⟨skin⟩.

2.55

path/o/logy
path **ol′** ō gē

Great! Now try this: **path/o** is a combining form meaning disease. Path/o/logy
is the study of disease. A path/o/logist is a physician specializing in diagnosing
(discovering) diseases. A pathologist usually works in the hospital laboratory
department called clinical ⟨path / o / logy⟩.

2.56

INFORMATION FRAME

Color is used in labeling cell and tissue types as well as describing observable
signs such as skin color changes. Skin might appear pale yellow, pink, reddened,
blue, darkened, or blotchy. These observations assist in making a correct
assessment of the patient's condition.

Echocardiogram
(Prepared by Lynne Schreiber, BS, RDMS, RT[R])

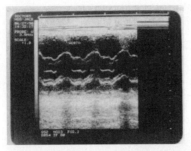

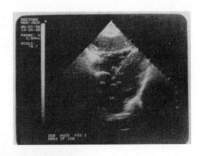

Echocardiograph *(Photo by Marcia Butterfield, courtesy of W. A. Foote Memorial Hospital, Jackson, MI)*

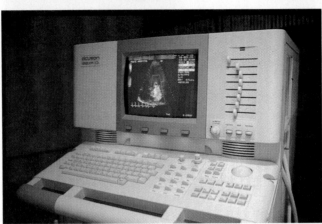

2.57

Jaundice is not a color change of the actual skin pigment, but a reflection of bright yellow through the blood plasma. When a person has a high blood bilirubin level, it gives the plasma a bright yellow color. This occurs, for example, as hepatitis B affects the liver. The patient's eyes, skin, and nailbeds appear yellow. This type of yellow look to the patient is called _____.

jaundice
jawn′ dis

2.58

Other liver conditions such as cancer or cirrhosis also cause a yellow or _____ appearance to the skin.

jaundiced

2.59

Derma is a word itself. It is a noun meaning skin. Cyan/o/derma is a compound word. It means ** _____ and is a (choose one) _____ (noun/adjective).

blue skin or bluish
  discoloration of the skin
  (due to low O_2 levels)
noun

PROFESSIONAL PROFILES

Registered radiologic technologists (RT[R]) use ionizing radiation (x-rays) to create images for diagnostic interpretation by physicians called radiologists. Knowledge of positioning patients for exposure, operation of the x-ray equipment and developers, anatomy, pathology, and human relations is essential. Education may be hospital or college based ranging from certificates to advanced degrees. The American Society of Radiologic Technologists (ASRT) and the American Registry of Radiologic Technologists (ARRT) monitor education standards and registration in this profession.

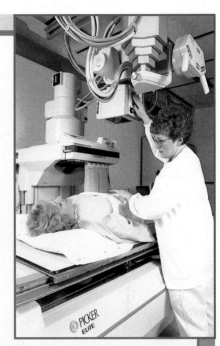

Radiographer positioning patient for x-ray *(Photo by Marcia Butterfield, courtesy of W. A. Foote Memorial Hospital, Jackson, MI)*

ANSWER COLUMN

NOTE: Most of these word parts are used as prefixes (e.g., leukocyte). An exception is **cyan/o**, which may be used either as a prefix (cyanoderma) or as a word root within a word (acrocyanosis).
Use this information for building words involving color:
(frames 2.64–2.94)

leuk/o	white
melan/o	black (dark pigment)
erythr/o	red
cyan/o	blue
chlor/o	green
xanth/o	yellow

2.60

cyan/o is used in words to mean blue or blueness. When photographers want to say something about how a film reproduces the color blue, they use _____.

cyan/o or cyan

Structures of the Skin

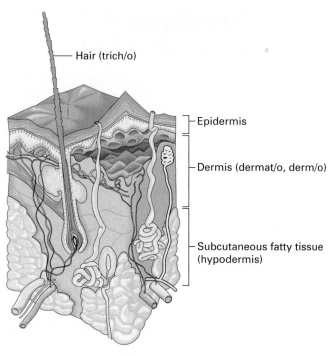

Hair (trich/o)

Epidermis

Dermis (dermat/o, derm/o)

Subcutaneous fatty tissue (hypodermis)

Structures of the Skin

2.61

-osis is a suffix,
forms a noun, and
means disease, condition, status, or process.
Build a word that means

condition of blueness _____/_____

cyan/osis
sī ə nō′ sis

condition of the skin _____/_____

dermat/osis
dûr mə tō′ sis

condition of blueness of the skin _____/_____/_____

cyan/o/derma
sī′ ənō **dûr**′ mə

or

dermat/o/cyan/osis
dûr **mat**′ ō sī ən **ō**′sis

2.62

-tic changes **-osis** from a noun to an adjective. Build the term that means
pertaining to a condition of blueness: _____/_____.

cyan/otic
sī ə **no**′ tik

ANSWER COLUMN

2.63

cyan

-osis

Acr/o/cyan/osis means blueness of the extremities. The part of the word that tells you that the color blue is involved is _____.
The part of the word that tells you this is a condition is _____.

2.64

erythr/o/derma
e rith′ rō **der**′ mə
leuk/o/derma
loo kō **der**′ mə
xanth/o/derma
zan′tho′ **der**′ mə
melan/o/derma
mel′ an ō **der**′ mə

Cyan/o/derma means blue skin. Build a word meaning
red skin _____/____/_____

white skin (vitiligo) _____/_____/_____

yellow skin _____/_____/_____

abnormally dark pigmented skin _____/_____/_____.

2.65

melan/o/cyte
mel′ an ō sīt
leuk/o/cyte
loo kō sīt
erythr/o/cyte
e **rith**′ rō sīt

The suffix **-cyte** means cell. A chlor/o/cyte is a green cell (in plants). Build a word meaning
black cell (dark pigmented) _____/____/_____

white (blood) cell _____/____/_____

red (blood) cell _____/____/_____

Acrocyanosis *(blueness of the extremities)*

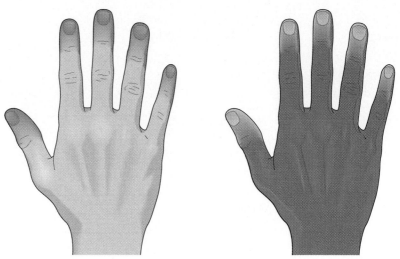

ANSWER COLUMN

2.66

The suffix **-blast** means embryonic or immature cell. A leuk/o/blast is an embryonic white cell. Build a word meaning an embryonic cell of the following colors

melan/o/blast

erythr/o/blast

(You pronounce)

black (dark pigment) _____/____/_____

red _____/____/_____

2.67

-emia is a suffix from the Greek word *hema*, for blood. **-emia** means blood condition. An/emia is lack of blood.

Build words involving the following colors when referring to blood conditions

xanth/emia

zan **thē′** mē ə

erythr/emia

e rith **rē′** mē ə

chlor/emia

klor **ē′** mē ə

yellow (jaundice) _____/_____

red (polycythemia) _____/_____

green (increased chlorine in the blood) _____/_____

NOTE: Chlorosis is a condition in which the skin takes on a greenish tinge due to anemia.

2.68

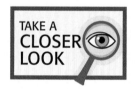
TAKE A CLOSER LOOK

Look at the following terms. Now look up each term in the dictionary. You will find that they are similar in spelling but different in meaning and use. Write the definitions below.

eryth/ema _____

erythr/emia _____

erythr/o/derma _____

From the word parts you have learned so far, see if you can analyze them without looking up the answers. Which one

erythr/emia

er ə **thrē′** mē ə

erythr/o/derma

er ə thrō **dûr′** mə

is a blood condition? _____ ;

is a skin condition? _____ .

2.69

green

yellow

red

white

black

chlor/o means _____ .

xanth/o means _____ .

erythr/o means _____ .

leuk/o means _____ .

melan/o means _____ .

ANSWER COLUMN

cyan/o/derma sī′ ə nēo **dûr′** mə or dermat/o/cyanosis	**2.70** Cyanoderma sometimes occurs when children swim too long in cold water. A person who has a bluish discoloration of the skin is described as having _____/____/_____.
leuk/o or leuk	**2.71** **leuk/o** means *white*. Pay attention to the "eu" spelling. There are many words in medicine that refer to white. To say something is white, use _____.
white skin, abnormally white skin, lack of pigment of the skin, vitiligo	**2.72** Leuk/o/derma means *_____ _____.
leuk/o/derma	**2.73** A disease in which people have patchy white areas on their skin is called vitiligo (vit i **lī′** gō). Sometimes these white areas are also called _____/____/_____.

2.74

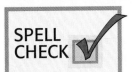

You may notice that some medical terms are particularly unusual and difficult to spell correctly. From time to time in this program you will be given a Spell Check frame which includes spelling hints that may be of assistance. Notice the unusual diphthong (two vowels together) in the combining form **leuk/o**. The "eu" is pronounced like a long "u" sound, but do not forget the e first, even though it is silent. The correct spelling is l-e-u-k-o, as in leukocyte and leukoderma.

PRONUNCIATION NOTE

WORD ORIGINS

As a general rule in Greek origin medical words, when two vowels are together, the second vowel's long sound is used, as in:
Examples
ea says ā;
ae says ē;
ie says ē;
ei says ī.

cyt/o	**2.75** **cyt/o** refers to cells. A cell is the smallest structural unit of all living things. To refer to this smallest part of the body, the combining form _____/____ is used.

ANSWER COLUMN

2.76

cyt/o
cells

Cytology is the study of cells. The part of cyt/o/logy that means cells
is _____/____.
A cyt/o/lo/gist studies _____.

2.77

cyt/o/logy

-logy is a suffix that means the study of. Build a word that means the study
of cells. _____/____/_____

2.78

path/o/logy
path **ol**′ ō gē or
eti/o/logy
e tē **ol**′ ō jē

Cyt/o/logists study diseases of the cell, like leukemia. The study
of the cause of disease is _____/____/_____.

2.79

cyt/o/meter
sīt **om**′ et er
cyt/o/metry
sīt **om**′ et rē

-meter is a suffix meaning an instrument used to measure or count something.
The instrument used to count cells is called a _____/____/_____. **-metry**
is a suffix meaning the process of measuring or counting something. The
process of counting cells is called ____/____/____.

2.80

instrument
process

The word cyt/o/meter refers to the _____ used to
measure or count. The word cyt/o/metry refers to the _____
of measuring or counting.

2.81

cyt/o/techn/o/logist
sī tō tek **nol** ō jist

A technician that prepares and screens slides
is a _____/____/_____/____/_____.

2.82

cell
sel

Of the several types of cells in blood, one is a leuk/o/cyte (refer to illustration).
A leukocyte is a white blood _____ (WBC).

2.83

leuk/o/cyte
l oo′ kō sīt

When physicians want to know how many leukocytes there are, they ask
for a _____/____/_____ count.

PROFESSIONAL PROFILE

Cytotechnologists prepare and screen tissue (cell) slides to detect abnormalities. They may issue results on normal tissues and work with pathologists to conclude final analysis of abnormal findings. A baccalaureate degree and clinical training will qualify the individual to take the Board of Registry of the American Society of Clinical Pathology (ASCP) certification exam to become a certified cytotechnologist, or CT (ASCP).

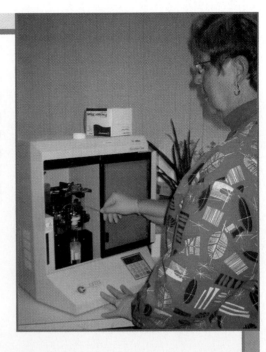

ANSWER COLUMN

	2.84
	There are several kinds of leukocytes in the blood. When physicians want to know how many of each type of leukocyte, they ask for a differential
leuk/o/cyte	_____/____/_____ count.
	2.85
	-penia is the Greek word (suffix) for poverty. The word that means decrease in or not enough white blood cells
leuk/o/cyt/o/penia loo′ kō sī′ tō **pē**′ nē ə	is _____/____/_____/____/_____.
	2.86
	Leuk/o/cyt/o/penia (leukopenia) means a decrease in white blood cells.
-penia	The part of the word that means decrease in is _____.
	2.87
	If the body does not produce enough white blood cells, the patient suffers
leukocytopenia	from _____.

ANSWER COLUMN

Blood cells *(leukocytes, erythrocytes, and thrombocytes)*

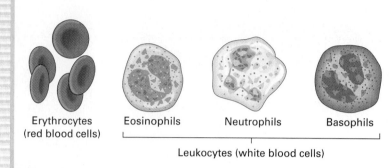

Erythrocytes (red blood cells)   Eosinophils   Neutrophils   Basophils

Leukocytes (white blood cells)

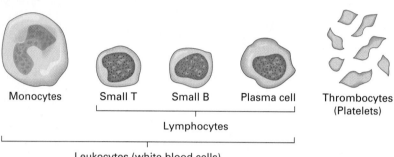

Monocytes   Small T   Small B   Plasma cell   Thrombocytes (Platelets)

Lymphocytes

Leukocytes (white blood cells)

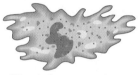

Wandering macrophage

Wright's stained blood smear

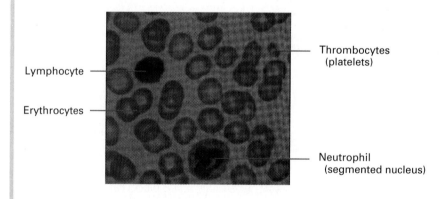

Lymphocyte

Erythrocytes

Thrombocytes (platelets)

Neutrophil (segmented nucleus)

2.88

You have heard of leuk/emia, popularly called "blood cancer." **-ia** is a noun suffix meaning condition. **-em** comes from the Greek word *hema*, meaning blood. A noun meaning, literally, a condition of white blood is _____/_____.

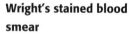

leuk/emia
l o͞o **kē**′ mē ə

2.89

In leukemia the blood is not really white. A laboratory finding of this disease is the presence of too many immature white cells (leukocytes) in the blood. This finding was used to name the disease _____.

leukemia

2.90

Look at the table of values that follows. A WBC of 25,000 would be abnormally high. **-osis** may be used to indicate an increase in numbers of blood cells. Build a word that means an increase in

white blood cells _____/____/_____/_____;

leuk/o/cyt/osis
loo′ kō sī **tō**′ sis

erythr/o/cyt/osis
e rith′ rō sī **tō**′ sis

red blood cells _____/____/_____/_____.

COMPLETE BLOOD COUNT (CBC)

Test	Normal Average Values
Specimen: Whole blood	
Hgb (Hb)—hemoglobin	12–16 grams/100 milliliters
Hct—hematocrit	36–48% formed elements
RBC—red blood cell count	4.2–6.2 million/mm^3
WBC—white blood cell count	5,000–10,000/mm^3
Platelet (thrombocyte) count	350,000–450,000/mm^3

Diff—white blood cell differential count—Wright's stained smear analysis based on 100 WBCs:

Neutrophil (bands): 3–5%	Neutrophil (segs): 54–62%
Lymphocytes: 25–33%	Monocytes: 3–7%
Eosinophils: 1–3%	Basophils: 0–1%

2.91

lymph/o, from the Latin word *lympha*, meaning water or liquid, is used to refer to lymph/atic system structures. A lymph/o/cyte is a type of WBC produced by the _____/_____ system.

lymph/atic
lim **fa**′ tik

ANSWER COLUMN

Cytometer—Automated instrument for analysis and counting blood cells

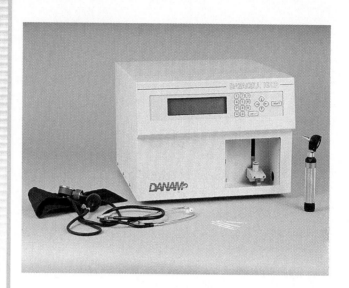

2.92

A type of leukocyte produced by the lymphatic system is

lymph/o/cyte
lim′ fō sīt

a _____/____/_____.

2.93

Acute lymphocytic leukemia (ALL) is a disease involving

lymph/o/cytes

the _____/____/_____.

2.94

erythr/o means red. Cells that contain a red substance (hemoglobin) are called

erythr/o/cytes
e **rith**′ rō sīts

red blood cells (RBCs) or _____/____/_____.

2.95

Look at the CBC values in the table on page 47. An RBC count of 2 million would be abnormally low. **-penia** is a suffix indicating deficiency in number. A patient who lacks red blood cells suffers

erythr/o/cyt/o/penia
e rith′ rō sīt′ ō **pē**′ nē ə

from _____/____/_____/____/_____.

2.96

Another type of blood cell is the thromb/o/cyte. Thrombocytes prevent excessive bleeding by allowing the blood to clot. An abnormal decrease

ANSWER COLUMN

thromb/o/cyt/o/penia
thromb′ ō sīt′ ō **pē**′ nē ə

in the number of these clot-forming cells

is _____/____/_____/____/_____.

2.97

thrombocytes

Blood-clotting cells (thrombocytes) are also called platelets. A platelet count would be done to obtain the number of _____.

2.98

thromb/o/cytes
throm′ bō sīts or
platelets
plāt′ lets

thromb/o means blood clot. The blood cells that help form blood clots are _____/____/_____.

2.99

thromb/o/cyt/osis
thromb′ ō sī **tō**′ sis
erythr/o/cyt/osis
e rith′ rō sī **tō**′ sis

-osis, used as a suffix with blood cells, indicates a condition characterized by increase in number. Build a term meaning increase in number of platelets (thrombocytes) _____/____/_____/_____;
red blood cells (erythrocytes) _____/____/_____/_____.

2.100

blast/o

A blast/o/cyte is an embryonic or immature cell. The combining form for embryonic or immature is _____/____.
Think of this . . . when you have a "blast," you may act immature!

2.101

blast

A cell in its embryonic stage is called a _____.

2.102

cell
sel

-cyte may be used as a suffix to indicate a type of cell. A leuk/o/cyte is a term referring to a type of white blood _____.

2.103

immature or embryonic

-blast may be used at the end of a word to indicate an immature or embryonic cell. A hist/o/blast is a group of tissue cells that are *_____.

ANSWER COLUMN

2.104

hist/o/blast
his′ tō blast
hist/o/logy
his **tol**′ ō jē
hist/ō/logist
his **tol**′ ō jist
hist/ ō /cyte
his′ tō sīt

Hist/o means tissues. Build a word that means:

immature tissue _____/____/_____;

the study of tissues _____/____/_____;

one who studies tissues _____/____/_____;

a tissue cell _____/____/_____.

2.105

INFORMATION
FRAME

Remember, your best friend is your medical dictionary. Look up the new terms you have learned for in-depth definitions.

2.106

megaly

In the word acr/o/megaly, the suffix for enlarged is _____.

2.107

megal/o

The combining form for enlarged is _____/____.

2.108

enlarged heart or
enlargement of the heart

cardi/o is the combining form for words about the heart. Cardi/o/megaly is a noun that means *_____

_____.

2.109

megal/o/cardia
meg′ ə lō **kär**′ dē ə

Megal/o/cardia also means enlargement or overdevelopment of the heart. When something causes an increase in the size of the
heart, _____/____/_____ exists.

2.110

megal/o/cardia
meg′ ə lō **kär**′ dē ə
or
cardi/o/megaly
kär′ dē ō **meg**′ ə lē

Megalocardia refers to heart muscle. When any muscle exercises, it gets larger. If the heart muscle has to overexercise, _____/____/_____
will probably occur.

ANSWER COLUMN

	2.111
megalocardia	Cardiac enlargement (CE) may be caused by prolonged, severe asthma that can cut down the supply of oxygen to the body and make the heart work harder. Another word for CE is _____.
	2.112
gastr	Megal/o/gastria means large or enlarged stomach. The word root for stomach is _____.
	2.113
megal/o/gastria meg′ ə lō **gas**′ trē ə	**megal/o** means large; gastr, from the Greek *gaster*, is the word root for stomach, and **-ia** is a noun suffix. Form a noun that means large or enlargement of the stomach: _____/____/_____.
	2.114
gastr/o/megaly gas′ trō **meg**′ ə lē megal/o/gastria meg′ ə lō **gas**′ trē ə	Another word for enlargement of the stomach is gastr/o/megaly. When the stomach is so large that it crowds other organs, _____/____/_____ or _____/____/_____ exists.
	2.115
gastromegaly	Enlargement of the stomach is called megalogastria or _____.
	2.116
condition	**-ia** is a noun suffix for condition. When megalogastria occurs, an undesirable _____ exists.
	2.117
mania	Mania is an English word that comes directly from the Greek word *mania*, which means madness. Many mental disorders are designated by compound words that end in this word, _____, meaning a condition of madness or excessive preoccupation.
	2.118
-ia	Mania is a noun for condition. The condition is madness or, more properly, mental disorder. The suffix that tells you mania is a noun and shows a condition is _____.

ANSWER COLUMN

2.119

megal/o/mania
meg′ ə lō **mā**′ nē ə

Megal/o/mania is a symptom of a mental disorder in which the patient has delusions of grandeur. Patients who have greatly enlarged opinions of themselves suffer from _____/____/_____.

2.120

megalomania

People with megalomania are often treated in mental health centers. Many such centers have a patient who claims to be a king or president. These patients are diagnosed with _____.

2.121

megalomania

Many people think Adolf Hitler suffered from delusions of grandeur
or _____.

2.122

enlargement of the heart
heart

Megal/o/cardia means *_____.
cardi is the word root for _____.

INFORMATION FRAME

2.123

Recall that **-ic** and **-ac** are adjective suffixes that mean pertaining to.
The following are adjectival forms of the words you have just learned:

leukemic   leukocytic
dermic   cyanotic
manic   melanic
gastric   xanthemic
cardiac   erythroblastic

For review use the material in the following chart to work the next frame.

WORDS ARE FORMED BY

I. Word root + suffix
   (a) dermat/itis
   (b) cyan/osis
   (c) duoden/al
II. Combining form + suffix
   (this can be a word itself)
   (a) acr/o/cyan/osis
   (b) leuk/o/cyte
III. Any number of combining forms + word root + suffix
   (a) leuk/o/cyt/o/pen/ia
   (b) electr/o/cardi/o/graphy

ANSWER COLUMN

word root	
suffix	
word root	
suffix	
duoden	
-al	
combining form	
word root	
suffix	
combining form	
suffix	
combining form	
combining form	
suffix	
electr/o	
cardi/o	
-graphy	

2.124

In I(a), dermat is the * _____;
    -itis is the _____.
In I(b), cyan is the * _____;
    -osis is the _____.
In I(c), the word root is _____;
    the suffix is _____.
In II(a), **acr/o** is the * _____;
    cyan is the * _____;
    -osis is the _____.
In II(b), **leuk/o** is the * _____;
    -cyte is the _____.
In III(a), **leuk/o** is a * _____;
    cyt/o is a * _____;
    -penia is a _____.
In III(b), the first combining form is _____/___;
the second combining form is _____/___;
the suffix is _____.
Good job!

Take five minutes and study the list of abbreviations in the following table.

Abbreviation	Meaning
ACVD	acute (or atherosclerotic) cardiovascular disease
ALL	acute lymphocytic leukemia
ARRT	American Registry of Radiologic Technologists
ARDMS	American Registry of Diagnostic Medical Sonography
ASRT	American Society of Radiologic Technologists
CBC	complete blood count
CCU	cardiac care unit (coronary care unit)
CE	cardiac enlargement
CPK	creatine phosphokinase (cardiac enzyme)
CT, CAT scan	computed tomography (scan)
CT(ASCP)	Cytotechnologist (American Society of Clinical Pathology)
DMS	diagnostic medical sonography
ECHO	echocardiogram
EKG, ECG	electrocardiogram
ER	emergency room
GA	gastric analysis
GI	gastrointestinal

(continues)

ANSWER COLUMN

Abbreviation	Meaning
Hb, Hgb	Hemoglobin
LDH	lactic dehydrogenase (cardiac enzyme)
MRI	magnetic resonance imaging
Ra	radium
RATx (RT)	radiation therapy
RBC	red blood cell (count)
RDCS	Registered Diagnostic Cardiac Sonographer
RT(R)	registered radiologic technologist
RVT	Registered Vascular Technologist
WBC	white blood cell (count)
XR	x-ray

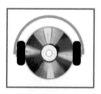

To complete your study of this unit, work the **Review Activities** on the following pages. Also, listen to the audio CD that accompanies *Medical Terminology: A Programmed Systems Approach*, 9th edition, and practice your pronunciation.

Additional practice exercises for this unit are available on the Learner Practice CD-ROM found in the back of the textbook.

REVIEW ACTIVITIES

CIRCLE AND CORRECT

Circle the correct answer for each question. Then check your answers in Appendix A.

1. Combining form for extremities
   a. acr
   b. acro
   c. arc
   d. arco

2. Word root for stomach
   a. gastro
   b. gastric
   c. stomat
   d. gastr

3. Compound word
   a. duodenum
   b. microscope
   c. dermatitis
   d. subglossal

4. Suffix for incision
   a. -ex
   b. -de
   c. -tomy
   d. -ectomy

5. Suffix for enlarged
   a. -ex
   b. -sub
   c. -megaly
   d. -hyper

6. Noun for first part of the small intestine
   a. colon
   b. duodenal
   c. enteric
   d. duodenum

REVIEW ACTIVITIES

7. Verb for removed
   a. excision
   b. excised
   c. ectomy
   d. exeresis

8. Adjective for heart
   a. cardiac
   b. cardious
   c. cardium
   d. cranial

9. Suffix for condition
   a. -es
   b. -ia
   c. -itis
   d. -o

10. Pronunciation symbol for accent
    a. —
    b. ə
    c. ′
    d. ^

11. Suffix meaning instrument used to cut slices
    a. -tome
    b. -tomy
    c. -meter
    d. -graph

12. Adjective for condition of blueness:
    a. cyanosis
    b. xanthotic
    c. cyanous
    d. cyanotic

13. Word root for x-ray
    a. tom
    b. graph
    c. echo
    d. radi

14. Suffix for making a new opening
    a. -itis
    b. -ectomy
    c. -ostomy
    d. -tomy

15. Erythro means
    a. green
    b. red
    c. white
    d. blue

SELECT AND CONSTRUCT

Select the correct word parts (some may be used more than once) from the following list and construct medical terms that represent the given meaning.

-ac	acro	-al	-algia	-blast	cardi(o)
chlor	cyano	cyt(e)(o)	derm(a)o	dermato	duodeno
echo ectomy	electro	-emia	-er	erythro	gastr/o(ia)
-gram	-graph	-graphy	-ia	-ic	-itis
leuko	-logy	mania	megal(o)(y)	melano	osis
-ostomy	paralysis	-pathy	penia	radio	sono
thrombo	tom(e)(o)	-tomy	um	xantho	

1. excision of the stomach _____

2. make a new opening (connection) between the stomach and the duodenum _____

3. blueness of the skin _____

4. disease condition of the skin _____

5. red blood cell _____

6. embryonic dark pigmented cell _____

7. decrease in the number of platelets _____

8. enlargement of the stomach _____

9. overenlarged (delusional) opinion of self _____

10. instrument used to make a recording of heart activity _____

REVIEW ACTIVITIES

11. incision into the first part of the small intestine _____

12. adjectival form of the word for heart _____

13. the process of obtaining an image from reflected sound _____

14. the picture (record) of sound reflected through the heart _____

15. one who takes x-rays _____

16. increase in WBCs _____

17. enlarged extremities _____

18. x-ray picture made through slices of the body _____

19. condition of yellow skin _____

20. the study of cells _____

DEFINE AND DISSECT

Give a brief definition and dissect each listed term into its word parts in the space provided. Check your answers by referring to the frame listed in parentheses and to your medical dictionary. Then listen to the CD to practice pronunciation.

Key: rt (word root), v (vowel)

1. duodenectomy (2.1)

_____/_____
rt   suffix

_____
definition

2. pathologist (2.55)

_____/_____/_____
rt   v   suffix

3. acrocyanosis (2.63)

_____/_____/_____/_____
rt   v   rt   suffix

4. cyanotic (2.62)

_____/_____/_____
rt   v   suffix

5. dermatome (2.4)

_____/_____/_____
rt   v   suffix

6. erythroderma (2.64)

_____/_____/_____
rt   v   suffix

7. melanocyte (2.65)

_____/_____/_____
rt   v   rt/suffix

REVIEW ACTIVITIES

8. echocardiography (2.50)

_____/____/_____/____/_____
rt   v   rt   v   suffix

9. leukocytopenia (2.85)

_____/____/_____/____/_____
rt   v   rt   v   suffix

10. thrombocytes (2.98)

_____/_____/_____
rt   v   suffix

11. cardiomegaly (2.108)

_____/_____/_____
rt   v   suffix

12. megalogastria (2.113)

_____/_____/_____
rt   v   rt/suffix

13. electrocardiograph (2.44)

_____/____/_____/____/_____
rt   v   rt   v   suffix

14. radiologist (2.53)

_____/_____/_____
rt   v   suffix

15. gastrectomy (2.3)

_____/_____
rt   suffix

16. gastroduodenostomy (2.10)

_____/____/_____/____/_____
rt   v   rt   v   suffix

17. erythrocytosis (2.90)

_____/_____/_____/_____
rt   v   rt   suffix

18. sonographer (2.48)

_____/_____/_____
rt   v   suffix

19. radiographer (2.52)

_____/_____/_____
rt   v   suffix

20. cytometer (2.79)

_____/_____/_____
rt   v   suffix

REVIEW ACTIVITIES

21. erythremia (2.67)

_____/_____
          rt   suffix

_____

22. cardialgia (2.36)

_____/_____
          rt   suffix

_____

23. duodenotomy (2.14)

_____/_____/_____
     rt   v   suffix

_____

24. tomography (2.33)

_____/_____/_____
   rt   v   suffix

_____

25. cardiologist (2.40)

_____/_____/_____
   rt   v   suffix

_____

ABBREVIATION MATCHING

Match the following abbreviations with their definition.

_____ 1. ALL	a. registered radiologic technologist
_____ 2. EKG	b. cardiac care unit
_____ 3. CT	c. echocardiogram
_____ 4. CCU	d. computed tomography
_____ 5. DMS	e. cardiac telogram
_____ 6. GI	f. gastric contents
_____ 7. ACVD	g. gastrointestinal
_____ 8. GA	h. diagnostic medical sonography
_____ 9. Ra	i. radium
_____ 10. ECHO	j. cardiac block catheter
	k. electrocardiogram
	l. acute lymphocytic leukemia
	m. acute cardiovascular disease
	n. gastric analysis

ABBREVIATION FILL-IN

Fill in the blanks with the correct abbreviation.

11. The WBC count and RBC count are part of the _____.

12. The CBC includes the _____ and the _____, which count the white and red blood cells.

13. Magnetic resonance imaging and radiography produce films of structures inside the body in a noninvasive way. The RT(R) with specialized training may perform either an _____ or an _____.

14. The _____ can assist the patient as they perform an MRI or x-ray.

REVIEW ACTIVITIES

15. Echocardiography is one type of sonography that is specifically used to view the heart. A _____ program can train individuals to perform _____ for diagnosis of heart disease.

16. A patient suffering from chest pain may be admitted to the _____. A cardiologist may order an _____ to understand the electrical changes in the heart and an _____ to see the efficiency of blood flow through the heart. LDH and CPK may also be performed as blood tests for cardiac enzymes.

17. When the heart muscle is damaged, the level of cardiac enzymes _____ and _____ could rise.

CASE STUDIES

The following case study is taken from an actual medical record. The patient name has been changed to protect confidentiality. By reading the case in each unit and studying the medical terms, you will gain a deeper understanding of the meaning and especially of the use of these terms. You will notice that several words are in color. These are key medical terms that you may have learned through the word-building system.

Write the term next to its meaning given below. Then draw slashes to analyze the word parts. You will also note the use of medical abbreviations. Look these up in your dictionary or find them in Appendix B. If you have any questions about the answers, refer to your medical dictionary or check with your instructor for the answers in Appendix A.

CASE STUDY 2-1

Discharge Summary

Pt: Age 76

Dx: **Acute** chest pain—**etiology** unknown

Mr. Harry Hart, a 76-year-old Caucasian male, was admitted through the emergency room (ER) where he presented via **ambulance** with **substernal** chest pain. Mr. Hart was also seen by Dr. Rick Cardio in **cardiac** consultation, and a dictated note is available on his chart.

Serial **electrocardiograms** were obtained during the course of Mr. Hart's hospitalization. These failed to reveal any acute injury. An **echocardiogram** was performed and interpreted by Dr. Cardio and found to be within normal limits. The chest **x-ray** was performed revealing no active **cardiopulmonary** disease with aortic arteriosclerosis being present. Radionuclide (isotope) cardiac **angiography** was performed and read as negative. The laboratory results were normal with a slightly elevated LDH.

Mr. Hart was admitted to CCU on routine **coronary** care orders. **Cardiac** consultation was obtained and after we ruled out any **acute cardiac** event, he was transferred to Stepdown with continuous cardiac **telemetry**. By 19 June his condition was stable enough to warrant discharge.

1. severe and short term _____

2. pertaining to the heart _____

3. sonography of the heart _____

4. below the sternum _____

5. electronic data transmission _____

6. hardening of the arteries _____

7. x-ray of a vessel _____

REVIEW ACTIVITIES

8. pertaining to heart and lungs

   _____

9. transport vehicle

   _____

10. study of cause

    _____

11. EKG

    _____

12. radiograph

    _____

CROSSWORD PUZZLE

Check your answers by going back through the frames or checking the solution in Appendix C.

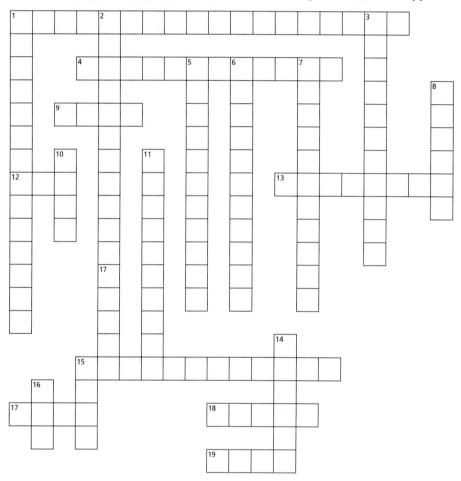

Across

1. instrument: makes an image (tracing) of heart activity
4. red skin
9. suffix: incision into
12. complete blood count (abbr.)
13. image made using ultrasound
15. enlarged stomach
17. suffix: condition in the blood
18. combining form for tissue
19. _____cardiography

Down

1. increase number of red blood cells
2. low platelet count
3. physician specialist in study of disease
5. physician specialist in imaging (x-ray)
6. study of the skin
7. embryonic pigment cell
8. suffix: new surgical opening
10. acute cardiovascular disease (abbr.)
11. technologist who studies cells
14. combining form for yellow
15. suffix: image or picture
16. diagnostic medical sonography (abbr.)

REVIEW ACTIVITIES

GLOSSARY

blastocyte	immature cell	erythrocytopenia	low numbers of erythrocytes
cardialgia	heart pain	erythrocytosis	high numbers of erythrocytes
cardiologist	physician specialist in heart disease	erythroderma	redness of the skin
cardiomegaly	enlarged heart	etiology	the study of the origin of disease
cyanoderma	blueness of the skin	gastralgia	stomach pain
cyanosis	condition of blueness	gastrectomy	excision of the stomach
cytologist	a technologist who studies cellular disease	gastric	pertaining to the stomach (adj.)
cytology	the science of studying cells	gastroduodenostomy	making a new opening between the stomach and duodenum
cytometer	instrument used to count cells		
cytometry	process of using a cytometer	gastromegaly	enlarged stomach
dermatology	the science of studying the skin	gastrostomy	making a new opening in the stomach
dermatome	instrument used to cut slices of skin tissue	histoblast	immature tissue cells
		histology	the science of studying tissues
duodenal	pertaining to the duodenum (adj.)	jaundice	yellow appearance due to high bilbin level in the blood
duodenotomy	incision into the duodenum	leukemia	blood cancer involving leukocytes
duodenum	first part of the small intestine		
echocardiography	sonography of the heart	leukocyte	white blood cell
electrocardiogram	picture (tracing) representing the electrical activity of the heart during the cardiac cycle	leukocytopenia	low numbers of leukocytes
		leukocytosis	high numbers of leukocytes
		leukoderma	abnormally white skin (vitiligo)
electrocardiograph	instrument that produces the electrocardiogram	lymphatic	pertaining to the lymph system
electrocardiography	process of using the electrocardiograph	lymphocyte	lymphatic system white blood cell
erythremia	abnormally red blood due to too many erythrocytes		
		megalomania	abnormally enlarged self-image
erythroblast	immature red blood cell		
erythrocytes	red blood cells	melanoblast	immature melanocyte

REVIEW ACTIVITIES

melanocyte	pigment cell
melanoderma	dark patches of skin
pathologist	physician specialist in the study of disease
pathology	the science of studying disease
radiogram	x-ray picture (film) (radiograph)
radiograph	instrument used to produce the radiogram or the x-ray film
radiography	process of producing radiograms (radiographs)
radiologist	physician specialist in the interpretation of radiograms and other diagnostic imaging modalities
sonogram	image of the body produced by computerized reflected sound
sonograph	instrument that reflects sound waves through the body, picks them up with a transducer, and uses a computer to create an image of body structures

sonographer	technologist who performs sonography
sonography	process of using a sonograph (ultrasonography)
thrombocytes	platelets, blood-clotting cell fragments
thrombocytopenia	low numbers of thrombocytes
thrombocytosis	high numbers of thrombocytes
tomogram	picture made by a tomograph
tomograph	instrument that uses x-ray to produce images through planes (slices) of the body
tomography	the process of using a tomograph
xanthemia	yellow condition of the blood (carotenemia)

UNIT 3

Oncology and the Central Nervous System

3.1

You can form words without even knowing their meaning. In the next three frames use what is needed from **encephal/o** + **-itis** to form a word: _____/_____.

encephal/itis

3.2

Use what is needed from **encephal/o**,
malac/o, and
-ia
_____/_____/_____/_____.

encephal/o/malac/ia
en sef′ ə lō mal **ā**′ shə

3.3

Use what is needed from **encephal/o**,
mening/o, and
-itis
_____/____/_____/_____.

encephal/o/mening/itis
en sef′ ə lō men′ in **jī** tis

3.4

Use what is needed from **encephal/o**,
myel/o, and
-pathy
_____/____/_____/____/_____.

encephal/o/myel/o/pathy
en sef′ ə lō mi′ əl **op**′ ə thē

3.5

A prefix goes in front of a word to change its meaning. In the words hyper/trophy, hyper/emia, and hyper/emesis, **hyper-** changes the meaning of **-trophy**, **-emia**, and emesis. **hyper-** is a _____.

prefix

3.6

hyper- is a prefix that means above or more than normal. In common slang, someone who is overactive is hyper. To say that a person is overly critical, you would use the word _____/critic/al.

hyper-

3.7

TAKE A CLOSER LOOK

hyper-

Our bodies do not work well when imbalanced by excesses. Look up the following conditions that are all caused by excesses. Write the substance or nature of the excess next to the term.

hypercholesterolemia _____

hypertoxicity _____

hyperflexion _____

hyperactivity _____

hyperlipidemia _____

hyperproteinuria _____

3.8

hypo- is a prefix that is just the opposite of hyper-. The prefix for below or less than normal is _____.

hypo-

3.9

TAKE A CLOSER LOOK

hypo-

Below normal levels of substances, sizes, or activity may also produce critical imbalance. Use your dictionary to discover the nature of each condition and write your answer next to the term.

hypocalcemia _____

hypodactylia _____

hyposensitive _____

hypothermia _____

hypokalemia _____

hypothyroidism _____

hypodermic _____

3.10

Hypo/trophy (atrophy) means progressive degeneration. When an organ or tissue that has developed properly wastes away or decreases in size, it is undergoing _____/_____.

hypo/trophy
or hí **pot′** rə f
a/trophy
a trō fē

ANSWER COLUMN

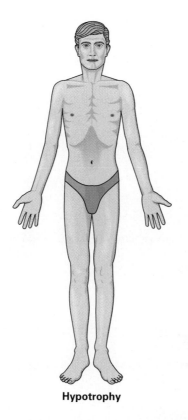

Hypotrophy

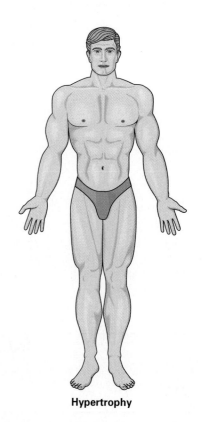

Hypertrophy

3.11

Hyperemesis gravidarum is a complication of pregnancy that can require hospitalization. The part of the disorder that tells you excessive vomiting occurs is _____.

hyperemesis
hī pûr **em′** ə sis

3.12

Gallbladder attacks can cause excessive vomiting. This, too, is called _____.

hyperemesis

3.13

Hypertrophy means overdevelopment. **-trophy** comes from the Greek word *trophe*, for nourishment. See the connection between nourishment and development? Overdevelopment is called _____/_____.

hyper/trophy
hī **pûr′** trə fē

ANSWER COLUMN

Blood pressure is measured using a sphygmomanometer.

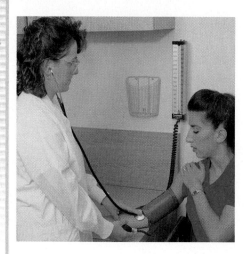

3.14

hypertrophy

Many organs can hypertrophy. If the heart overdevelops, the condition
is _____ of the heart.

3.15

hyper/tension
hī pûr **ten**′ shən

Abnormally high blood pressure (BP) (tension) is
called _____/_____.

3.16

high blood pressure

Essential hypertension and nonessential hypertension are both conditions of
* _____.

3.17

hypo/tension
hī pō **ten**′ shun

If hypertension is elevated BP, then hypo/tension indicates lowered BP.
A blood pressure of 120/80 mmHg is a normal average. A BP of 90/60 mmHg
may indicate _____/_____.

NOTE: mmHg means millimeters of mercury.

3.18

hypertension

Diuretic medications may be prescribed to lower the blood pressure (BP)
in patients with _____ by increasing excretion of fluids.

3.19

aden
aden/o

aden/o is used in words that refer to glands. The word root is _____.
The combining form is _____/____.

ANSWER COLUMN

3.20

aden/itis
ad ə **ni′** tis

Build a word that means inflammation of a gland (word root + suffix rule):
_____/_____.

3.21

-ectomy
aden-
aden/ectomy
ad ə **nek′** t ə mē

Aden/ectomy means excision or removal of a gland. The part that means
excision is _____. The part that means gland is _____. The word for
removal of a gland is _____/_____.

3.22

adenectomy

An adenectomy is a surgical procedure. If a gland is tumorous, part or all of it
can be excised. This operation is an _____.

3.23

aden/oma
ad ə **nō′** mə

A tumor is an abnormal growth of cells, also referred to as a neoplasm.
-oma is the suffix for tumor. Form a word that means tumor of a
gland: _____/_____
Note: Not all tumors are cancerous.

3.24

adenoma

Sometimes the thyroid gland develops an adenoma. In this case, a patient's
history might read, ". . . hyperthyroidism noted—due to presence of a thyroid
_____."

3.25

adenoma
adenectomy
or thyroidectomy
thī roid **ek′** tō mē

When a thyroid _____ (tumor of a gland) is found, a
partial _____ (excision of gland)
may be performed.

3.26

word root
vowel
aden/o/pathy
ad ə **nop′** ə thē

Recall **-pathy** is a suffix meaning disease. Aden/o/pathy means any disease
of a gland. In this word you have a *_____ plus
a _____ and suffix to form the word
_____/___/_____.

3.27

adenopathy

Adenopathy means glandular disease in general. When the diagnosis is made
of a diseased gland but the disease is not specifically known or stated, the
word used is _____.

ANSWER COLUMN

3.28

Adenopathy
adenoma
adenectomy

_____ (glandular disease) could be diagnosed as
an _____ (glandular tumor). If so, the surgeon may advise
that an _____ (excision of a gland) be performed.

3.29

lymph/aden/o/pathy
lim fad′ ə **nop**′ ə thē

Recall **lymph/o** refers to lymphatic tissue. Any disease of the lymph
glands could be called _____/_____/____/_____.

3.30

adenitis
adenectomy

When a gland is found to have a mild _____ (inflammation),
no _____ (surgery) is indicated.

3.31

tumor **too** mer
fat

An adenoma is a glandular tumor. **-oma** is the suffix for _____. A lip/oma
is a tumor containing fat. **lip/o** is the combining form for _____.

3.32

lip/oma
lip **ō**′ mə

A lip/oma is usually benign (noncancerous). A fatty tumor is called
a _____/_____.

3.33

lymph/oma
lim **fō**′ mə

A tumor composed of lymph tissue is called a _____/_____.

3.34

TAKE A CLOSER LOOK

Lesion, ulcer, tumor, and growth. We often hear these terms used, but are they
the same? How do we know when and how to use them?

lesion
lē′ zhun

A lesion may be one of many possible types of abnormal tissue conditions
including macules, vesicles, papules, ulcers, abscesses, and tumors, just to
name a few.

ulcer
ul′ ser

Ulcers are a more specific type of lesion. They are open sores on the skin or
mucous membranes.

tumor
too mer

A tumor is an abnormal growth in numbers and/or types of cells and may
be cancerous.

The term "growth" is a common term that is nonspecific and used less often
in formal diagnosis. Look up these terms in your dictionary and you will find
several pages of interesting information.

Malignant melanoma
(Courtesy of Robert A. Silverman, MD, Pediatric Dermatology, Georgetown University)

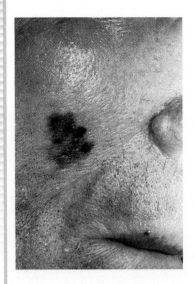

3.35

carcin/o, from the Greek word *carcinos*, meaning crab, is the combining form for cancer (CA). A carcin/oma is a *_____.

cancerous tumor or
malignant tumor

3.36

A carcinoma may occur in almost any part of the body. A stomach cancer is called gastric _____.

carcinoma

3.37

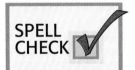

Make sure you use and say the correct form:

metastasis	singular noun	me **ta**′ sta sis
metastases	plural noun	me **ta**′ sta sēs
metastatic	adjective	me ta **sta**′ tik
metastasize(d)	verb	me **ta**′ sta sízd

3.38

Metastasis is the transfer of a disease from one organ to another not connected to it. Carcinoma may metastasize (spread to other parts of the body) through the lymphatic system. The intestine has a rich blood supply. For this reason, intestinal _____/_____ is extremely dangerous, as it may metastasize to the liver.

carcin/oma
kär sin **ō**′ mə

NOTE: meta- means beyond and **-stasis** means in one place (staying). Metastasis (met., metas., mets.) means spreading beyond the original place.

ANSWER COLUMN

meta/stasis me **ta**′ sta sis	**3.39** A carcinoma may spread to another body part. The portion that grows in a new location is called a _____/_____.
carcinoma	**3.40** Carcinoma may be confined to the site (from the Latin *situs*; think of *situ*ation) of its origin. In this case, it is called _____ in situ.
aden/o/carcin/oma ad′ ə nō kär sin **ō**′ mə	**3.41** Form a word that means cancer of glandular tissue: _____/____/_____.
sarc/oma sär **kō**′ mə	**3.42** Carcinoma indicates the cancer originated from epithelial tissue. When cancer of connective tissue is found, it is called sarc/oma. Bone cancer is a type of _____/_____.
connective	**3.43** From what you have just learned, draw a conclusion about this. Kaposi's sarcoma is a condition many people with acquired immunodeficiency syndrome (AIDS) develop. Sarcoma indicates this is a cancerous condition of _____ tissue.
black melan/oma mel ə **nō**′ mə	**3.44** **melan/o** means _____. Melan/osis means black pigmentation. A word that means black tumor is _____/_____.

Squamus cell carcinoma
(Courtesy of Robert A. Silverman, MD, Pediatric Dermatology, Georgetown University)

TUMOR TERMINOLOGY

Combining Form	Meaning	Tumor
Epithelial Tissue		
Benign		
aden/o	gland	adenoma
melan/o	dark pigmented	melanoma
papill/o	small elevation of tissue	papilloma
fibr/o	fibrous tissue	fibroadenoma
Malignant		
aden/o	gland, glandular tissue	adenocarcinoma
melan/o	dark pigmented	melanocarcinoma (malignant melanoma)
carcin/o	squamous cell (skin)	squamous cell carcinoma
carcin/o	basal cell (skin)	basal cell carcinoma
Connective-Hematopoietic-Nerve Tissue		
Benign		
oste/o	bone	osteoma
chondr/o	cartilage	chondroma
leiomy/o	smooth muscle	leiomyoma
lip/o	fat	lipoma
ather/o	fatty, porridgelike	atheroma
hem/angi/o	blood vessel	hemangioma
neur/o	nerve	neuroma
Malignant		
oste/o	bone	osteosarcoma
chondr/o	cartilage	chondrosarcoma
leiomy/o	smooth muscle	leiomyosarcoma
lip/o	fat	liposarcoma
angi/o	vessel	angiosarcoma
leuk/o	white	leukemia
myel/o	bone marrow	myeloma
lymph/o	lymphatic	lymphosarcoma
neur/o	nerve	neurosarcoma

3.45

Melanin is the pigment that gives dark color to the hair, skin, and choroid (dark pigmented area) of the eye. A black pigmented cell is a _____/____/_____.

melan/o/cyte
mel′ ə nō sĭt
mə **lan**′ ə sĭt

ANSWER COLUMN

Kaposi's sarcoma *(Courtesy of Robert A. Silverman, MD, Clinical Associate Professor, Department of Pediatrics, Georgetown University)*

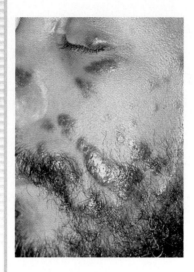

3.46

black or dark skin coloring (pigmentation) (literally, black skin)

Melanoderma means *_____.

3.47

melan/o/carcin/oma
mel′ ə nō kär si **nō**′ mə

You have already learned that a carcin/oma is a form of cancer.
A darkly pigmented cancer is _____/____/_____/_____.

3.48

melanocarcinoma

When a dark hairless mole on the skin grows or changes, a physician should be consulted for there is the possibility of black-mole cancer
or _____.

3.49

Plural Formation

Recall from the word-building section in Unit 1 that medical words often have special suffixes for plural formation. Words that end in **-oma** form a plural by using **-mata** as the suffix. In the list below, the first plural is done for you; *you* form the rest.

Singular	Plural
carcinoma	carcinomata
lipoma	_____
sarcoma	_____
atheroma	_____

lipomata
sarcomata
atheromata

ANSWER COLUMN

adenomata	adenoma _____
melanomata	melanoma _____

NOTE: Although these plural forms are proper medical terminology, you will see (and hear dictated) carcinomas, lipomas, melanomas, and so on. These have become accepted forms in many places.

3.50

onc/o from the Greek word *oncos,* meaning mass, is a combining form meaning tumor. The study of tumors is onc/o/logy. A specialist who studies

onc/o/logist
on **kol**′ ō jist

tumors is called an _____/____/_____.

3.51

A hospitalized patient with a disease caused by a malignant tumor might

onc/o/logy
on **kol**′ ō jə

be treated in the _____/____/_____ unit.

3.52

lip/o
lip/oid
lip′ oid

The combining form for fat is _____/_____. **-oid** is a suffix that means like or resembling. Build a word that means fatlike or resembling fat: _____/_____.

3.53

fat
lipoid

The word lipoid is used in both chemistry and pathology. It describes a substance that looks like fat, dissolves like fat, but is not _____. A word that means resembling fat is _____.

3.54

lipoid

In proper amounts cholesterol is essential to health, but too much may cause atherosclerosis (hardening of blood vessels due to fatty deposits). Cholesterol is an alcohol that resembles fat; therefore, it is _____.

3.55

ather/o is the combining form for fatty or porridgelike. A tumorlike thickening and degeneration of the blood vessel walls that is caused by fatty deposits

ather/oma
ather **ō**′ mə
atheró/scler/osis
a′ ther ō skler **ō**′ sis

is called an _____/_____. Hardening of vessel walls due to fatty deposits is called _____/_____/_____/_____.

ANSWER COLUMN

	3.56
tissue	The combining form that refers to tissue is **hist/o**. Hist/o/lysis is the destruction of _____.
	3.57
tissue	A hist/o/genous substance is a substance that is made of _____.
	3.58
hist/o/logy his **tol′** ə jē hist/o/log/ist his **tol′** ə jist	Build words meaning the study of tissue _____/___/_____; one who studies tissues _____/___/_____/_____.
	3.59
hist/o/blast **his′** tō blast hist/o/cyte **his′** tō sīt hist/oid **his′** toid	Build words meaning an embryonic tissue (cell) _____/___/_____; a tissue cell _____/___/_____; resembling tissue _____/_____.
	3.60
new	**neo-** from the Greek *neos* means new. Neo/genesis means generation of _____ tissue.
	3.61
new new	Neo/natal refers to the _____ born. A neo/plasm is a tumor or _____ growth (formation—plasm/o).
	3.62
neo/natal nē ō **nāt′** əl	A special unit for the newborn is the _____/_____ intensive care unit.
	3.63
neo/plasm **nē′** ō plaz əm	Neo/plasm refers to any kind of tumor or abnormal growth of cells. A nonmalignant tumor is called a benign _____/_____.

PROFESSIONAL PROFILES

Medical technologists (MTs [ASCP]), medical laboratory technicians (MLTs), and certified laboratory assistants (CLAs) physically and chemically analyze and culture urine, blood, and other body fluids and tissues to determine the presence of all types of diseases. They work closely with physician specialists such as oncologists, pathologists, and hematologists. Knowledge of specimen collection, anatomy and physiology, biochemistry, laboratory equipment, asepsis, and quality control is essential. The American Society of Clinical Pathology (ASCP) is a professional organization that oversees credentialing and education in the medical laboratory professions.

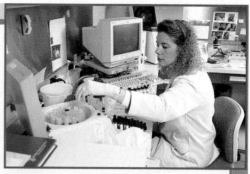

Medical technologist performing blood analysis *(Photo by Marcia Butterfield, courtesy of W. A. Foote Memorial Hospital, Jackson, MI)*

ANSWER COLUMN

3.64

neoplasm
neoplasm
neoplasms

A neoplasm may be a malignant tumor. Carcinoma is a malignant
_____. A melanoma can be a malignant
_____. An onc/ologist is a physician who studies
_____ (plural).

3.65

neoplasm
neoplasm

A sarcoma is a malignant _____ of connective tissue.
Oste/o/sarcoma is a malignant _____ of the bone.

3.66

anti/neo/plastic
an' ti nē' ō **plas**' tik

anti/tumor/i/genic
an' ti tōo/môr ə **jen**' ik

anti/tumor/i/genesis
an' ti tōo/môr ə **jen**' ə sis

anti- is a prefix meaning against. **–plast/ic** is an adjective suffix for abnormal growth. A therapeutic agent that works against cancerous neoplasms is called an _____/_____/_____ agent.

-genesis refers to development. An agent that inhibits the development of tumors is an _____/_____/____/_____ (adjective) agent.

The process of inhibiting development of a tumor is _____/_____/____/_____ (noun).

ANSWER COLUMN

Four types of tissue and their function

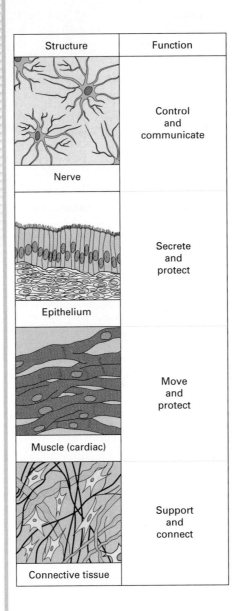

Structure	Function
Nerve	Control and communicate
Epithelium	Secrete and protect
Muscle (cardiac)	Move and protect
Connective tissue	Support and connect

3.67

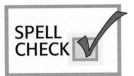

SPELL CHECK ✓

Watch out for these similar combining forms:
ather/o—porridgelike, fatty;
arteri/o—arteries;
arthr/o—joint.

3.68

Muc/oid means resembling mucus. **-oid** is a suffix
meaning *_____. The word root for mucus
is _____ and its combining form is _____/____.

like or resembling

muc

muc/o

ANSWER COLUMN

Mucous and serous membranes

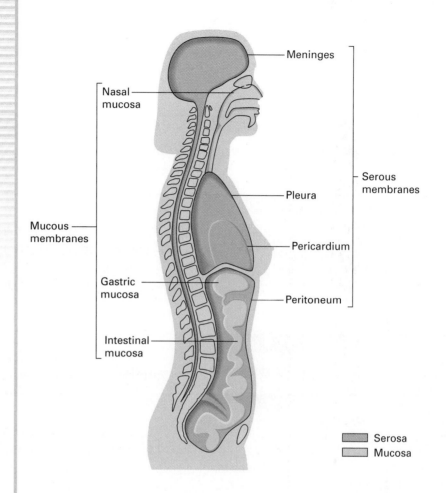

Nasal mucosa

Meninges

Mucous membranes

Serous membranes

Pleura

Pericardium

Gastric mucosa

Peritoneum

Intestinal mucosa

Serosa
Mucosa

3.69

Mucoid is an adjective that means resembling or like mucus. There is a substance in connective tissue that resembles mucus. This is a _____/_____ substance.

muc/oid
my\overline{oo} koid

3.70

Muc/us is a secretion of the muc/ous membrane. **-us** is a noun suffix. **-ous** is an adjectival suffix. The muc/ous membrane secretes _____/_____.

muc/us
my\overline{oo} kəs

3.71

Mucus is secreted by cells in the nose. It traps dust and bacteria from the air. One of the body's protective devices is _____.

mucus

ANSWER COLUMN

3.72

mucus
muc/ous
myōō kəs

The mucous membrane secretes _____. The tissue that secretes mucus is the _____/_____ membrane or muc/osa.

3.73

mucus
mucous

The noun (the secretion) built from **muc/o** is _____. The adjective (pertaining to) built from **muc/o** is _____.

3.74

muc/osa
myōō **kō′** sə

The mucous membrane or mucosa is found lining the open body cavities. This protective, mucous membrane can also be called the _____/_____.

NOTE:The digestive system is considered an open body cavity because it is essentially open from mouth to anus.

3.75

mucosa

The stomach lining is the gastric _____.

3.76

mucus
mucoid
mucosa or
mucous membrane

The mucosa secretes _____. Anything that resembles mucus is _____. Mucoid substances are not mucus; therefore, they are not secreted by the *_____.

3.77

ser/osa
se **rō′** sə

The serous membranes line the closed body cavities and cover the outside of organs such as the intestines. Serosa is the noun form. The intestinal _____/_____ is a membrane that covers the intestine.

3.78

ser/ous
ser′ us

The mucous membranes line the open body cavities and the _____/_____ (adjective) membranes line the closed cavities.

3.79

cephal

At this stage of word building, learners sometimes find that they have one big pain in the head. The word for pain in the head is cephal/algia (often shortened to cephalgia). The word root for head is _____.

ANSWER COLUMN

Structures of the head

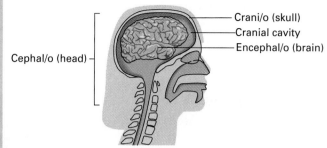

Cephal/o (head)

Crani/o (skull)
Cranial cavity
Encephal/o (brain)

3.80

-algia

One suffix for pain is _____.

3.81

cephal/algia
sef ə **lal**′ jē ə

If you are suffering from cephal/algia, persevere, for later this gets to be fun.
Any pain in the head may be called _____/_____.

3.82

cephalalgia

The combining form for head is cephal/o. The word for pain in the
head is _____.

3.83

cephal/o/dynia
sef ə lō **din**′ ē ə
cephal/algia

Odyne is a Greek word for pain. Another word for pain in the head is
cephal/o/dynia. This word shows the combining form plus a suffix. If this
seems a headache, relax. Either word, _____/____/_____ or
_____/_____, will do for headache.

NOTE: Cephalgia is also correct spelling.

3.84

word root
combining form

Recall the suffixes **-algia** and **-dynia**. They are usually interchangeable.
When **-algia** is used as a suffix it is preceded by a (choose one)
*_____ (combining form/word root). When **-dynia**
is used, it is preceded by a (choose one) *_____
(combining form/word root).

3.85

cephal/o/dynic
sef ə lō **din**′ ik

-dynia can take the adjectival form **-dynic**. An adjective that means
pertaining to head pain is _____/____/_____.

ANSWER COLUMN

3.86

cephalodynic

To say medically that headache (HA) discomfort exists, use the
adjective _____ for headache.

3.87

cephalalgia
cephalodynia
cephalodynic

Two nouns for head pain are _____
and _____. The adjective used for head pain
is _____.

3.88

adjective
-ic

Cephal/ic means pertaining to or toward the head. Cephal/ic is
a(n) _____ (noun/adjective). This is evident because
cephalic ends in _____.

3.89

cephal/ic
s ə **fal**′ ik

Cephalic is an adjective. A case history reporting head cuts due to an accident
might read, "_____/_____ lacerations present."

3.90

cephalic

In the phrase "lack of cephalic orientation," the adjective is _____.

3.91

encephal/itis
en sef′ ə **lī**′ tis

*In*side the head, *en*closed in bone, is the brain; **encephal/o** is used in
words pertaining to the brain. Build a word meaning inflammation
of the brain: _____/_____.

3.92

-oma
encephal/oma
en sef ə **lō**′ mə

The suffix for tumor is _____. Use what is necessary from encephal/o
to build a word for brain tumor: _____/_____.

3.93

brain

The Greek word for hernia is *kele*, indicating an abnormal protrusion or swelling;
the suffix is **-cele**. Encephal/o/cele is a word meaning herniation
of _____ tissue.

3.94

encephal/o/cele
en **sef**′ ə lō sēl

An encephalocele occurs when brain tissue protrudes through a cranial fissure
(see illustration). The word for herniation of brain tissue is
_____/____/_____.

ANSWER COLUMN

Encephalocele

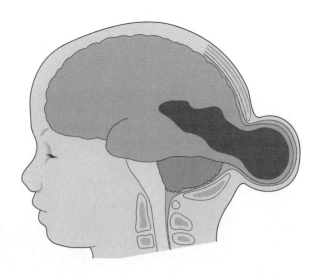

3.95

Any hernia is a projection of a part from its natural cavity. Herniation is indicated by **-cele**. A projection of brain tissue from its natural cavity

encephalocele

is an _____.

3.96

Brain herniation is sometimes a finding in hydrocephaly. This condition, in

encephalocele

medical language, is called an _____.

3.97

Malacia is a word meaning softening of a tissue. Encephal/o/malac/ia means

softening of brain tissue

* _____.

3.98

-tomy is used as a suffix for making an *incision* or temporary opening.

encephal/o/tomy
en sef′ ə **lot**′ ō mē

An incision into the brain is an _____/___/_____.

3.99

Using what is necessary from malac/o with the suffix **-tomy**, form a word that

malac/o/tomy
mal ə **kot**′ ə mé

means incision of soft areas: _____/___/_____.

ANSWER COLUMN

Sagittal section of the brain

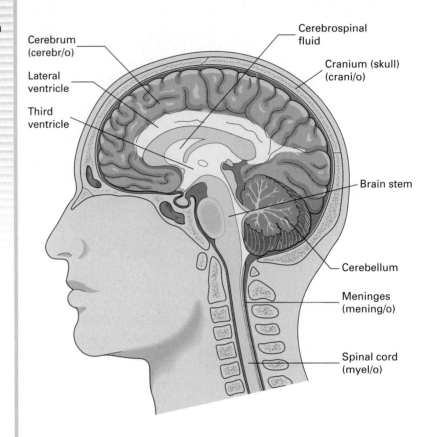

Sagittal section of the brain

- Cerebrum (cerebr/o)
- Lateral ventricle
- Third ventricle
- Cerebrospinal fluid
- Cranium (skull) (crani/o)
- Brain stem
- Cerebellum
- Meninges (mening/o)
- Spinal cord (myel/o)

3.100

encephal/o/malac/ia
en sef′ ə lō mə **lā**′ shə

Encephal/o/malac/ia ends in **-ia**, which is a suffix that forms a noun and indicates a condition. A noun meaning softening of brain tissue is _____/_____/_____/_____.

3.101

encephalomalacia

An accident causing brain injury could result in the softening of some brain tissue, or _____.

3.102

electr/o/encephal/o/gram
e lek′ trō en sef′ ə lō gram

From your knowledge of the word parts **electr/o**, **encephal/o**, and **-gram** build a term meaning picture of the electrical activity of the brain: _____/____/_____/____/_____ (EEG).

3.103

electr/o/encephal/o/graphy
e lek′ trō en sef ə **log**′ ra fē

The process of recording electrical brain activity is called _____/____/_____/____/_____. The instrument used to

PROFESSIONAL PROFILES

Electroneurodiagnostic (END) technologists are allied health professionals who perform electroencephalography (EEG), evoked potentials (EP), polysomnography (PSG), nerve conduction studies (NCS), and electronystagmography (ENG). The END technologist works under the supervision of a physician who is responsible for interpretation and clinical correlation of the results. Individuals entering the END profession may be graduates of a Committee on Accreditation of Allied Health Education Programs (CAAHEP) accredited associate degree program and may take a national certification exam in electroneurodiagnostic technology developed by the American Board of Registration of EEG and EP Technologists.

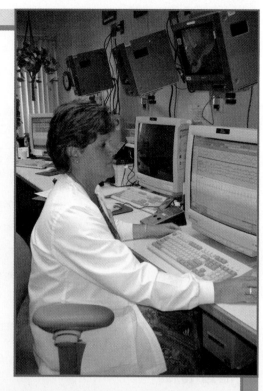

ANSWER COLUMN	
electr/o/encephal/o/graph e lek′ trō en **sef**′ ə lō graf	record the EEG is an _____/____/_____/____/_____.
	3.104
electr/o/neur/o/diagnos/tic ē lek′ trō nōō rō di əg **nos**′ tik	The study of brain wave activity, whether awake or asleep, is the work of physicians assisted by the _____/____/_____/____/_____/_____ (END) technologist.
	3.105
surgical repair of the skull or cranium	**crani/o** is used in words referring to the crani/um or skull. **-plasty** is the suffix for surgical repair. Crani/o/plasty means *_____.
	3.106
crani/o/malac/ia krā nē ō mə **lā**′ shə	The word for softening of the bones of the skull is _____/____/_____/_____.

ANSWER COLUMN

Right lateral view of the cranium

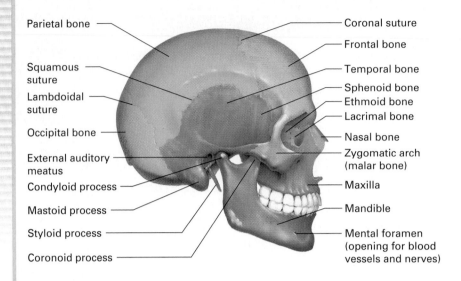

Parietal bone
Coronal suture
Frontal bone
Squamous suture
Temporal bone
Sphenoid bone
Lambdoidal suture
Ethmoid bone
Lacrimal bone
Occipital bone
Nasal bone
External auditory meatus
Zygomatic arch (malar bone)
Condyloid process
Maxilla
Mastoid process
Mandible
Styloid process
Mental foramen (opening for blood vessels and nerves)
Coronoid process

---

crani/ectomy
krā′ nē **ek**′ tə mē

3.107

The word meaning excision of part of the cranium is _____/_____.

---

crani/o/tomy
krā nē **ot**′ ə mē

3.108

The word for incision into the skull is _____/____/_____.

---

crani/o/meter
krā′ nē **om**′ ə tər

3.109

-meter is the suffix for instrument used to measure. An instrument used to measure the cranium is the _____/____/_____.

---

cranial
cranial

3.110

There are cranial bones. There are also _____ nerves. There are grooves and furrows called _____ fissures.

---

adjectival

3.111

Crani/al is the (choose one) _____ (noun/adjectival) form of cranium.

---

cerebr/um
ser′ ə brəm, sə **rē**′ brəm

3.112

Crani/o/cerebr/al refers to the skull and the cerebr/um. The cerebr/um is a part of the brain. **Cerebr/o** is used to build words about the _____/_____.

ANSWER COLUMN

	3.113
cerebrum	The cerebrum is the part of the brain in which thought occurs. When you think, you are using your _____.
	3.114
cerebrum	Feeling is interpreted in the cerebrum. Motor impulses also arise in the _____.
	3.115
cerebrum	Thinking, feeling, and movement are controlled by the gray matter of the _____. (Were you ever told to use your gray matter? This is why.)
	3.116
cerebr/al **ser**′ ə brəl, s ə **rē**′ brəl	The adjectival form of cerebrum is _____/_____.
	3.117
cerebral	There is a cerebral reflex. There are cerebral fissures. You have probably heard of _____ hemorrhage (bleeding).
	3.118
inflammation of the cerebrum	Cerebr/itis means *_____ _____.
	3.119
a cerebral tumor	A cerebr/oma is *_____.
	3.120
cerebr/o/tomy ser ə **brot**′ ə mē	An incision into the cerebrum to drain an abscess is a _____/____/_____.
	3.121
cerebrum (brain)	The vascular system refers to the blood vessels. A cerebr/o/vascular accident (CVA; stroke) occurs because a vascular lesion within the _____ either blocks blood flow or causes a hemorrhage.

ANSWER COLUMN

3.122

cerebr/o/vascul/ar
ser ē′ brō **vas**′ kū lär

People with hypertension are at high risk for a CVA or
_____/____/_____/_____ accident.

3.123

high blood pressure
vessels of the heart
abnormal function

Use what you have learned to analyze the following condition by writing its
meaning in the blank.
hyper/tensive *_____
cardi/o/vascul/ar *_____
dis/ease*_____
Abbreviation: HCVD

3.124

cerebr/o/spin/al
ser ē′ brō **spi**′ nəl

Cerebr/o/spin/al refers to the brain and spinal cord. There is fluid that bathes
the cerebrum and spinal cord. It is _____/____/_____/_____
fluid (CSF).

3.125

cerebrospinal

A spin/al puncture is sometimes done to remove _____ fluid.

3.126

cerebrospinal

There is even a disease called _____ meningitis.

3.127

mening/es
me **nin**′ jēz

Meninx is a Greek word for membrane. **mening/o** is the combining form for the
meninges, a three-layered membrane that covers the brain and spinal cord.
These three layers include the pia mater, arachnoid, and dura mater. The
protective covering of the brain and spinal cord is the _____/_____.

3.128

mening/o/cele
me **nin**′ gō sēl

A herniation of the meninges is a _____/____/_____.

3.129

meninges

A mening/o/cele is a herniation of the _____.

3.130

meninges

Mening/o/malac/ia means softening of the _____.

Meningocele and
myelomeningocele

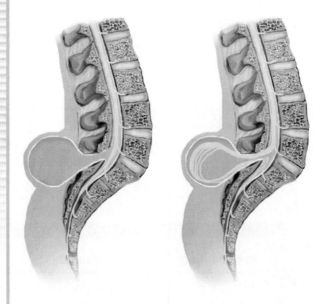

(A) Meningocele **(B) Myelomeningocele**

**Exterior left lateral view of
the brain**

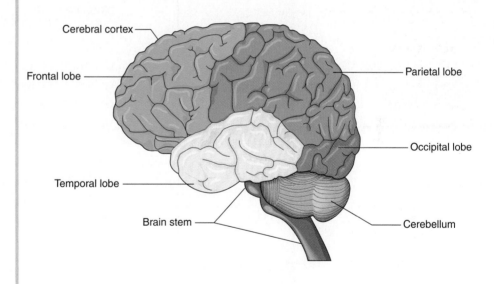

Cerebral cortex

Frontal lobe

Parietal lobe

Occipital lobe

Temporal lobe

Brain stem

Cerebellum

3.131

Mening/itis can occur as cerebr/al meningitis, spin/al meningitis,
or cerebr/o/spin/al _____/_____.

mening/itis
men in **jī′** tis

ANSWER COLUMN

3.132

meningitis

There are many kinds of meningitis. The tubercle bacillus can cause tuberculous meningitis. Mening/o/cocci are bacteria that cause epidemic _____.

PRONUNCIATION NOTE

When g is followed by e, i, y it is usually pronounced like a "j" (soft g) as in ginger. When g is followed by a, o, u it is pronounced like a hard "g" sound as in goat, gate, and gut. Practice saying: meningitis, meningocele j (soft g) (hard g).

Abbreviation	Meaning
AIDS	acquired immunodeficiency syndrome
ASCP	American Society of Clinical Pathology
BX	Biopsy
BCC	basal cell carcinoma
BP	blood pressure
CA	calcium
CA	cancer
CIS	carcinoma in situ
CLA	certified laboratory assistant
CP	cerebral palsy
CSF	cerebrospinal fluid
CV	cardiovascular
CVA	cerebrovascular accident (stroke)
EEG	electroencephalography
END	Electroneurodiagnostic
ENG	electronystagmomgraphy
EP	evoked potential
HA	headache
HCVD	hypertensive cardiovascular disease
MBD	minimal brain dysfunction
met., metas., mets.	metastasis/metastases
MLT	medical laboratory technician
mmHg	millimeters of mercury (pressure)
MT	medical technologist
NCS	Nerves conduction studies
PSG	Polysomnography
TIA	transient ischemic attack

ANSWER COLUMN

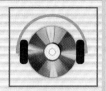

To complete your study of this unit, work the **Review Activities** on the following pages. Also, listen to the audio CDs that accompany *Medical Terminology: A Programmed Systems Approach,* 9th edition, and practice your pronunciation.

Additional practice exercises for this unit are available on the Learner Practice CD-ROM found in the back of the textbook.

REVIEW ACTIVITIES

CIRCLE AND CORRECT

Circle the correct answer for each question. Then check your answers in Appendix A.

1. Word root for development
   a. troph
   b. tropic
   c. tome
   d. path

2. Combining form for gland
   a. glandul
   b. adreno
   c. adeno
   d. glando

3. Prefix for below or less than normal
   a. hyper-
   b. hypo-
   c. ology-
   d. en-

4. Suffix for disease condition
   a. -pathy
   b. -patho
   c. -tropho
   d. -ic

5. Combining form for cancer
   a. cancerous
   b. situ
   c. carcino
   d. neoplasm

6. Suffix for one who studies
   a. -logy
   b. -ist
   c. -logist
   d. -er

7. Suffix for instrument that records
   a. -phonogram
   b. -graph
   c. -gram
   d. -graphy

8. Word root for head
   a. myel
   b. cephal
   c. encephal
   d. crani

9. Suffix for herniation
   a. -itis
   b. -malacia
   c. -cytes
   d. -cele

10. Combining form for brain
    a. myelo
    b. encephalo
    c. cerebr
    d. meningo

11. The membrane surrounding the closed cavities
    a. mucosa
    b. dermal
    c. serosa
    d. meninges

12. Suffix for like or resembling
    a. -oid
    b. -oma
    c. -ous
    d. -ible

13. Combining form for skull
    a. cephal/o
    b. occipital
    c. crani/o
    d. oste/o

14. Word root for tumor
    a. oma
    b. onc
    c. sarc/o
    d. carcin

15. Suffix for pain
    a. -cele
    b. -oid
    c. -alic
    d. -dynia

16. Combining form for tissue
    a. cyt/o
    b. hyper
    c. neo
    d. hist/o

REVIEW ACTIVITIES

SELECT AND CONSTRUCT

Select the correct word parts from the following list and construct medical terms that represent the given meaning.

aden(o)	anti	blast	carcin(o)	cele
cephal(o)	cerebr(o)	crani(o)	cyte	ectomy
electr(o)	encephal(o)	epitheli(o)	genesis	graph
graphy	histo	hyper	hypo	itis
lip(o)	logist	logy	lymph(o)	malac(ia)
mening(o)	muc(o)	mucosa	neo	nat/al
oid	oma	onc(o)	pathy	plasm (plastic)
plasty	sarc(o)	spinal	tension	tomy
trophy				

1. herniation of the brain   _____

2. instrument for recording brain function   _____

3. surgical repair of the skull   _____

4. brain and spinal cord (adjective)   _____

5. malignant tumor of a gland   _____

6. resembling mucus   _____

7. fatty tumor   _____

8. softening of the skull   _____

9. incision into the cerebrum   _____

10. inflammation of the meninges   _____

11. one who studies tumors   _____

12. connective tissue tumor   _____

13. tumor involving lymph glands   _____

14. overdevelopment   _____

15. low blood pressure   _____

16. specialist in study of tissues   _____

17. new growths (tumors)   _____

18. agent that works against tumors   _____

19. immature tissue cell   _____

20. pertaining to the newborn   _____

REVIEW ACTIVITIES

DEFINE AND DISSECT

Give a brief definition and dissect each listed term into its word parts in the space provided. Check your answers by referring to the frame listed in parentheses and to your medical dictionary. Then listen to the CD to practice pronunciation.

1. encephalomalacia (3.2)

   _____/_____/_____/_____
         rt   v   rt   suffix

   _____
            definition

2. hypertrophy (3.13)

   _____/_____
       pre   suffix

3. hyperemesis (3.11)

   _____/_____
       pre   rt/suffix

4. adenectomy (3.21)

   _____/_____
       rt   suffix

5. hypertension (3.15)

   _____/_____
       pre   rt/suffix

6. carcinoma (3.35)

   _____/_____
       rt   suffix

7. lipoid (3.52)

   _____/_____
       rt   suffix

8. oncology (3.51)

   _____/_____/_____
       rt   v   suffix

9. mucosa (3.74)

   _____/_____
       rt   suffix

10. cephalalgia (3.81)

    _____/_____
        rt   suffix

11. encephalocele (3.94)

    _____/_____/_____
        rt   v   suffix

REVIEW ACTIVITIES

12. electroencephalogram (3.102)

_____/_____/_____/_____/_____
   rt   v   rt   v   suffix

13. craniomalacia (3.106)

_____/_____/_____
   rt   v   rt/suffix

14. cerebrotomy (3.120)

_____/_____/_____
   rt   v   suffix

15. meningitis (3.131)

_____/_____
   rt   suffix

16. cerebrospinal (3.124)

_____/_____/_____/_____
   rt   v   rt   suffix

17. histology (3.58)

_____/_____/_____
   re   v   suffix

18. atheroma (3.55)

_____/_____
   rt   suffix

19. cerebrovascular (3.122)

_____/_____/_____/_____
   rt   v   rt   suffix

20. metastasis (3.39)

_____/_____
   pre   suffix

21. serous (3.78)

_____/_____
   rt   suffix

22. craniometer (3.109)

_____/_____/_____
   rt   v   suffix

23. neoplasm (3.63)

_____/_____
   pre   suffix

REVIEW ACTIVITIES

24. electroneurodiagnostic (3.104)

_____/____/_____/____/_____/_____

       rt   v   rt   v   rt   suffix

25. melanocarcinoma (3.47)

_____/____/_____/_____

      rt   v   rt   suffix

ART LABELING

Label the following structures of the head and neck by placing the number in front of the correct combining form below.

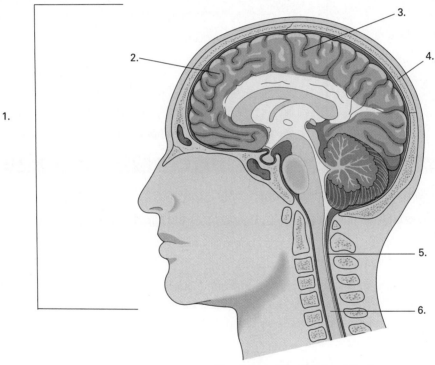

Structures of the Head and Neck

Write the body part represented by

_____   myel/o   _____

_____   crani/o   _____

_____   mening/o   _____

_____   cerebr/o   _____

_____   encephal/o   _____

_____   cephal/o   _____

REVIEW ACTIVITIES

ABBREVIATION MATCHING

Match the following abbreviations with their definition.

_____ 1. ASCP

_____ 2. EEG

_____ 3. MBD

_____ 4. met., metas., mets.

_____ 5. TIA

_____ 6. CP

_____ 7. CSF

_____ 8. CIS

_____ 9. HA

_____10. CA

a. basal cell carcinoma

b. cancer

c. metastasis/metastases

d. American Society of Clinical Pathology

e. electrocardiogram

f. heart and chronic venereal disease

g. minimal brain dysfunction

h. cerebrospinal fluid

i. carcinoma in situ

j. myocardial infarction

k. cerebral palsy

l. electroencephalogram

m. headache

n. transient ischemia attack

ABBREVIATION FILL-INS

Fill in the blanks with the correct abbreviations.

11. The medical laboratory technician (_____) prepared the blood sample for testing.

12. Having blood pressure (_____) that is abnormally high (200/100 _____) and blood vessel disease is serious for the patient with _____.

13. The patient has experienced several episodes of blurred vision, dizziness, and fatigue brought on by a loss of blood flow to the brain. A _____ could be a precursor to a stroke or _____, which is followed by paralysis, loss of consciousness, and possibly death.

14. The biopsy indicated a basal cell carcinoma (_____).

REVIEW ACTIVITIES

CASE STUDIES

Write the term next to its meaning given below. Then draw slashes to analyze the word parts. Note the use of medical abbreviations. Look these up in your dictionary or find them in Appendix B. If you have any questions about the answers, refer to your medical dictionary or check with your instructor for the answers in Appendix A.

CASE STUDY 3-1

Present Illness from History and Physical Report

Pt: Female, age 45, **gravida 4**, **para 4**

Dx: **Carcinoma** in situ, uterine cervix

Ms. Sally Pingo was seen on August 28 after approximately an eight-year absence from this **gynecology** office. She had a **Pap** smear done in Dr. Lapar's office on August 4, which described squamous cell carcinoma in situ. An in-office **colposcopy** was done on the same day with minimal abnormalities noted by visualization of the cervix. Appropriate **biopsies** were taken, and the pathology report described severe **dysplasia** and/or squamous carcinoma in situ, possible **poikilocytotic atypia** from cervical biopsies. Also the **endocervical** curettings had strips of squamous epithelium exhibiting severe dysplasia and/or carcinoma in situ with glandular atypia. We decided to offer Ms. Pingo a **D&C** and laser **conization** to further delineate the extent of the pathology. All risks and benefits of this procedure were discussed with the patient and her family. Informed consent was obtained, and the procedure was scheduled.

1. dilation and curettage _____
2. inside the neck of the uterus _____
3. different cell shapes _____
4. abnormal (poor) development _____
5. not typical _____
6. four pregnancies, four living children _____
7. cancerous tumor _____
8. process of using a colposcope _____
9. excision of a cone of tissue _____
10. specialty—females _____
11. Papanicolaou test _____
12. excision of tissue for study _____

REVIEW ACTIVITIES

CROSSWORD PUZZLE

Check your answers by going back through the frames or checking the solution in Appendix C.

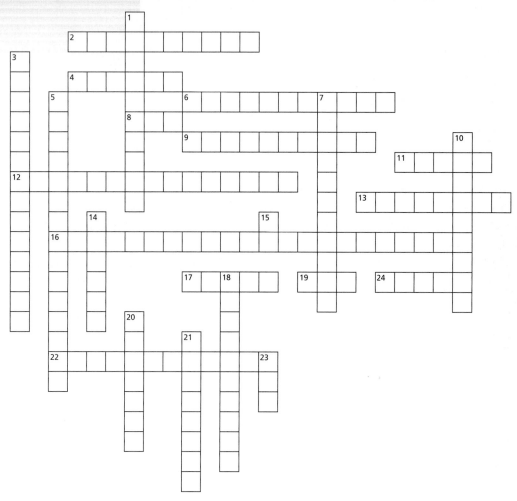

Across

2. remove a gland
4. usually benign fat tumor
6. hernia of the meninges
8. suffix for tumor
9. loss in structure size
11. suffix for instrument used to measure
12. hardening of a vessel caused by fat
13. tumor of melanocyte
16. process of producing EEG
17. watery substance produced by mucosa
19. carcinoma in situ (abbreviation)
22. high blood pressure
24. a new growth is a Neo_____.

Down

1. tumor physician
3. glandular cancer
5. disease of lymph glands
7. synonym cephalodynia
10. muscle tissue tumor (fibroid)
14. membrane covering closed cavities
15. blood pressure
18. incision into the skull
20. connective tissue cancer
21. inside the head, brain (word root)
23. a newborn is a _____nate.

REVIEW ACTIVITIES

GLOSSARY

adenectomy	excision of a gland
adenitis	inflammation of a gland
adenoma	tumor of a gland or glandular tissue
adenopathy	disease condition of a gland or glandular tissue
antineoplastic	agent that works against tumor growth
atheroma	fatty (porridgelike) tissue tumor found in blood vessels
atherosclerosis	hardening of blood vessels caused by fatty growths
carcinoma	cancer of epithelial tissue
cephalalgia	head pain (synonym for cephalodynia)
cephalic	pertaining to the head
cephalodynic	pertaining to head pain (adjective)
cerebral	pertaining to the cerebrum (adjective)
cerebritis	inflammation of the cerebrum
cerebroma	tumor of the cerebrum
cerebrospinal	pertaining to the cerebrum and spine
cerebrovascular	pertaining to the cerebrum and blood vessels
cerebrum	largest part of the brain includes the frontal, temporal, and occipital lobes
craniectomy	excision of part of the skull
craniomalacia	softening of the skull

craniometer	instrument used to measure the size of the skull
cranioplasty	surgical repair of the skull
craniotomy	incision into the skull
cranium	skull
electroencephalogram	tracing (picture) showing brain wave activity
electroencephalograph	instrument used to turn brain waves into electrical patterns showing a picture of changes in activity
encephalitis	inflammation of the brain
encephalomalacia	softening of brain tissue
encephalomeningitis	inflammation of the brain and meninges
encephalomyelopathy	disease condition of the brain and spinal cord
electroneurodiagnostic	electrical diagnostic testing (imaging) of nervous system function
glandular	pertaining to a gland
histology	study of tissues
hypertension	high blood pressure
hypertrophy	overdevelopment, increase in size
hypotension	low blood pressure
hypotrophy	underdevelopment, decrease in size
lipoid	resembling fat
lipoma	fatty tissue tumor

REVIEW ACTIVITIES

lymphadenopathy	disease condition of the lymph glands	mucosa	mucous membrane (noun)
lymphoma	lymph tissue tumor	mucus	watery substance secreted by mucous membranes
melanocarcinoma	malignant (cancerous) melanoma	neonatal	pertaining to newborn
		neoplasm	new growth (tumor)
melanoma	tumor involving growth of melanocytes	neurodiagnostic	pertaining to diagnostic studies performed to examine the nervous system by detecting electrical changes
meninges	three-layered membrane surrounding the brain and spinal cord		
		oncologist	physician specialist in diseases involving tumors
meningitis	inflammation of the meninges		
meningocele	herniation of the meninges	oncology	the science that studies tumors
metastasis	tumor that spreads beyond its origin (noun) pl. metastases	sarcoma	cancer of connective tissue
metastasize	to spread beyond its origin (verb)	serosa	serous membrane
		tumor	abnormal growth of tissue
metastatic	pertaining to a metastasis or metastases		

UNIT 4

Orthopedics, Osteopathy, and Body Regions

PRONUNCIATION NOTE

Now that you are learning more complex terms, it is time to suggest a way to remember some of the commonly mispronounced words. Begin with the suffixes **-scope** and **-scopy**. The suffix **-scope** is pronounced just as it looks (skōp) as in arthroscope (**är′** thrō skōp), endoscope (**en′** dō skōp).

But **-scopy** is not pronounced as it looks. The "o" from the combining form blends with the suffix and is a short "o" sound as in os' trich or op'era. The accent is also placed on this vowel-suffix blend (**os′** ko pē) arthroscopy (arthr **os′** ko pē), endoscopy (en **dos′** ko pē)

Many other suffixes follow a similar pronunciation pattern.

Try the first few familiar terms and apply the pattern to the rest.

Suffix	Pronunciation	Example
o/graphy	**og′** ra fē	photography
o/meter	**om′** ə ter	thermometer
o/metry	**om′** ə trē	geometry
o/logy	**ol′** ə gē	biology
o/stomy	**os′** tō mē	colostomy
o/pathy	**op′** ə thē	dermatopathy
o/lysis	**ol′** ə sis	cytolysis
o/stasis	**os′** st ə sis	hemostasis
o/trophy	**ot′** trō fē	hypotrophy
o/clysis	**ok′** l ə sis	rectoclysis
o/tomy	**ot′** ə mē	gastrotomy

Refer back to this list as you learn these suffixes.

4.1

Osteon is a Greek word meaning bone. Oste/o/pathy means disease of the bones. From this word, form the combining form for bone:

oste/o

_____/_____.

99

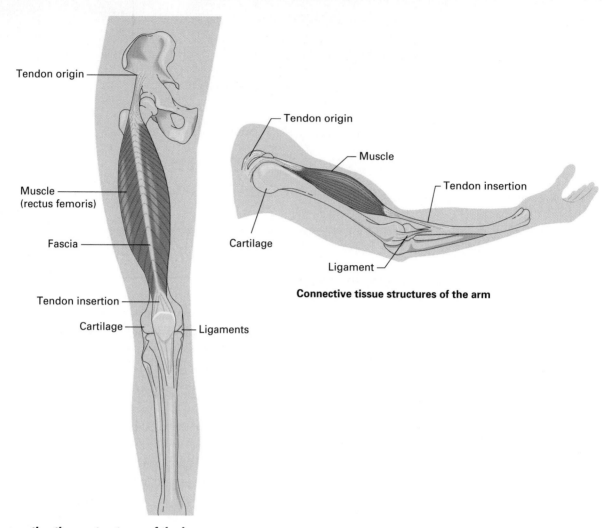

Connective tissue structures of the leg

Connective tissue structures of the arm

ANSWER COLUMN	
	4.2
oste/itis	A word meaning inflammation of the bone is ____/____.
os tē **ī**′ tis	NOTE: The "e" in oste is part of the word root.
	4.3
	Oste/o/malac/ia means softening of the bones. To say that bones have lost a detectable amount of their hardness, use the noun
oste/o/malac/ia	_____/____/_____/____.
os′ tē ō m ə **lā**′ shə	

ANSWER COLUMN

	4.4
	The eti/o/logy of oste/o/malacia (adult rickets) includes vitamin D deficiency, phosphate deficiency, and abnormal excretion of calcium by the kidneys. A contributing factor is use of tobacco products. Whatever the cause, softening
oste/o/malac/ia eti/o/logy et ē **ol**′ ə gē	of the bone is called _____/____/_____/___. The study of the cause of a disease is _____/____/_____.
	4.5
osteomalacia	A disorder of the parathyroid glands (hyper/parathyroid/ism) can cause calcium to be withdrawn from the bones. When this occurs, _____ results.
	4.6
oste/o/pathy os′ tē **op**′ ə thē	Recall **-pathy** means any disease. Form a word that means disease of bone: _____/____/_____.
	4.7
oste/o/path/ic os tē ō **path**′ ik	A doctor of osteopathy (DO) receives special training about the skeleton and its relationship to disease. Using the adjectival form, we call this special type of doctor an _____/____/_____/_____ physician.
	4.8
oste/oma os tē **ō**′ m ə oste/o/mata os′ tē **ō**′ m ə ta	A hard outgrowth on a bone may be a bone tumor or _____/_____. Build the plural form: _____/____/_____.
	4.9
joint	**-pathy** means disease. Oste/o/arthr/o/pathy is a noun that means any disease involving bones and joints. **arthr/o** is used in words to mean _____.
	4.10
oste/o arthr/o pathy oste/o/arthr/o/pathy os′ tē ō är **throp**′ ə thē	Oste/o/arthr/o/pathy is a compound noun. Analyze it: _____/____ bone (combining form); _____/____ joint (combining form); _____ disease (suffix). Now put these together and form the term meaning bone and joint disease. _____/____/_____/____/_____

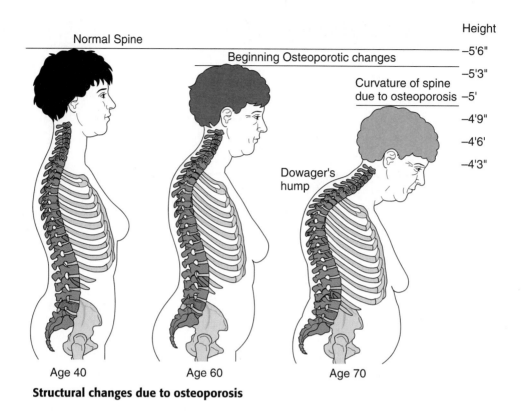

Normal Spine

Beginning Osteoporotic changes

Curvature of spine
due to osteoporosis

Height
−5'6"
−5'3"
−5'
−4'9"
−4'6'
−4'3"

Dowager's
hump

Age 40   Age 60   Age 70

Structural changes due to osteoporosis

ANSWER COLUMN

4.11

Poros is a Greek word meaning passageway. Oste/o/por/osis is a disease condition of the bone in which there is deterioration of the bone matrix causing pores and weakness. Calcium deficiency and hormone changes associated with menopause in women along with a hereditary predisposition can lead to

oste/o/por/osis
os' tē ō por ō' sis
bone

_____/____/_____/_____.
Oste/o/penia is a condition of *bone* loss.

4.12

A proper diet that includes adequate calcium in addition to weight-bearing exercise such as walking may help to prevent porosity of the bones, called

osteoporosis
oste/o/penia
os' tē ō pē nē ə

_____. Bone loss is
called _____/____/_____.

4.13

Recall *sarcoma* is used to indicate cancer of connective tissue. Bone is connective

oste/o/sarc/oma
os' tē ō sar **cō**' m ə

tissue; therefore, bone cancer is called _____/____/_____/____.

PROFESSIONAL PROFILES

Doctor of Osteopathy (DO): Osteopathic physicians are fully licensed to practice medicine, performing the same duties as a medical doctor (MD, allopathic doctor). Because of the original philosophy of osteopathic medicine, founded by Dr. Andrew Still in 1874, they identify the musculoskeletal framework as a key element to health. They also believe that the body has a natural ability to heal itself given a favorable environment and good nutrition and so act as teachers to help patients take a responsible role in their own well-being and to change unhealthy patterns. In addition, osteopathic manipulative therapy (OMT) is incorporated in the training and practice of osteopathic physicians. Although 60% practice primary care, osteopathic physicians may specialize in surgery, obstetrics, anesthesiology, internal medicine, psychiatry, and other medical specialties. The American Osteopathic Association (AOA) is the national professional organization that oversees education and licensure of Doctors of Osteopathy.

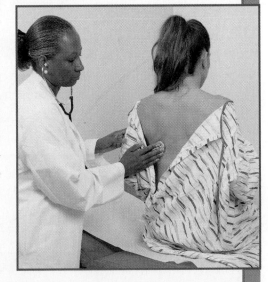

Osteopathic physican performing an exam

ANSWER COLUMN

4.14

myel/o is a combining form used to mean either the bone marrow or the spinal cord. A condition characterized by increased and abnormal bone marrow or spinal cord development is myel/o/dys/plasia:

myel/o—bone marrow or spinal cord

dys-—prefix for difficult or poor

-plasia—suffix for growth and development

When you see **myel/o**, read further to see whether it

spinal cord,   refers to *_____

bone marrow   or *_____.

ANSWER COLUMN

4.15

encephal/o/myel/o/pathy
en sef′ ə lō mī el **op**′ ə thē
oste/o/myel/itis
os′ tē ō mī′e **li**′ tis
myel/o/dys/plasia
mī′ el ō dis **plā**′ zha

Any disease of the brain and spinal cord is
called _____/____/_____/____/_____.
Inflammation of the bone and marrow is
called _____/____/_____/_____.
Defective formation of the spinal cord is
called _____/____/_____/_____.

4.16

arthr/o/scope
är′ thrō skōp

arthr/o is the combining form for joint. An instrument used to look at something
is a **-scope**. An instrument used to look into a joint is
an _____/____/_____.

4.17

bone marrow germ cell
myel/o

Find the word myeloblast in your dictionary. Write the meaning here.
*_____
The combining form of myel is _____/____.

4.18

myel/o/cyt/ic
mī′ el ō **sit**′ ik
myel/o/cele
mī′ el ō sēl
mening/o/myel/o/cele
menin′ gō **mī**′ el ō sēle

Use your dictionary to help build a word meaning
pertaining to myelocytes _____/____/_____/_____;
herniation of the spinal cord _____/____/_____.
herniation of the spinal cord and meninges
_____/____/_____/____/_____

4.19

defective (poor or
abnormal) formation
defective formation
of a joint

-plasia means development or formation. This kind of formation occurs naturally
instead of being done by a plastic surgeon. Hyper/plasia is an
increase in the number of cells in a tissue (i.e., tumor). **dys-** means defective.
Dys/plasia means *_____.
Arthr/o/dys/plasia means
*_____.

4.20

myel/o/dys/plasia
mī′ ə lō dis **plā**′ zhə

Build a term that means defective (abnormal) formation of the spinal
cord: _____/____/_____/_____ (body part + disorder).

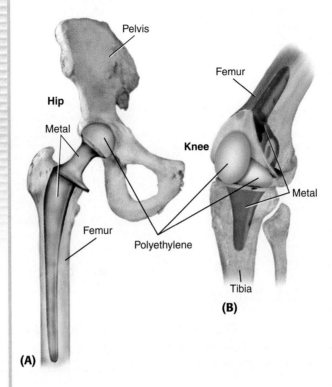

ANSWER COLUMN

Arthroplasty: (A) total hip replacement; (B) total knee replacement. A strong polyethylene plastic replaces the articular (joint) cartilage and a metallike stainless steel or titanium is used to replace bone.

Arthroscope in use

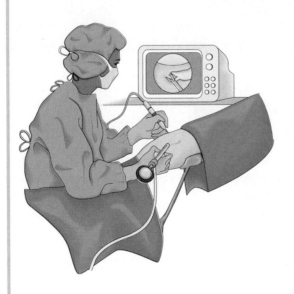

4.21	

a/plasia means failure of an organ to develop. A word that means overgrowth or too much development is _____/_____.

hyper/plasia
hī per **plā**′ zhə

Internal view of of knee through arthroscope

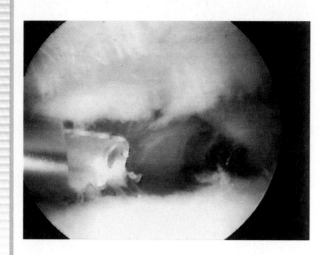

4.22

hypo/plasia
hī pō **plā**′ zhə
a/plasia
ā **plā** zhə

Hypo- is the opposite of **hyper-**. If excessive development is hyperplasia, deficient development is expressed as _hypo_ / _plasia_____.
Complete lack of development is ____/_____.

4.23

arthr/o/scopy
är **thros**′ kō pē

arthr/o is the combining form for joint. The name of the procedure for examining the joints by looking with an arthroscope is called _arthr_/ _o_ / _scopy_.

4.24

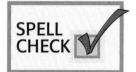

As you learn the medical terms about joints, watch the spelling of the word root arthr and combing form **arthr/o** for joint. They are easily confused with two other word parts that look similar but have quite different meanings.

arthr/o   joint (an "r" before the "t" and no "e")
ather/o   fatty or porridgelike (no "r" before the "t" and an "e" after the "h")
arteri/o   artery (no "h" following the "t")

4.25

Arthr/o/plasty
är′ thrō plas′ tē

arthr / _o_ / _plasty_ means surgical repair of a joint. **-plasty** means surgical repair.

USE THE FOLLOWING TABLE TO MAKE A DISTINCTION BETWEEN VARIOUS TERMS RELATED TO DEVELOPMENT AND GROWTH.

-plasia	refers to changes in number and form of cells
a/plasia, a/plastic	lack of or decreased cell growth (syn: hypoplasia)
ana/plasia	abnormal growth of undifferentiated cells
dys/plasia	production of abnormally formed cells or tissues
hyper/plasia	abnormal increase in number of cells
hypo/plasia	abnormal decrease in number of cells or tissues
-trophy	refers to changes in size of cells and organs
a/trophy	decrease in size of tissues, wasting
hyper/trophy	increase in size of cells, tissues, or organs
hypo/trophy	progressive degeneration (syn: atrophy)
-genesis	refers to original growth of cells and organs
a/genesis	absence of original development
hyper/genesis	repeated creation of body parts or organs (extra organs)
hypo/genesis	congenital underdevelopment of organs

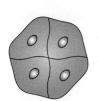 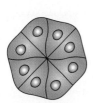 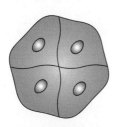 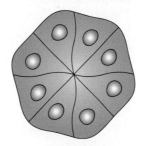 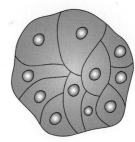

| Normal (size and number normal) | Hyperplasia (increased numbers) | Hypertrophy (increased size) | Hypertrophy and hyperplasia (increase in size and number) | Dysplasia (abnormal cells and increase in numbers) |

Hyperplasia, hypertrophy, dysplasia

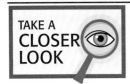

TAKE A CLOSER LOOK

surgical repair or reconstruction

4.26

Plastic surgery has nothing to do with plastic (the material). The word root plast means form, mold, or rebuild. Think of a plast/ic surgeon building a new nose or molding a face. This is surgical reconstruction. The suffix **-plasty** means *_____.

ANSWER COLUMN

	4.27
arthroplasty	Arthr/o/plasty may take many forms. When a joint has lost its ability to move, movement can sometimes be restored by an _____.
	4.28
arthr/itis är **thrī**′ tis arthr/itic är **thrī**′ tik	Arthr/itic means pertaining to a joint. Form a word that means inflammation of a joint: _____/_____. A medication used to treat arthritis is an anti/_____/_____ agent.
	4.29
oste/o/arthr/itis os′ tē ō är **thrī**′ tis	Arthritis characterized by inflammation and destruction of bone and joint tissue is called _____/____/_____/_____ (OA).
	4.30
arthritis	Rheumatoid arthritis (RA) Rheumatoid is Greek for resembling discharge or fluid. Affects the softer tissues of the joint often accompanied by fluid in the joints. RA still causes inflammation of the joint or _____.
	4.31
arthr/o/tomy är **throt**′ ə mē	You're getting to be pretty good at this, aren't you? Form a word that means incision into a joint: _____/____/_____.

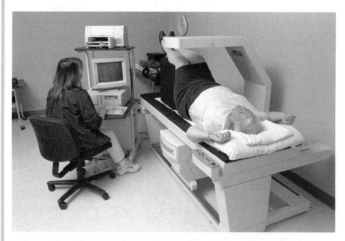

A bone density scan is performed to determine a baseline and a client's fracture risk. The patient is positioned, the scanner aligned, and a computer image created. A physician then interprets the results.

ANSWER COLUMN

INFORMATION FRAME

4.32

In Latin *tendo* means to stretch. Tendons are made of connective tissue and attach muscle to bone. Ligaments attach bone to bone and fascia attaches muscle to muscle.

4.33

ten/o, **tend/o**, and **tendin/o** are all combining forms for tendon. Use your dictionary to help you. Build three terms meaning repair of the tendons:

tend/o/plasty
ten′ dō plas tē
ten/o/plasty
ten′ ō plas tē
tendin/o/plasty
ten′ din ō plas tē

_____/____/_____,

_____/____/_____, and

_____/____/_____.

4.34

tendin/o is used to build words about inflammation of the tendons.
Inflammation of a tendon is _____/_____.

tendin/itis
ten′ din **ī′** tis

NOTE: Tendinitis is the proper term, but tendonitis is accepted.

4.35

ten/o is used to build the terms for pain in a tendon. Two terms for tendon pain are

ten/algia
ten **al′** jē ə
ten/ō/dynia
ten′ ō **din′** ē ə

_____/_____ and

_____/____/_____.

4.36

Bursa in Latin means purse or bag. A bursa is a small serous sac between a tendon and a bone. **burs/o** refers to the *bursae* (plural) of the body. Build words meaning:

burs/itis
bûr **sī′** tis
burs/ectomy
bûr **sek′** tə mē
burs/ae
bûr′ sē

inflammation of a bursa _____/_____;

excision of a bursa _____/_____;

more than one bursa _____/_____.

4.37

The word oste/o/chondr/itis means inflammation of bone and cartilage.
The combining form for cartilage is _____/____.

chondr/o

ANSWER COLUMN

Rib cage and shoulder joint

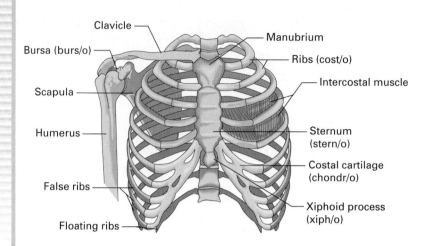

Clavicle

Manubrium

Bursa (burs/o)

Ribs (cost/o)

Scapula

Intercostal muscle

Humerus

Sternum (stern/o)

Costal cartilage (chondr/o)

False ribs

Xiphoid process (xiph/o)

Floating ribs

4.38

cartilage
kär ti ləg

Cartilage is a tough, elastic connective tissue found in the ear, nose tip, and rib ends. The lining, of joints also contain _____.

4.39

chondr/algia
kon **dral**′ gē ə
chondr/o/dynia
kon′ drō **din**′ ē ə

Form two words meaning pain in or around cartilage:
_____/_____
(word root)   (suffix)
_____/_____/_____.
(combining form)   (suffix)

4.40

ten/o/plasty
ten′ ō plast tē
ten/o/dynia
ten′ ō **din**′ ē ə

Use **ten/o** to build words meaning:
repair of tendons ____/____/_____;

pain in tendons ____/____/_____.

4.41

excision of cartilage

Chondr/ectomy means * ~~Excision of cartilage~~ _____.

4.42

ribs

Chondr/o/cost/al means pertaining to ribs and cartilage. **cost/o** is used in words about the _____.

4.43

cost/ectomy
kos **tek**′ t ə mē

Form a word that means excision of a rib or ribs:
_____/_____.

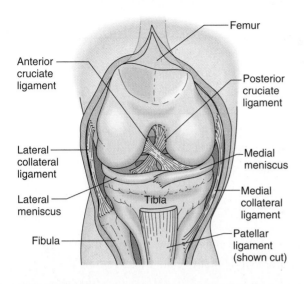

(A) Major ligaments of the knee, anterior view

Femur

Anterior cruciate ligament

Posterior cruciate ligament

Lateral collateral ligament

Medial meniscus

Lateral meniscus

Tibia

Medial collateral ligament

Fibula

Patellar ligament (shown cut)

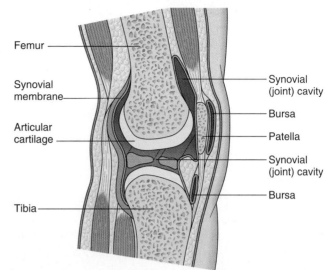

(B) Synovial joint and bursa, right lateral view

Femur

Synovial membrane

Articular cartilage

Tibia

Synovial (joint) cavity

Bursa

Patella

Synovial (joint) cavity

Bursa

ANSWER COLUMN

	4.44
adjective	Chondr/o/cost/al is an adjective. This is evident because **-al** is the ending for an _____.
	4.45
chondr/o cost al chondr/o/cost/al kon′ drō **kos**′ t ə l pertaining to cartilage and ribs	Analyze chondr/o/cost/al: _____/____ cartilage; _____ rib; _____ suffix. Now put them together: _____/____/_____/_____. This means *_____.
	4.46
cost/al **kos**′ t ə l	Form a word that means pertaining to the ribs: _____/_____.
	4.47
inter-	Inter/cost/al means between the ribs. The prefix for between is _____. **EXAMPLE:** International means between nations.
	4.48
inter/chondr/al in′ t ə r **kon**′ dr ə l	Hypo/chondr/iac means below the cartilage. Form an adjective that means between cartilages: _____/_____/al.

ANSWER COLUMN

4.49

Inter/cost/al means between the ribs. **inter-** is the prefix that

between

means _____.

4.50

Inter/cost/al may refer to the muscles between the ribs. The muscles that

inter/cost/al
inter **kos**′ t ə l

move the ribs when breathing are the _____/_____/_____

muscles.

4.51

The external intercostal muscles assist with inhalation by enlarging the rib cage.
The internal intercostal muscles assist with breathing out by decreasing the size

intercostal

of the rib cage. Breathing is assisted by the _____ muscles.

4.52

dent

Inter/dent/al means between the teeth. The word root for tooth is _____.

4.53

dent/al
den′ t ə l

Form an adjective that means pertaining to the teeth: _____/_____.

4.54

dent/algia
den **tal**′ jē ə

Pain in the teeth, or a toothache, is called _____/_____.

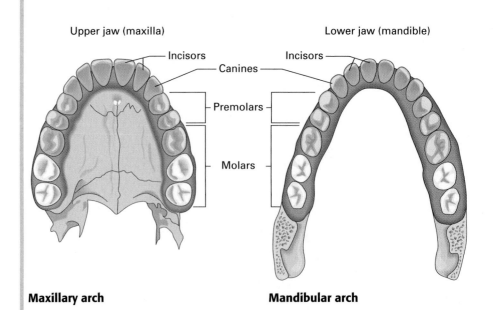

Maxillary arch   **Mandibular arch**

ANSWER COLUMN

	4.55
dent/oid **den**′ toid	Great! Try this: **-oid** is the suffix that means like or resembling. Form a word that means tooth shaped or resembling a tooth: _____/_____.
	4.56
teeth teeth	A dent/ist (Doctor of Dental Surgery DDS) takes care of _____. A dent/ifrice is used for cleaning _____.
	4.57
orth/odont/ist ôr′ thō **don**′ tist	**orth/o** is a combining form taken from the Greek word *orthos*, meaning straight. **odont/o** means shaped like a tooth. A dentist who specializes in straightening abnormally positioned teeth is called an _____/_____/_____.
	4.58
around or near	**peri-** is a prefix meaning around or near. Peri/odont/al disease is diseased tissue *_____ the teeth.
	4.59
peri/odont/al pair′ ē ō **don**′ tal	A periodontist may perform surgery of the gums or tissues around the teeth. This is _____/_____/_____ surgery.
	4.60
peri/oste/um pair′ ē **os**′ tē əm peri/chondr/ium pair′ ē **kon**′ drē əm peri/cardi/um pair′ ē **kar**′ dē əm	Build terms meaning the membrane around the bone: _____/_____/um; the membrane around the cartilage: _____/_____/ium; the membrane around the heart: _____/_____/um.
	4.61
orth/o	An orth/o/ped/ist (ōr thō **pēd**′ ist) is a physician who specializes in the prevention and treatment of musculoskeletal disorders. The combining form indicating that "straightening" may be done is _____/___.
	4.62
orth/o/ped/ist ôr thō **ped**′ ist	A broken bone is called a fracture (Fx). Often the fracture must be manipulated so that the bone will heal straight. An _____/___/_____/_____ is the specialist who treats fractures.

ANSWER COLUMN

TAKE A CLOSER LOOK

4.63

Orth/o/tics is the science that studies and develops mechanical appliances used as supportive devices. The specialist who designs and fits these devices is called an orth/o/tist. This practice is closely related to the prosthet/ists who work with patients in need of replacing an amputated limb. The appliance the prosthet/ist produces is called a prosthesis. Look in the "ortho" and "prosth" sections of your dictionary to find the word that means

orth/o/sis, orth/o/tic
ôr **thō**′ sis, ôr **tho**′ tik

devices used to stabilize or prevent deformity

_____/_____/_____;

prosthet/ist
pros′ the tist

specialist in making artificial body parts:

_____/_____;

prosthet/ic
pros **the**′ tik

pertaining to (adjective) a prosthesis:

_____/_____.

4.64

lumb/o builds words about the lower back. Lumb/ar is the adjectival form.

lumb/ar
lum′ b ə r, **lum**′ bär

An adjective meaning pertaining to the lower back is _____/_____.

4.65

lumbar

There are five lumbar vertebrae. Low back pain is called _____ pain.

4.66

lumbar

L_1, L_2, L_3, L_4, and L_5 are the five _____ vertebrae.

4.67

adjective
pertaining to the chest
and lower back or
something near these areas

thorac/o is the combining form for chest or thorax. Thorac/o/lumb/ar is a(n) (choose one) _____
(noun/adjective) meaning ** _____.

NOTE: T_1–T_{12} are the twelve thoracic vertebrae.

4.68

INFORMATION FRAME

supra- is a prefix that means on, higher in position, over, or above.

4.69

supra

Supra/lumb/ar means above the lumbar region. A prefix that means above is _____.

Orthotic device used to straighten the wrist, holding it firmly

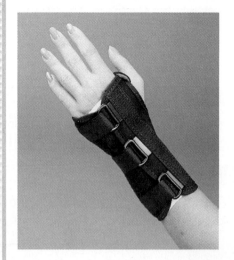

Thorax and regions of the abdomen

Direction	Prefix	Word root/ Suffix
below	hypo	chondr/iac
upon	epi	gastr/ic
above	supra	lumb/ar
below	hypo	gastr/ic

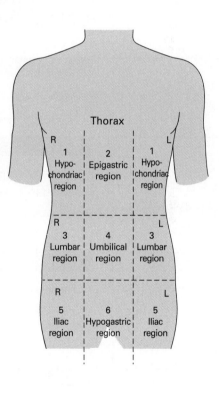

4.70

above the lumbar region or above the lower back

Supra/lumb/ar means *_____.

4.71

above the ribs

Supra/cost/al means *_____.

ANSWER COLUMN

	4.72
on top of	Supra/crani/al refers to the surface of the head * _____on top of_____ the skull.
	4.73
noun	The pubis is a bone of the pelvis. Pub/is is a (choose one) _____ (noun/adjective).
	4.74
pubis pyōo bis pubic pyōo bik	From **pub/o** form a noun _____; an adjective _____. (See the illustration of the pelvic bones in Unit 14.)
	4.75
pub/is pyōo′ bis	The pub/ic bone is also called the _____/_____.
	4.76
pubis	Supra/pub/ic means above the pubis. **pub/o** is used in words about the _____.
	4.77
supra/pub/ic s ōo pr ə **pyōo′** bik	The suprapubic region is above the arch of the pub/is. When the urinary bladder is incised above the pubis, an incision is made in the _____/_____/_____ region.
	4.78
suprapubic incision region	"The incision is made in the suprapubic region." From this sentence pick out the adjective _____; two nouns _____ _____.
	4.79
anything close to incision of bladder from the suprapubic region	Try to figure out what surgery is done in a supra/pub/ic cyst/o/tomy *_____ _____.
	4.80
pelv/is **pel′** vis	The pelv/is is formed by the pelv/ic bones. **pelv/i** refers to the _____/_____ (noun).

ANSWER COLUMN	
pelves **pel**′ vēs	The plural of pelvis is _____.

4.81

Pelv/i/metry is done during pregnancy to determine the measurements of the pelvis. To find a woman's pelvic size, the physician does _____/____/_____.

pelv/i/metry
pel **vim**′ ə trē

4.82

Look up pelvimetry or pelvis in your dictionary. Taking pelvic measurements is called _____.

pelvimetry

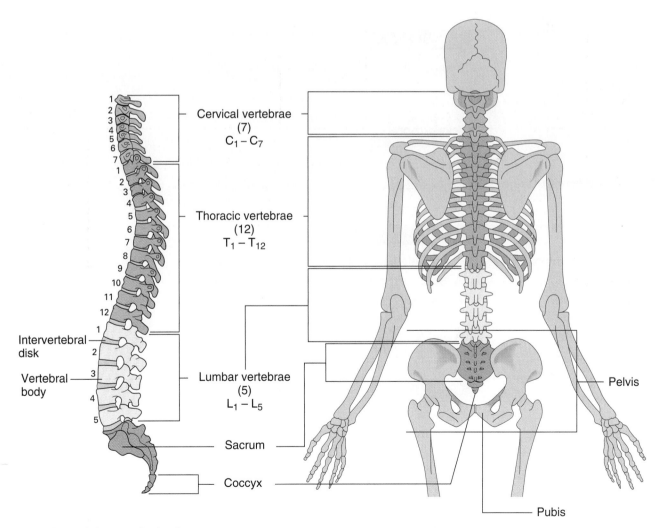

Divisions of the vertebral column

ANSWER COLUMN

4.83

Cephal/o/pelvic disproportion (CPD) can lead to serious complications during delivery. A physician may determine whether a woman will have trouble during labor by doing _____.

pelvimetry

4.84

Look in the dictionary for a word that names the device used for pelvimetry.
It is a _____/____/_____.

pelv/i/meter
pel vim′ ə tər

4.85

A pelvimeter measures the diameter of the pelvis. When the head (**cephal/o**) of the fetus is larger than the diameter of the mother's pelvis (**pelv/o**), this is called _____/____/_____/_____ disproportion (CPD).

cephal/o/pelv/ic
cef′ əl ō pel′ vik

4.86

The adjective meaning *above* the pelvis is
_____/_____/_____.

supra/pelv/ic
sōō prə pel′ vik

4.87

-meter is a suffix meaning an instrument used to measure. A speed/o/meter is an _____ to measure speed. A pelv/i/meter is an _____ to measure the pelvis.

instrument
instrument

4.88

A cyt/o/meter _____ cells.
A cephal/o/meter _____ the head.
A thorac/o/_____ measures the chest.

A cardi/o/_____ measures the heart.

measures (counts)
measures
thorac/o/meter
thôr′ ə kom′ ə tər
cardi/o/meter
kär′ dē om′ ə tər

4.89

Ab/norm/al is a word that means deviating (turning away) from what is normal.
ab- is a _____/fix that means from or away from.

pre

4.90

away from
or not

Abnormal is used as an ordinary English word. Abnormal means
*_____ normal.

4.91

from or away from

ab- is a prefix that means *_____.

4.92

wandering from (the
normal course of events)

Ab/errant uses the prefix **ab-** before the English word (errant) for wandering.
Ab/errant means *_____.

NOTE: Think of an error or something gone wrong.

4.93

ab/errant
ab **air′** ənt or
ab′ air ənt

Ab/errant is used in medicine as a term to describe a structure that wanders
from the normal path. When some nerve fibers follow an unusual route,
they form an _____/_____ nerve.

4.94

aberrant

Aberrant nerves wander from the normal nerve track. Blood vessels that follow
a path of their own are _____ vessels.

4.95

aberrant

Lymph vessels may be found in unexpected areas of the body. They follow
an _____ course.

4.96

ab/duct/ion
ab **duk′** shun

In Latin *ducere* (word root: duct) means to lead or move. Ab/duct/ion means
movement away from a midline. When the arm is raised away from the side
of the body, _____/_____/_____ has occurred.

4.97

abduction

Abduction can occur from any midline. When the fingers of the hand are spread
apart, _____ has occurred in four fingers.

ANSWER COLUMN

4.98

abducted
ab **duk**′ tad

A child who has been kidnapped and taken away from home has
been _____ (past tense verb).

4.99

ad/duct/ion
ə **duk**′ shən
ad/duct
a **dukt**′

ad- is a prefix meaning toward. Movement toward a midline
is _____/_____/_____ (noun). When a patient is asked to
move his arm toward his body, he is asked to _____/_____ (verb) his arm.

NOTE: In medical dictation, the physician may emphasize a-b duct (abduct) or
a-b duction (abduction) and a-d duct (adduct) or a-d duction (adduction), to
avoid misunderstanding. This would be a good time for you to make a note of the
difference as well.

4.100

ad/dict/ion
ə **dik**′ sh ə n

Ad/diction means being drawn toward some habit. The person who takes
drugs habitually suffers from drug _____/_____/_____.

4.101

addiction

Addiction implies habit. Alcoholism is an _____ to alcohol.

4.102

addict

A person addicted to drugs is a drug addict. A person addicted to cocaine is a
cocaine _____.

4.103

ad/hes/ion
ad **hē**′ zh ə n

An ad/hes/ion is formed when two normally separate tissues join together.
They adhere to each other. Adhering to another part forms
an _____/_____/_____.

Abduction/Adduction

Abduction

Adduction

4.104

adhesions

Patients are usually encouraged to ambulate soon after surgery to help prevent postoperative _____.

4.105

adhesions

Pain or intestinal obstruction may be caused by abdominal _____.

4.106

ab/domen
ab′ də mən

abdomin/o is used to form words about the abdomen. When you see **abdomin/o** any place in a word, you think about the _____/_____.

4.107

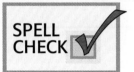

SPELL
CHECK ✓

In the spelling of the combining form for abdomen, the "e" changes to "i"—**abdomin/o**.
EXAMPLE: The abdominal incision was made in the RLQ of the abdomen.

4.108

pertaining to the
abdomen

Abdomin/al is an adjective that means
* _____.

NOTE: For descriptive reference the abdomen may be divided into four quadrants including the right upper quadrant (RUQ), the left upper quadrant (LUQ), the right lower quadrant (RLQ), and the left lower quadrant (LLQ).

**Abdomen divided into
quadrants**

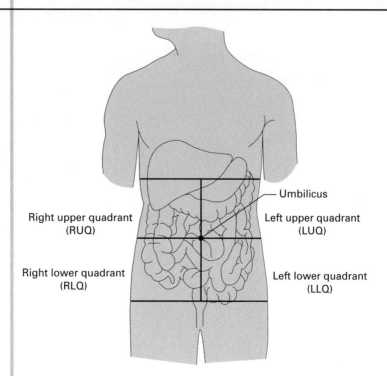

Right upper quadrant
(RUQ)

Umbilicus

Left upper quadrant
(LUQ)

Right lower quadrant
(RLQ)

Left lower quadrant
(LLQ)

ANSWER COLUMN

4.109

the insertion of a needle
into a body cavity for
the purpose of
aspirating fluid

Look up the words *paracentesis* and *centesis* in your dictionary. Write the
definition here: ** _____

_____ .

NOTE: p. abdominal is paracentesis of the abdomen or abdominocentesis.

4.110

abdomin/o/centesis
ab dom' i nō sen **tē'** sis

Abdomin/o/centesis means tapping or puncturing of the abdomen. This is a
surgical puncture for the removal of fluid. The word for surgical puncture of
the abdomen is _____/____/_____ .

4.111

abdominocentesis

Centesis (surgical puncture) is a word in itself used as a suffix. Build a word
meaning surgical puncture, or tapping of the abdomen: _____ .

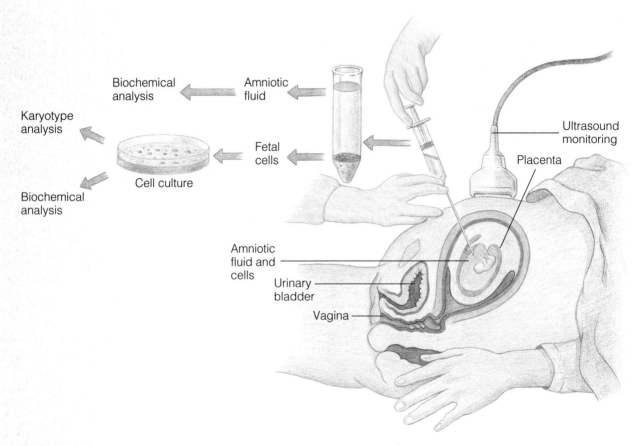

Amniocentesis

ANSWER COLUMN	
	4.112
	amni/o refers to the amnion, the protective sac that surrounds the fetus. Tapping or puncturing this sac to remove cells for genetic testing is called
amni/o/centesis am′ nē ō sen **tē**′ sis	_____/____/_____.
	4.113
amniocentesis	During amniocentesis, fluid and cells are removed from the amnion. Surgical puncture of the amnion is called _____.
	4.114
cardi/o/centesis kär′ dē ō sen **tē**′ sis	The word for surgical puncture of the heart is _____/____/_____.
	4.115
	Abdomin/o/cyst/ic means pertaining to the abdomen and urinary bladder. Analyze abdomino cystic:
abdomin/o	_____/_____ combining form;
cyst	_____ word root;
ic	_____ suffix.
abdomin/o/cyst/ic ab dom′ i nō **sis**′ tik	Now put them together to form the word ____/____/____/____.
	4.116
cyst	From abdomin/o/cyst/ic you see that the word root for urinary bladder is _____.
	4.117
bladder	**cyst/o** is used to form words that refer to the urinary _____.
	4.118
cyst/o/tomy sis **tot**′ ə mē	The word for incision into the urinary bladder is _____/____/_____.
	4.119
cyst/ectomy sis **tek**′ t ə mē	The word for excision of the urinary bladder is _____/_____.
	4.120
cyst/o/scopy sis **tos**′ cō pē	Recall that **-scopy** is a suffix for the procedure used to look into an organ or body cavity. The process of examining by looking with an instrument into the urinary bladder is _____/____/_____.

ANSWER COLUMN

Cystoscopy

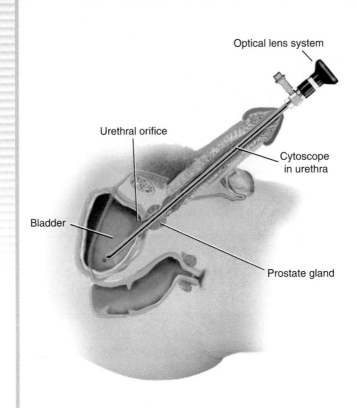

Optical lens system

Urethral orifice

Cytoscope in urethra

Bladder

Prostate gland

---

urinary bladder

4.121

A cyst/o/scop/ic exam (cysto) is used to look inside the
*_____.

---

cyst/o/plasty
sis′ tō plas′ tē

4.122

Surgical repair of the bladder is _____/___/_____.

---

cystocele

4.123

When the bladder herniates into the vagina, a _____ is formed.

---

thorac/ic
thô **ras**′ ik

4.124

thorac/o is used to form words about the thorax or chest. A word that means pertaining to the chest is _____/_____. See the illustration of body cavities.

---

thoraces
thôr′ ə sēs

4.125

The plural form of thorax is _____.

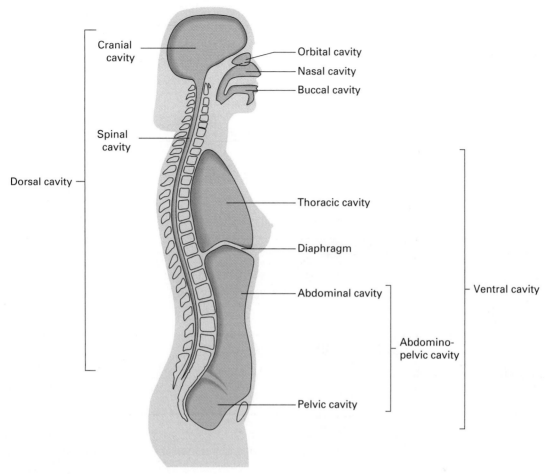

Body cavities

4.126

Abdomin/o/thorac/ic means pertaining to the abdomen and thorax. The thorax is the chest. Supply the word parts for

abdomin/o

thorac

ic

_____/_____ abdomen;

_____ thorax;

____ suffix—pertaining to.

Now put them together to form

abdomin/o/thorac/ic

abdom′ i nō thô **ras**′ ik

_____/____/_____/_____.

4.127

Abdomin/o/thorac/ic pain means, literally, pain in the abdomen and chest. A physician who describes lesions in these areas could call them

abdominothoracic

_____ lesions.

4.128

An incision may be made into the chest to insert a chest tube for the purpose of draining blood and fluid from the lung. A word that means incision of the chest is _____/_____/_____.

thorac/o/tomy
thôr′ ə **kot**′ ə mē

4.129

A word that means surgical tapping (puncture) of the chest to remove fluids is _____/_____/_____.

thorac/o/centesis
thôr′ ə kō sen **tē**′ sis

4.130

SPELL CHECK ✓

Usually, thoracocentesis is shortened to thoracentesis (thôr′ ə sen **tē**′ sis). Find out which form is used by your local hospital.

4.131

A word that means any chest disease is _____/_____/_____.

thorac/o/pathy
thôr′ ə **kop**′ ə thē

4.132

Build a term meaning pertaining to the thoracic and lumbar vertebrae:
_____/_____/_____.

thorac/o/lumbar
thôr′ ak ō **lum**′ bar

4.133

TAKE A CLOSER LOOK 👁

Take a closer look at terms referring to cysts and bladders. A cyst (**-cyst**) may be used as a word or as a suffix. The terms cyst and bladder both refer to any fluid-filled, saclike structure, and describe the urinary bladder, the gallbladder, or an abnormality such as an ovarian cyst are all fluid-filled, sac like structures. If **cyst/o** is used at the beginning of a word, it usually refers to the urinary bladder, i.e., cyst/o/scopy. If **-cyst** is used as a suffix, it indicates a less specific fluid-filled saclike structure, i.e., hydrocyst. To indicate the gallbladder, use the word root cholecyst/, i.e., cholecyst/itis.

4.134

A hydro/cyst is a sac (or bladder) filled with watery fluid. **hydro-** is used as a prefix in words to mean *_____.

NOTE: Think of a fire hydrant.

water or fluid or
watery fluid

Hydrocele

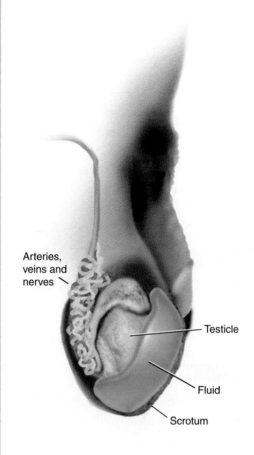

Arteries,
veins and
nerves

Testicle

Fluid

Scrotum

4.135

An accumulation of fluid in a saclike cavity, especially in the scrotum, is called
a hydro/cele. Two- to five-year-old boys often develop this fluid-filled saclike
swelling in the scrotum called a _____/_____.

hydro/cele
hī′ drō sēl

4.136

A hydrocyst and a hydrocele are both fluid-filled sacs. The more specific term
used to name the condition often found in infant and young boys is

_____.

hydrocele

ANSWER COLUMN

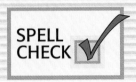

SPELL CHECK ✓

4.137

It is easy to get confused when terms seem to have the same meaning, are spelled similar, but have quite different practical uses. Look up the following terms in your medical dictionary to be sure of their use.

cyst/o/cele—urinary bladder herniation, most common in women; a cystocele is usually a weakened anterior vaginal wall with the urinary bladder bulging into the vagina

hydr/o/cyst—may be found almost anywhere in the body this is a sacklike structure with watery contents

hydr/o/cele—collection of fluid in a herniated cavity, most often related to a congenital condition; fluid-filled peritoneum herniated into the scrotum

4.138

Hydro/cephalus is characterized by an enlarged head due to increased amount of fluid in the skull. A collection of fluid in the head is called _____/_____.

hydro/cephal/us
hī′ drō **sef′** ə ləs

4.139

Hydrocephalus, unless arrested, results in deformity. The face seems small. The eyes are abnormal. The head is large. _____ also causes brain damage.

Hydrocephalus

4.140

Because of the damage to the brain children with _____ are usually mentally challenged.

hydrocephalus

4.141

Hydrocephalus is the noun. The adjectival suffix is **-ic**.
_____/_____/_____ children may attend schools for the mentally impaired.

Hydro/cephal/ic
hī′ dro se **fal′** ik

4.142

-phobia, from the Greek word for fear, is used as a suffix meaning any
*_____. Build a word meaning abnormal fear of water: _____.

abnormal fear
hydrophobia

4.143

Find the word phobia in a dictionary. It may list more than 100 definitions. How many phobias do you recognize already? **_____.
An abnormal fear of water is _____/_____.

between three and twelve
hydro/phobia
hī′ drō **fō′** bē ə

	4.144
hydrophobia	If a person is bitten by a dog with rabies, he or she may contract rabies, which is also called _____ (so named because rabid animals are afraid of choking while drinking and will not drink water).
	4.145
hydro/therapy hī′ drō **ther′** ə pē	Therapy means treatment. Treatment by water (H_2O) is _____ / _____.
	4.146
hydrotherapy	Physical therapists (PT) use swirling water baths to increase ease of movement. This is called _____.

Abbreviation	Meaning
AOA	American Osteopathic Association
C_1–C_7	cervical vertebrae 1–7
CPD	cephalopelvic disproportion
CXR	chest x-ray
cysto	cystoscopy
DDS	doctor of dental surgery (dentist)
DO	doctor of osteopathy
DTs	delirium tremens
FAS	fetal alcohol syndrome
Fx	fracture
H_2O	water
L_1–L_5	lumbar vertebrae 1–5
LLQ	left lower quadrant (abdomen)
LUQ	left upper quadrant (abdomen)
OA	osteoarthritis
OMT	osteopathic manipulative therapy
ORTHO (ORTH)	orthopedics (orthopedist)
PT	physical therapy (therapist)
RA	rheumatoid arthritis
RLQ	right lower quadrant (abdomen)
RUQ	right upper quadrant (abdomen)
T_1–T_{12}	thoracic vertebrae 1–12

ANSWER COLUMN

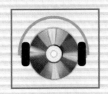

To complete your study of this unit, work the **Review Activities** on the following pages. Also, listen to the audio CDs that accompany *Medical Terminology: A Programmed Systems Approach,* 9th edition, and practice your pronunciation.

Additional practice exercises for this unit are available on the Learner Practice CD-ROM found in the back of the textbook.

REVIEW ACTIVITIES

CIRCLE AND CORRECT

Circle the correct answer for each question. Then check your answers in Appendix A.

1. Word root for bone
   a. calci
   b. ortho
   c. oste
   d. osteo

2. Combining form for joint
   a. arther
   b. artero
   c. arthero
   d. arthro

3. Suffix for instrument used to look
   a. -scope
   b. -scopy
   c. -graph
   d. -scopic

4. Combining form for tendon
   a. chondro
   b. teno
   c. tendonitis
   d. tendon

5. Word root for rib
   a. costal
   b. chondr
   c. cost
   d. ribo

6. Prefix for between
   a. inter-
   b. intra-
   c. peri-
   d. endo-

7. Combining form for tooth
   a. toid
   b. dentin
   c. dontia
   d. dento

8. Combining form for straight
   a. oto
   b. ortho
   c. donto
   d. oligo

9. Prefix for above
   a. inter-
   b. hypo-
   c. supra-
   d. infra-

10. Suffix for the process of measuring
    a. -metro
    b. -meter
    c. -metr
    d. -metry

11. Prefix meaning toward
    a. ab-
    b. hyper-
    c. in-
    d. ad-

12. Adjective for bladder or sac
    a. cystosis
    b. cystic
    c. cytic
    d. cystal

13. Word root for move or lead
    a. mor
    b. domin
    c. duct
    d. go

14. Adjective suffix
    a. -ous
    b. -ia
    c. -us
    d. -sis

15. Combining form for abdomen
    a. abdomen/o
    b. stomat/o
    c. stomach/o
    d. abdomin/o

REVIEW ACTIVITIES

SELECT AND CONSTRUCT

Select the correct word parts from the following list and construct medical terms that represent the given meaning.

a (an)	ab	abdomin(o)	ad	al
amni/o	arthr(o)	cele	centesis	cephal(ic)(o)
chondr(o)	cost(o)	cyst	dent(o)	dont(o)
duct	dys	errant	hydro	hyper
hypo(o)	inter	ist	itis	lumb(o)(ar)
malacia	metr/o(y)(ic)(er)	oma	orth(o)	oste(o)
osteo	pathy	ped	pelv/i(o)	peri
phobia	plasia	plasty	pubo(is)(ic)	sarc(o)
scope(y)(ic)	supra tendin(o)	tendon	tendin/o	ten/o, tend/o
therapy	thorac(o)(ic)	(t)ion	troph/y/ic	

1. softening of the bone _____

2. movement away from the body _____

3. water-filled sac _____

4. water on the head (brain) (adjective) _____

5. above the pubic bone _____

6. between the ribs _____

7. surgical puncture of the abdomen _____

8. process of looking into a joint _____

9. wandering in an abnormal path _____

10. specialist in straightening teeth _____

11. inflammation of the cord that connects muscle to bone _____

12. instrument to measure the pelvis _____

13. pertaining to the head and pelvis _____

14. bone and joint specialist _____

15. bone cancer _____

16. increase in size of tissues or an organ _____

17. abnormally formed cells _____

18. defective development of cartilage _____

19. surgical puncture for removal of cells from the amniotic sac _____

20. just above the lower back _____

REVIEW ACTIVITIES

DEFINE AND DISSECT

Give a brief definition and dissect each term listed into its word parts in the space to provided. Check your answers by referring to the frame listed in parentheses and to your medical dictionary. Then listen to the CD to practice pronunciation.

1. osteomalacia (4.3)

_____/___/_____/_____
      rt   v   rt   suffix

_____
                definition

2. osteoarthropathy (4.10)

_____/___/_____/___/_____
      rt   v   rt   v   suffix

_____

3. arthroscopy (4.23)

_____/_____/_____
         rt   v   suffix

_____

4. tendoplasty (4.33)

_____/_____/_____
         rt   v   suffix

_____

5. chondralgia (4.39)

_____/_____
           rt   suffix

_____

6. intercostal (4.50)

_____/_____/_____
        rt   rt   suffix

_____

7. orthodontist (4.57)

_____/_____/_____
       rt   rt   suffix

_____

8. suprapubic (4.77)

_____/_____/_____
         pre   rt   suffix

_____

9. thoracolumbar (4.67)

_____/_____/_____/____
      rt   v   rt   suffix

_____

10. pelvimetry (4.81)

_____/_____/_____
        rt   v   suffix

_____

11. aberrant (4.93)

_____/_____
     pre   rt

_____

REVIEW ACTIVITIES

12. adduction (4.99)

_____/_____/_____
pre   rt   suffix

13. myelodysplasia (4.20)

_____/___/_____/_____
rt   v   pre   suffix

14. abdominocentesis (4.110)

_____/_____/_____
rt   v   suffix

15. thoracotomy (4.128)

_____/_____/_____
rt   v   suffix

16. periosteum (4.60)

_____/_____
pre   rt/suffix

17. hydrophobia (4.143)

_____/_____
pre   rt/suffix.

18. orthopedist (4.62)

_____/_____/_____/_____
rt   v   rt   suffix

19. hypochondriac (4.48)

_____/_____/_____
pre   rt   suffix

20. cephalopelvic (4.85)

_____/_____/_____/_____
rt   v   rt   suffix

21. cystoscopy (4.120)

_____/_____/_____
rt   v   suffix

22. adhesion (4.103)

_____/_____/_____
pre   rt   suffix

23. bursectomy (4.36)

_____/_____
rt   suffix

24. tendinitis (4.34)

_____/_____
rt   suffix

REVIEW ACTIVITIES

25. osteosarcoma (4.13)

_____ / ____ / _____ / _____
rt   v   rt   suffix

_____

26. orthotic (4.63)

_____ / _____ / _____
rt   v   suffix

_____

27. prosthetist (4.63)

_____ / _____
rt   suffix

_____

28. hydrocele (4.135)

_____ / _____
pre   suffix

_____

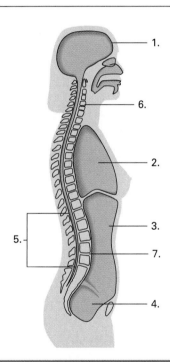

1.

6.

2.

3.

5.

7.

4.

ART LABELING

Label the diagram by placing the number in front of the correct combining form.

Write the body part name.

_____	pelv/o/i	_____
_____	crani/o	_____
_____	thorac/o	_____
_____	abdomin/o	_____
_____	lumb/o	_____
_____	oste/o	_____
_____	arthr/o	_____

REVIEW ACTIVITIES

ABBREVIATION MATCHING

Match the following abbreviations with their definition.

_____	1. CPD	a. cerebropulmonary disease
_____	2. LLQ	b. fracture
_____	3. OA	c. fetal alcohol syndrome
_____	4. H_2O	d. cephalopelvic disproportion
_____	5. DO	e. left upper quadrant
_____	6. Fx	f. hydrogen
_____	7. cysto	g. orthopedist
_____	8. RA	h. osteoarthritis
_____	9. PT	i. right abdomen
_____	10. FAS	j. bladder
		k. rheumatoid arthritis
		l. physician therapist
		m. cystoscopy
		n. left lower quadrant
		o. physical therapist
		p. water
		q. doctor of dental surgery
		r. doctor of osteopathy

ABBREVIATION FILL-IN

Fill in the blanks with the correct abbreviations.

11. An alcoholic experiencing withdrawal symptoms may get the _____.

12. The liver is located in the _____ of the abdomen.

13. DOs may use _____ as treatment to relieve back pain.

14. A dentist is indicated by the abbreviation _____.

15. The department that cares for patients with bone fractures is _____.

CASE STUDIES

Write the term next to its meaning given below. Then draw slashes to analyze the word parts. Note the use of medical abbreviations. Look these up in your dictionary or find them in Appendix B. If you have any questions about the answers, refer to your medical dictionary or check with your instructor for the answers in Appendix A.

REVIEW ACTIVITIES

CASE STUDY 4–1

REPORT SUMMARY

Preoperative diagnosis: Septic **arthritis** of the left knee

Orthopedic procedure: **Arthroscopic** examination, culture, **arthroplasty** left knee

A large bore cannula was introduced from the upper and **medial** quadrant of the knee joint through a stab **incision (arthrotomy)**. The trocar was removed and **pyorrhea** was observed. A swab was sent for culture. All pus was aspirated and the knee joint irrigated then inflated with 3 L of saline. The **arthroscope** was introduced through the inferior lateral quadrant of the knee through a similar stab incision. The knee was inspected and the entire field looked inflamed. The **patella** showed grade 2 **chondromalacia**, and the patella was tilted only in contact with the lateral condyle at about 30 degrees suggesting chronic patellar malalignment. The medial meniscus showed evidence of much more **inflammation** than the condyle, the margins thick, and fraying. . . . The scope was moved to the **mediolateral** side and inspected. . . . A motorized synovial cutter was introduced, and a partial synovectomy was performed; the soft cartilage of the patellar facets were shaved. The ends of the meniscus were trimmed (**meniscectomy**). The wound was irrigated with saline, Maracaine instilled, and a hemovac drain inserted through one of the cannulas before the instruments were removed. A padded dressing and knee immobilizer was applied and hemovac attached to its bag. The patient was transferred to the recovery room in excellent condition.

1. reddened and swollen _____

2. instrument used to look into a joint _____

3. pertaining to the middle and side _____

4. excision of the meniscus _____

5. softening of the cartilage _____

6. inflammation of a joint _____

7. pertaining to the use of an arthroscope _____

8. kneecap _____

9. pertaining to bone specialty _____

10. middle _____

11. discharge of pus _____

12. cut into _____

13. incision into a joint _____

14. surgical repair of a joint _____

REVIEW ACTIVITIES

CROSSWORD PUZZLE

Check your answers by going back through the frames or checking the solution in Appendix C.

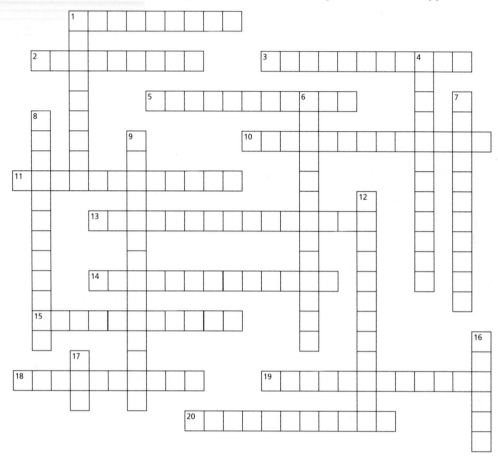

Across

1. tissues growing together that normally do not
2. pertaining to the abdomen
3. tissue around the teeth
5. physician (DO)
10. synonym for tenoplasty
11. excision of cartilage
13. surgical puncture to remove fluid from chest
14. pertaining to ribs and cartilage
15. area above the lower back or waist
18. inflamed tendon
19. bone cancer
20. person who develops artificial limbs

Down

1. raising arm to the side away from the middle
4. used to measure chest circumference
6. enlarged head due to fluid (congenital)
7. process of examining a joint with a scope
8. specialist in straightening teeth
9. defective development of bone marrow
12. condition of porous bones
16. suffix for development
17. dentist (abbreviation)

REVIEW ACTIVITIES

GLOSSARY

abdomen	belly area, cavity below the thorax	chondralgia, chondrodynia	cartilage pain
abdominocentesis	surgical puncture of the abdomen to remove fluid	chondrectomy	excision of cartilage
abduct	move away from the midline (verb)	chondrocostal, costochondral	pertaining to cartilage and rib
abduction	movement away from the midline, e.g., arm abducted from side	costectomy	excision of a rib
		cystocele	herniation of the urinary bladder (into the vagina)
aberrant	wandering from normal location, process, or behavior	cystoplasty	surgical repair of the urinary bladder
abnormal	deviating from the average or expected	cystoscopy	process of examining the bladder using a scope
addiction	habitual attraction, may include physical dependence	cystotomy	incision into the urinary bladder
adhesions	tissues grown together that are normally separate	dentalgia	tooth pain
		dentist	specialist in care of teeth
amniocentesis	surgical puncture of the amnion to obtain cells for testing	dentoid	resembling a tooth
		dysplasia	poor or defective development
arthritis	inflammation of a joint	etiology	study of the origin of a disease
arthroplasty	surgical repair or reconstruction of a joint	fascia	tissue that connects muscle to muscle
arthroscope	instrument used to look into a joint		
arthroscopy	process of using an arthroscope to examine a joint	hydrocele	serous fluid accumulation in a saclike cavity (Example: testicular hernia)
arthrotomy	incision into a joint	hydrocephalus	fluid in the skull causing deformity and brain damage
bursa	serous sac between a tendon and bone (pl. bursae)	hydrocyst	fluid-filled sac
bursectomy	excision of a bursa	hydrophobia	abnormal fear of water, rabies
bursitis	inflammation of a bursa	hydrotherapy	therapy using water
cardiocentesis	surgical puncture of the heart to remove fluid	hyperplasia	abnormally increased development referring to quantity of cells

REVIEW ACTIVITIES

interchondral	pertaining to between the cartilage (intercartilaginous)
intercostal	pertaining to between the ribs
interdental	pertaining to between the teeth
ligament	tissue that connects bone to bone and supports visceral organs
lumbar	pertaining to the lower back, between the thorax and sacrum
meniscectomy	excision of the meniscus of the knee
myelocytes	bone marrow cells
myelodysplasia	defective development of the bone marrow or spinal cord
orthodontics	dental practice of straightening teeth
orthodontist	dentist specializing in straightening teeth
orthopedist	physician specialist in treatment of skeletal and joint disorders
orthotics	pertaining to appliances used to support muscoloskeletal system
orthotist	specialist who develops and assists patients with orthotics
osteitis	inflammation of the bone
osteoarthritis	inflammation of the bone and joint
osteoarthropathy	disease of bone and joint
osteochondritis	inflammation of the bone and cartilage
osteoma	bone tumor

osteomalacia	softening of the bone
osteomyelitis	inflammation of the bone and bone marrow
osteopathic	pertaining to the practice of osteopathic physicians or bone disease
osteopathy	disease of the bones
osteopenia	loss of bone
osteoporosis	porous condition of the bone due to deterioration of bone matrix
osteosarcoma	cancer of the bone
pelvis	the bony structure including the ilium, ischium, pubis, sacrum, and coccyx
pericardium	around the heart (membrane)
perichondrium	around the cartilage (membrane)
periodontal	around the tooth
periodontist	dentist specializing in treatment of diseased tissue around the teeth
periosteum	around the bone (membrane)
prosthesis	artificial limb or other body part replacement
prosthetics	pertaining to prostheses
prosthetist	specialist who develops and assists patients with prostheses
pubic	pertaining to the pubis, bone in the lower anterior pelvis
supracostal	above the ribs
supracranial	above or on top of the skull
supralumbar	above the lumbar spine

REVIEW ACTIVITIES

suprapubic	above the pubis
tenalgia, tenodynia	tendon pain
tendinitis	inflammation of a tendon
tendon	tissue that connects muscle to bone
tendinoplasty, tenoplasty, tendoplasty	surgical repair of a tendon
thoracocentesis, thoracentesis	surgical puncture of the thorax to remove fluid

thoracolumbar	pertaining to the chest and lower spine
thoracometer	instrument used to measure the chest
thoracopathy	disease of the chest
thoracotomy	incision into the thorax
thorax	chest, area of the back posterior to the chest (pl. thoraces)

UNIT 5

Pathology, Otorhinolaryngology, and Prefixes dys-, brady-, tachy-, poly-, syn-

ANSWER COLUMN	
	5.1
TAKE A CLOSER LOOK	In words such as carcinoma and coccus, the first "c" is pronounced as a hard "c" with a "k" sound. When followed by o, u, a, or a consonant, "c" is pronounced with a "k" sound, e.g., coat, cut, cake, cluck.
	5.2
hard "c" or "k" (pronounce them aloud)	In the words colon and cardiac, the "c" is pronounced with a *_____ sound. NOTE: Listen to the audio CDs that accompany this text for coaching on pronunciation.
	5.3
TAKE A CLOSER LOOK	In the words cerebrum and incision, the "c" is pronounced with a soft "c" or "s" sound. When "c" is followed by i, e, or y, it is pronounced with a soft "c" or "s" sound, e.g., city, cereal, cycle.
	5.4
soft "c" or "s"	According to the "c" rule, in the words cystocele and encephalitis each "c" is pronounced with a *_____ sound.
	5.5
INFORMATION FRAME	Remember the "c" rule for those terms that follow.
	5.6
cocc	The Greek word *coccos* means grain or seeds. When building words about the spherically shaped family of bacteria, the cocc/i, use the word root _____.

BACTERIA

Cocci   Bacilli   Curved rods

Diplococcus   Staphylococcus   Bacillus   Diplobacillus   Spirochete

Streptococcus   Streptobacillus

VIRUSES

Virus

OTHER PATHOGENS

Filarial worms   Trichomonas   Yeast   Lice

Disease-producing microorganisms

ANSWER COLUMN	
	5.7
cocci **kok′** sī coccus **kok′**us	Pneumonia may be caused by a pneum/o/coccus such as *Streptococcus pneumoniae*. From this you know the bacteria responsible for pneumonia belong to the _____ (plural family). The singular form is _____.
	5.8
cocci	One form of meningitis is caused by the mening/o/coccus. It, too, is a member of the (plural family) _____.

ANSWER COLUMN

5.9

There are three main types of cocci. Cocci growing in pairs are
dipl/o/_____.

cocci
kok′ si

5.10

Gon/o/rrhea is a venereal disease caused by *Neisseria gonorrhoeae*.
This gon/o/coccus grows in pairs, so it is a _____/____/_____/_____.

dipl/o/cocc/us
dip′lō **kok**′ us

5.11

Cocci growing in twisted chains are strept/o/_____.
Cocci growing in clusters are staphyl/o/_____.

cocci
cocci

5.12

strept/o means twisted chains or strips. Streptococci
(strep) grow in twisted chains as shown here. If you
should see a chain of cocci when examining a slide
under the microscope, you would say they were
_____/____/_____/____.

Streptococcus

strept/o/cocc/i
strep′ tō **kok**′ sī

5.13

Name the type of coccus in the following statements. Sore throat may be
caused by β-hemolytic _____/____/_____/____. Some pus formation
is due to _____/____/_____/____ *pyogenes*.

strept/o/cocc/us
Strept/o/cocc/us

5.14

Staphyle is the Greek word for bunch of grapes. **staphyl/o** is used to build words
that suggest a bunch of grapes. Staphylococci (staph) grow in clusters like a
bunch of _____.

grapes

5.15

Staphylococci grow in clusters like grapes. If you should
see a cluster of cocci when using the microscope,
you would say they were
_____/____/_____/____.

Staphylococcus

staphyl/o/cocc/i
staf i lō **kok**′ sī

ANSWER COLUMN

Impetigo pustules caused by either streptococcus or staphylococcus *(Courtesy of Robert A. Silverman, MD, Clinical Associate Professor, Department of Pediatrics, Georgetown University)*

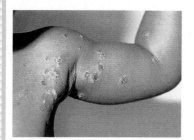

5.16

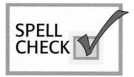
SPELL CHECK ✓

Proper genus and species names are used to identify bacteria and parasites. They are italicized with the genus name capitalized, for example: *Staphylococcus aureus*, *Escherichia coli*. When abbreviating, you may use the genus initial and the species name. The genus initial is capitalized but the phrase is not italicized, for example: S. aureus, E. coli.

5.17

In Latin *baculus* means staff or rod. A *bacillus* (plural *bacilli*) is a rod-shaped bacterium (plural *bacteria*). Use bacillus to form a term that means a rod-shaped double bacillus

Diplobacillus

dipl/o/bacill/us
dip′ lō ba **sil**′ us
strept/o/bacill/us
strep′tō ba **sil**′ us

_____/____/_____/____;

a rod-shaped bacillus growing in twisted chains

_____/____/_____/____.

Now, you've got it!

5.18

bacill/i
bə **si**′ lī

Klebsiella pneumoniae, a pneum/o/bacill/us, is another common cause of pneumonia. These rod-shaped bacteria are _____/____.

HINT: The word bacteria is plural, so the plural form is needed to complete this statement correctly.

5.19

bacterium
bak **ter**′ ē um
bacilli
bə **sil**′ ī

The plural term bacteria is normally used because we rarely find one bacterium. Remember the plural rule: **-um** is singular, **-a** is plural.
The singular of bacteria is _____.
Now try this one: If the plural of coccus is cocci, the plural of bacillus is _____.
Good.

ANSWER COLUMN

	5.20
staphylococci	The bacteria that cause carbuncles grow in a cluster like a bunch of grapes. Carbuncles are caused by _____.
	5.21
staphylococci	Most bacteria that form pus grow in a cluster. They are _____.
	5.22
staphyl/o/cocc/i	A common form of food poisoning is also caused by _____/____/_____/___.
	5.23
staphyl/o/cocc/us staf′ ə lō **ko′** kəs	A common skin bacterium that may contaminate food, causing toxins to be produced, is _____/____/_____/__.
	5.24
staphyl/o/plasty **staf′** i lō plas′ tē	Surgical repair of the uvula is _____/____/_____.

SEXUALLY TRANSMITTED DISEASES (STDS)

Causative Agent	Disease
Bacteria	
Chlamydia trachomatis	Chlamydia, urogenital infection
Neisseria gonorrhoeae	gonorrhea (clap)
Treponema pallidum	syphilis
Viruses	
hepatitis B virus (HBV)	hepatitis
human immunodeficiency virus (HIV)	HIV infection which converts to AIDS AIDS (acquired immunodeficiency syndrome)
human papilloma virus (HPV)	condylomata acuminata (venereal warts)
herpes simplex virus (HSV)	genital herpes lesions
Parasites	
Trichomonas vaginalis	trichomoniasis, urogenital infection
Phthirus pubis	lice, pediculosis pubis (crabs)
Sarcoptes scabiei	scabies (mites)
Fungi	
Candida albicans	candidiasis (yeast infection)

ANSWER COLUMN

	5.25
inflammation of the uvula	Staphyl/itis (uvul/itis) means *_____.
	5.26
excision of the uvula **yōo′** vyōo lə	Staphyl/ectomy (uvul/ectomy) means _____.
	5.27
staphyl/itis staf′ i **lī′** tis uvul/itis yōo′ vyōo **lī′** tis staphyl/ectomy staf′ i **lek′** tō mē uvul/ectomy yōo′ vyōo **lek′** tō mē	**Staphyl/o**, from the Greek means cluster of grapes. **uvul/o**, from the Latin word meaning cluster of grapes, is also used when referring to the palatine uvula. Build words meaning inflammation of the uvula _____/_____ or _____/_____; removal of the uvula _____/_____ or _____/_____.
	5.28
pus	**py/o** is the combining form used for words involving pus. A py/o/cele is a hernia containing _____.
	5.29
py/o/gen/ic pī′ ō **jen′** ik	**-genic** means producing or forming. Many staphylococci are pyogenic. Bacteria that produce pus are ____/____/_____/____.
	5.30
onc/o/gen/ic on′ kō **jen′** ik path/o/gen/ic pa′ thō **jen′** ik	Try this one. Remember that **onc/o** refers to tumors. If a condition or substance promotes tumor production, it is said to be _____/____/_____/____. If organisms produce disease, they are _____/____/_____/____. Good try.
	5.31
py/o/thorax pī′ ō **thôr′** aks	Py/o/thorax means an accumulation of pus in the thoracic cavity. When pus-forming bacteria invade the thoracic lining, ____/____/_____ results.

ANSWER COLUMN
Structures of the mouth

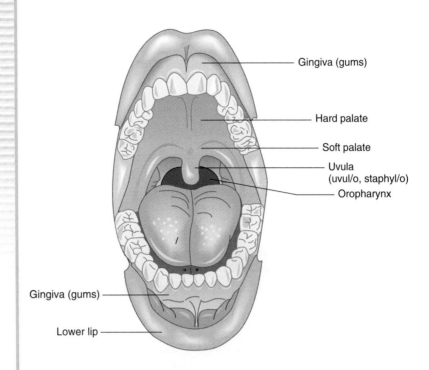

Gingiva (gums)

Hard palate

Soft palate

Uvula
(uvul/o, staphyl/o)

Oropharynx

Gingiva (gums)

Lower lip

5.32

Pneumonia (fluid and infection) and lung abcess are two other diseases
causing _____.

pyothorax

5.33

A py/o/gen/ic bacterium is one that forms pus. You may know the noun genesis,
meaning creation or beginning, as in the words generate and generation. The
adjective that means something that produces or forms pus is
_____/_____/_____/_____.

py/o/gen/ic
pī′ ō **jen**′ ik

5.34

Pyogenic bacteria are found in boils. Boils become purulent (contain pus).
This pus is formed by _____ bacteria.

pyogenic

5.35

Look up purulent in your medical dictionary. It means pus forming
or _____.

pyogenic

5.36

-rrhea is a suffix meaning flow or discharge. Think of diarrhea, which means to
flow through.
Py/o/rrhea means *_____.

flow or discharge of pus

ANSWER COLUMN

SPELL CHECK ✓

-rrhea

5.37

The "rrh" in **-rrhea** is an unusual spelling for English words. It comes from the Greek language.

There will be three more suffixes with "rrh" in their spelling in future frames. To indicate flow or discharge use the suffix _____.

---

py/o
pī′ō rē′ ə

5.38

Py/o/rrhea alveolaris is a disease of the teeth and gums. The part of this disease's name that tells you that pus is discharged is _____/_____.

---

pyorrhea

5.39

There is also a disease of a salivary gland for which there is a flow of pus. This is _____ salivaris.

---

ear
ear
ear

5.40

ot is a Greek word root meaning ear. Ot/o/rrhea means a discharge from the ear.
ot/o is the combining form for _____.
An ot/o/scope is used to examine the _____.
An ot/ic solution is prepared for treatment of the _____.

---

ot/o/scopy
ō tos′ kō pē
ot/ic
ō′ tik

5.41

The process of examining the ear using an otoscope is called
_____/_____/_____.

The term that means pertaining to the ear is _____/_____.

---

ot/o/rrhea
ō tō rē′ ə

5.42

Ot/o/rrhea is both a sign and a disease. No matter which is meant, the word
_____/_____/_____ is used for a discharge from the ear(s).

---

otorrhea

5.43

Otitis media involves discharge, inflammation, and deafness. One of the signs of this disease is discharge or _____.

---

inflammation of the ear

5.44

Otorrhea may be caused by ot/itis media (OM), an infection in the middle ear causing inflammation and discharge. Ot/itis means
* _____.

ANSWER COLUMN

Otoscope with different sized reusable specula

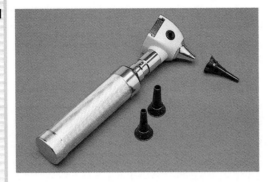

Structures of the Ear

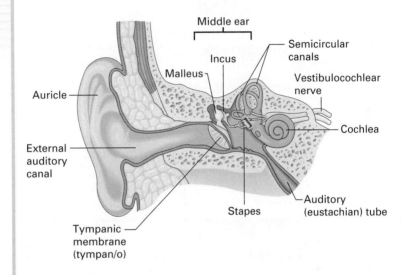

Middle ear

Semicircular canals

Incus

Malleus

Vestibulocochlear nerve

Auricle

Cochlea

External auditory canal

Stapes

Auditory (eustachian) tube

Tympanic membrane (tympan/o)

5.45

Auris sinistra (AS) refers to the left ear. Auris dextra (AD) refers to the right ear, and auris uterque (AU) to both ears. Ot/itis media causes pain in ears which are inflamed.

Ear pain is ____/_____ or _____/___/_____.

ot/algia
ō **tal′** jē ə
ot/o/dynia
ō tō **din′** ē ə

5.46

otodynia or otalgia

When otitis media is prolonged, there has usually been enough destruction of the tissue that _____ (ear pain) no longer occurs.

5.47

otodynia or otalgia

Small children often complain of earache. Medically, this could be called _____.

ANSWER COLUMN

5.48

eardrum

Recall that AS refers to the left ear and AD refers to the right ear. Membrana tympani dextra (MTD) refers to the right eardrum. Membrana tympani sinistra (MTS) refers to the left _____.

5.49

eardrum
tympan/o

Look up tympanum in your dictionary. The tympanum is the _____. One combining form for tympanum is _____/____.

5.50

tympan/ic
tim **pan**′ ik
tympan/o/tomy
tim′ p ə n **ot**′ ə mē
tympan/ectomy
tim′ p ə **nek**′ t ə mē

Build a word meaning:
pertaining to the eardrum _____/_____;

incision into the eardrum _____/____/_____;

excision of the eardrum _____/_____.

NOTE: A common synonym for tympan/o/tomy is myring/o/tomy (mī ring ot′ ə mē). Both are incisions for the purpose of inserting tubes in the eadrum.

5.51

tympan/o/metry
tim′ pən **om**′ ə trē

Recall that metr is the word root for measure. **-metry** indicates the process of measuring. The process of measuring the function of the eardrum is called _____/____/_____.

5.52

tympan/ites
tim′ pə **nī**′ tēz

In your dictionary, using the word root tympan, find a word that means distended with gas—as tight as a drum. The word is _____/_____.

5.53

tympanites

If a patient complains of a very bloated, gassy feeling and has a distended abdomen, the doctor may write _____ on the chart.

5.54

Study the following prefixes to be used to build words related to voice, speaking, breathing, heart rate, swallowing, and digestion.

PROFESSIONAL PROFILES

The audiologist, Certificate of Clinical Competency in Audiology (CCC-A),** performs diagnostic hearing tests, fits hearing aids, works with patients in rehabilitation of hearing loss, and makes appropriate medical referrals to physicians. In hospitals, audiologists work with a variety of patients including high-risk infants, and perform intraoperative monitoring during surgery. Audiologists receive a master of arts degree from a school accredited by the American Speech and Hearing Association (ASHA), which also administers the certification process for audiologists and speech pathologists.

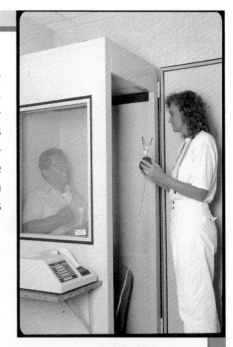

Audiologist performing audiometry

ANSWER COLUMN

Prefix	Meaning	Example
a-	not, lack of (before a consonant)	a/genesis
an-	not, lack of (before a vowel)	an/emia
brady-	abnormally slow	brady/phagia
dys-	difficult, abnormal, poor, painful	dys/pepsia
tachy-	abnormally fast	tachy/cardia

5.55

audi/o is a combining form for hearing. The study of hearing is audi/o/logy. Build terms that mean an instrument used to measure hearing

audi/o/meter
aw′ dē **om**′ ət ər

_____/____/_____;

the process of measuring hearing

audi/o/metry
aw′ dē **om**′ ə trē

_____/____/_____;

a record made by the instrument used to test hearing

audi/o/gram
aw′ dē ō gram

_____/____/_____.

NOTE: An audience listens in an auditorium.

ANSWER COLUMN	
	5.56
audi/o/log/ist aw′ dē **ol**′ ō jist	A hearing specialist is called an: _____/____/_____/_____.
	5.57
	phon/o means voice or vocal sounds. A/phonia means
unable to make sounds	*_____.
	Dys/phonia means
weak voice (poor, etc.)	*_____.
	5.58
	Brady/phasia means
slow speech	*_____.
	A/phasia means
absence of speech	*_____.
	Phon/ic means
pertaining to the voice	*_____.
	A phon/o/meter is
an instrument for measuring intensity of vocal sounds	*_____ _____.
	5.59
	Build terms that mean the study of: voice or vocal sounds
phon/o/logy fon **ol**′ ō jē audi/o/logy aw de **ol**′ ō jē phas/o/logy f ās **ol**′ ō jē	_____/____/_____; hearing _____/____/_____; speech _____/____/_____.
	5.60
nose flow or discharge	**-rrhea** is a suffix meaning flow or discharge. Rhinorrhea means discharge from the nose. rhin/o is used in words about the _____. **-rrhea** is used to indicate *_____.
	5.61
rhin/itis rī **nī**′ tis	Rhinoceros is from the Greek word meaning nose-horn. Using what is necessary from **rhin/o**, form a word that means inflammation of the nose: _____/_____.

ANSWER COLUMN

Hearing aid

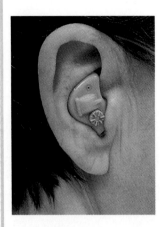

5.62

rhin/o/rrhea
rī nō **rē′** ə

Rhin/o/rrhea is a symptom. Drainage from the nose due to a head cold is a symptom called _____/____/_____.

5.63

rhinorrhea

A discharge from the sinuses through the nose is a form of _____.

5.64

rhinorrhea

Nasal catarrh (ka tär′) is another source of _____.

5.65

rhin/o/plasty
rī′ nō plas′ tē

Build a word that means surgical repair of the nose. _____/____/_____

5.66

rhin/o/tomy
rī **not′** ə mē

Form a word that means incision of the nose. _____/__/_____

5.67

calculus or stone

A rhin/o/lith is a calculus or stone in the nose. **lith/o** is the combining form for *_____.

5.68

calculi (calculus) or stones
lith/o/gen/ic
lith ō **jen′** ik

-genesis is used as a noun suffix meaning generating, producing, or forming. Lith/o/genesis means producing or forming
*_____. The adjectival form of lithogenesis is _____/____/_____/____.

ANSWER COLUMN

5.69

Lith/o/logy is the science of dealing with or studying

calculi or stones

* _____.

5.70

lith/o/tomy
li **thot′** ə mē
lith/o/meter
(You pronounce)

Using what is necessary from **lith/o**, build a word meaning an incision for the removal of a stone _____/____/_____.

Name an instrument for measuring size of calculi. _____/____/_____

5.71

gall or bile

Calculi or stones can be formed in many places in the body. A chol/e/lith means a gallstone. **chol/e** is the combining form for *_____.

5.72

chol/e/lith
kō′ lə lith

Chol/e/lith means gallstone. One result of gallbladder disease is the presence of a gallstone or _____/____/_____.

5.73

INFORMATION FRAME

-iasis is a suffix used to indicate a pathologic condition. **-iasis** may also be used when an infestation has occurred.

5.74

chol/e/lith/iasis
ko′ lē lith ī′ ə sis

Lith/iasis is a disease condition characterized by the presence of stones (calculi). The presence of gallstones in the gallbladder is called

_____/____/_____/_____.

5.75

trichomonas
yeast (monilia)
filarial worm or local
   inflammation of lymph
   nodes
giardia lamblia

Look up the following terms in your medical dictionary. What is the "organism" that causes each infestation?

trichomoniasis   _____

moniliasis   _____

elephantiasis   *_____

_____

giardiasis   *_____

Trichomonas vaginalis

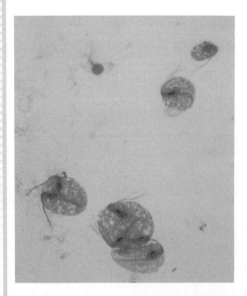

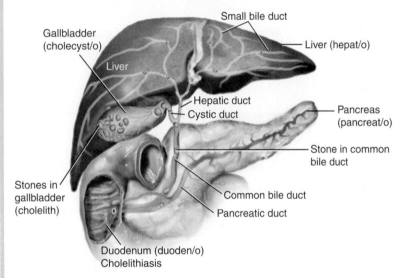

Small bile duct

Gallbladder
(cholecyst/o)

Liver (hepat/o)

Liver

Hepatic duct
Cystic duct

Pancreas
(pancreat/o)

Stone in common
bile duct

Stones in
gallbladder
(cholelith)

Common bile duct

Pancreatic duct

Duodenum (duoden/o)
Cholelithiasis

5.76

gallbladder

Bile (gall) is secreted by the gallbladder (GB). Chol/e/cyst is a medical name
for the _____.

5.77

Recall that **-gram** refers to a picture and **-graphy** refers to the process of taking
the picture or recording. Build terms from the following meanings:
an x-ray of the gallbladder

chol/e/cyst/o/gram
kō′ lē **sist**′ ō gram
chol/e/cyst/o/graphy
kō′ lē sist **og**′ raf ē

_____/____/_____/____/_____;

the process of taking a gallbladder x-ray

_____/____/_____/____/_____.

ANSWER COLUMN

5.78

Gallstones can result in inflammation of the gallbladder (chol/e/cyst). Medically, this is called _____/____/_____/_____.

chol/e/cyst/itis
kō′ lə sist ī′ tis

NOTE: Ultrasound (US) of the gallbladder (GB) is becoming a common procedure for diagnosing cholecystitis.

5.79

Cholecystitis is accompanied by pain and hyperemesis. Fatty foods aggravate these symptoms and should be avoided in cases of _____.

cholecystitis

5.80

Butter, cream, and even whole milk contain fat and may have to be avoided by patients with _____.

cholecystitis

5.81

When a cholelith causes cholecystitis, surgery may be needed. One surgical procedure is an incision into the gallbladder, called

chol/e/cyst/o/tomy
kō′ lə sist **ot**′ ə mē

a _____/____/_____/__/_____.

5.82

Usually the presence of a gallstone calls for the excision of the gallbladder. This is a _____/____/_____/_____.

chol/e/cyst/ectomy
kō′ lə sist **ek**′ tə mē

5.83

A calculus or stone in the nose is a _____/____/_____.

rhin/o/lith
rī′ nō lith

5.84

slow

brady- is used in words to mean slow. Brady/cardia means _____ heart action.

5.85

Brady/phag/ia means slowness in eating. Abnormally slow swallowing is also called _____/_____/____.

brady/phag/ia
brad ē **fā**′ jē ə

5.86

From brady/phagia you find the word root phag for eat. (More of phag/o later.) Slow eating is _____.

bradyphagia

Cholecystography showing
presence of many gallstones

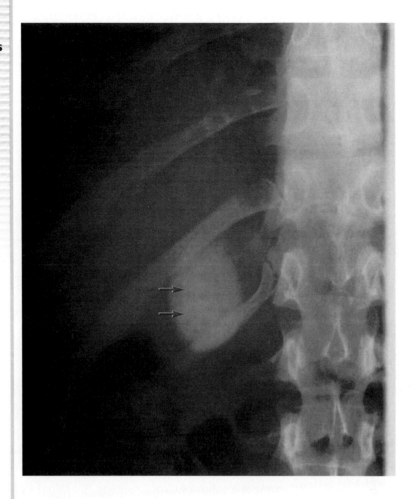

5.87	
bradyphagia	Elderly people who chew and swallow very slowly are exhibiting _____.

5.88	
brady/cardi/a brad ē **kär′** dē ə	Abnormally slow heart action is _____/_____/_____.

5.89	
fast or rapid	tachy- is used in words to show the opposite of slow. tachy- means * _____.

5.90	
rapid heart action	Tachy/cardia means * _____.

ANSWER COLUMN

5.91

tachy/phagia
tak ē **fā**′ jē ə

The word for fast eating is _____/_____.

5.92

tach/o/gram
tak′ ō gram

Tachos is a Greek word that means swiftness, as in tachometer. A record of the velocity of the blood flow is a _____/____/_____.

5.93

tachy/cardi/a
tak ē **kär**′ dē ə

An abnormally rapid heartbeat is called _____/_____/____.

5.94

respiration or breathing

pne/o comes from the Greek word *pneia*, meaning breath. **pne/o** any place in a word means *_____.

5.95

silent

When **pne/o** begins a word, the "p" is silent. When **pne/o** occurs later in a word, the "p" is pronounced. In pne/o/pne/ic, the first "p" is _____; the second is pronounced (nē op′ nē ik).

5.96

slow breathing
tachy/pnea
tak ip **nē**′ ə or
tak **ip**′ nē ə

-pnea is a suffix meaning breathing. Brady/pnea (brād ip nē′ ə) means
*_____. A word for rapid breathing is _____/_____.

5.97

tachypnea

The rate of respiration (R) is controlled by the amount of carbon dioxide (CO_2) in the blood. Increased carbon dioxide speeds up breathing and causes _____.

5.98

tachypnea

Muscle exercise increases the amount of CO_2 in the blood. This speeds respiration (R) and produces _____.

5.99

tachypnea

Running a race causes _____.

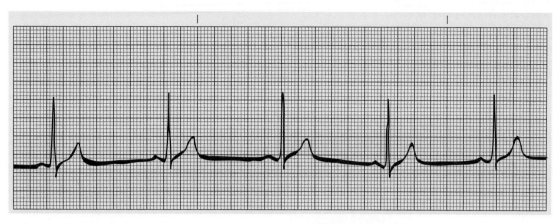

Brady cardia < 60 bpm

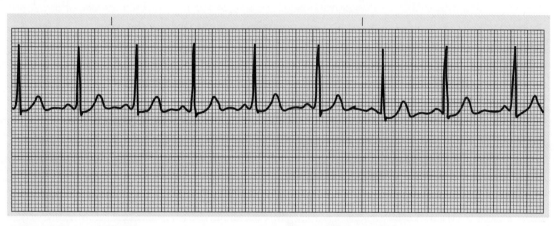

Tachycardia > 100 bpm

ANSWER COLUMN	
	5.100
without breathing	a- and an- are prefixes meaning without or lack of. A/pnea literally means *_____.
	5.101
a/pnea ap **nē′** ə, **ap′** nē ə	Apnea means cessation of breathing. If the level of carbon dioxide in the blood falls very low, ____/_____ results.
	5.102
apnea brady/pnea brad ip **nē′** ə or brad **ip′** nē ə	When breathing ceases for a bit, _____ results. If breathing is merely very slow, it is called _____/_____.

ANSWER COLUMN

5.103

a- and an-

The prefixes meaning without are *_____.

NOTE: **a-** and **an-** are prefixes meaning without or lack of. **a-** is used preceding a consonant. **an-** is used preceding a vowel.

5.104

without generation (origin)

Genesis is both a Greek and an English word. It means generation (origin or beginning). A/gen/esis means *_____.

5.105

a/gen/esis
ə **jen**′ ə sis

By extension, agenesis means failure to develop or lack of development. When an organ does not develop, physicians use the word
____/_____/_____.

5.106

agenesis

Agenesis can refer to any part of the body. If a hand does not develop, the condition is called _____ of the hand.

5.107

agenesis

When the stomach is not formed, _____ of the stomach results.

5.108

carcin/o/gen/esis
kär′ si nō **jen**′ ə sis

The development of cancer is called
_____/____/_____/_____.

5.109

carcin/o/gen/ic
kär′ si nō **jen**′ ic

A term that means pertaining to the development of cancer is
_____/____/_____/____.

5.110

INFORMATION FRAME

dys- is the prefix for painful, faulty, diseased, bad, or difficult. men is the word root for menstruation. **-rrhea** means flow or discharge.

5.111

dys/men/o/rrhea
dis′ men ō **rē**′ ə

Build words that mean
painful or difficult menstruation
_____/_____/____/_____;

ANSWER COLUMN	
ANSWER COLUMN a/men/o/rrhea ā′ men ō **rē**′ ə	absence of menstruation ___/_____/___/_____.
	5.112
dys/phag/ia dis **fā**′ jē ə difficult	Dysphagia means difficult swallowing. Analyze dysphagia: ___dys___/___phag___/___ia___ **dys-** in dysphagia means _____.
	5.113
dys/pnea disp **nē**′ ə, **disp**′ nē ə	Dys/trophy literally means poor development. The word for difficult breathing is ___dys___/___pnea___.
	5.114
digestion dī **jest**′ shun	*Pepsis* is the Greek word for digestion. From this you get the combining form **peps/o** and the adjective pept/ic to use in words about ___digestion___.
	5.115
digestion dys/peps/ia dis **pep**′ shə	Dys/peps/ia means poor ___digestion___. The result of food eaten too rapidly may be ___/___/___.
	5.116
dyspepsia	Dyspeps/ia is a noun. Eating under tension also may cause _____.
	5.117
a/peps/ia a **pep**′ shə brady/peps/ia brad i **pep**′ shə pept/ic **pep**′ tik	Cessation of digestion (without digestion) is ___/_____/___, while slow digestion is _____/_____/___, and stomach ulcers are _____/_____ ulcers.
	5.118
therm/o/meter thûr′ **mom**′ ə tər	Normal average body temperature is 37°C or 98.6°F. **therm/o**, from the Greek word *thermos*, is the combining form that means heat. An instrument to measure heat is a _____/___/_____, which may be calibrated in Celsius or Fahrenheit.

ANSWER COLUMN

Correlation between Celsius and Fahrenheit scales

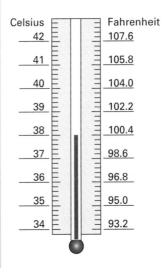

Celsius	Fahrenheit
42	107.6
41	105.8
40	104.0
39	102.2
38	100.4
37	98.6
36	96.8
35	95.0
34	93.2

To convert:
(9/5 x temperature in Celsius) + 32° = temperature in Fahrenheit

5/9 x (temperature in Fahrenheit – 32°) = temperature in Celsius

---

5.119

Build words meaning
pertaining to heat

therm/al or therm/ic
thûr′ mə l or **thur**′ mik
_____/____;

therm/o/esthesi/a
thûr′ mō es **thēs**′ ē ə
oversensitivity to heat
_____/____/esthes/ia;

therm/o/algesia
thûr′ mō al **jēs**′ ē ə
_____/____/algesia

therm/o/gen/esis
thûr′ mō **jen**′ ə sis
formation of (body) heat
_____/____/gen/esis.

5.120

Build a word meaning abnormal fear of heat

therm/o/phobia
thûr′ mō **fō**′ bē ə
_____/____/_____;

therm/o/plegia
thûr′ mō **plē**′ jē ə
heatstroke (paralysis)
_____/____/plegia;

dia/therm/y
di′ ə thûr mē
heating through tissue (treatment)
dia/_____/____.

5.121

Diarrhea literally means to flow through and refers to a watery bowel movement (BM). Dia/therm/y means generating heat through (tissues).

through
heat
suffix
dia- means _____;
therm means _____;
-y is a noun _____.

ANSWER COLUMN

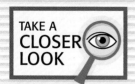

therm or therm/o
(Try it!)

5.122

Body temperature above 101°F can indicate fever. For information about temperature scales or variations in body temperature, look in the dictionary for words beginning with *_____.

5.123

hyper/therm/ia
hī′ per **thûr**′ mē ə
hypo/therm/ia
hī′ pō **thûr**′ mē ə

Using **hyper-** and **hypo-**, build a word that means

high body temperature (fever) _____/_____/_____;

low body temperature _____/_____/_____.

Vital Signs Normal Values*				
	Infant	**6-Year-Old**	**14-Year-Old**	**Adult**
Blood pressure (BP)	65–122 / 30–84	85–115 / 48–64	99–137 / 50–70	100–140 / 60–90
Respirations (R)	30–50	16–22	14–20	12–20
Pulse (P)	100–170	70–115	60–110	60–100
All Ages				
Temperature (T) Oral (PO)	98.6°F, 37°C			
Rectal (R)	99°F, 37.7°C			
Axillary (AX)	97.6°F, 36.4°C			

*Values taken from *Health Assessment and Physical Examination*, 2nd ed., by M. E. Z. Estes, 2002, Albany, NY: Delmar.

5.124

micro- means small. Hydro/cephal/us is a condition involving fluid in the head. A condition of an abnormally small head is called

micro/cephal/us
mī′ krō **sef**′ ə ləs

_____/_____/_____.

ANSWER COLUMN

5.125

Microcephalus limits the size of the brain. Most microcephalic people are mentally impaired. Occasionally a baby is born with an unusually small head,

microcephalus

or _____.

5.126

A cyst is a sac containing fluid.
A very small cyst is a

micro/cyst
mī′ krō sist

_____/_____.

A very small cell is a

micro/cyte
mī′ krō sīt

_____/_____.

micro/cardi/a
mī′ krō **kär′** dē ə

A condition of having a small heart is

_____/_____/_____.

micro/gram
mī′ krō gram

One thousandth of a milligram (0.001 mg) is

a _____/_____ (mcg) (0.000001 g one millionth of a gram).

5.127

Surgery performed on minute structures using a microscope and small

micro/surgery
mī′ krō **sûr′** jər ē

instruments is _____/_____.

5.128

large

macro- is the opposite of **micro-**. **macro-** is used in words to mean _____.

NOTE: **micro-** and **macro-** are combining forms used as prefixes.

5.129

macro/cyte(s)
mak′ rō sīt(s)

Things that are macro/scop/ic can be seen with the naked eye. Very large cells are called _____/_____.

5.130

macro/cephal/us
ma krō **sef′** ə ləs
macro/blast
ma′ krō blast
macro/cocc/us
ma′ krō **ko′** kus

An abnormally large head is a

_____/_____/____.

A large embryonic (germ) cell is a

_____/_____.

A very large coccus is a

_____/_____/____.

ANSWER COLUMN

	5.131
abnormally	Use your dictionary to help you define the following conditions.
large tongue	macro/gloss/ia *_____
large ear(s)	macrot/ia *_____
large nose	macro/rhin/ia *_____
large lips	macro/cheil/ia *_____

	5.132
dactyl	*Dactylos* is a Greek word meaning finger. Macro/dactyl/ia is a condition of abnormally large fingers or toes. The word root for fingers or toes is _____.

	5.133
dactyl/o	Another way of saying large fingers or toes is dactyl/o/megal/y. The combining form for finger or toe is _____/_____.

	5.134
	A finger or toe is also called a digit. (When you see digit, finger, or toe, use **dactyl/o**.) Build a word meaning
	inflammation of a digit
dactyl/itis	_____/_____;
dak ti **lī**′ tis	cramp or spasm of a digit
dactyl/o/spasm	_____/_____/_____ _____
dak ti lō spaz′ əm	a fingerprint
dactyl/o/gram	_____/_____/_____. (picture).
dak′ tilō gram	

	5.135
condition of having	Macro/dactyl/ia means *_____
abnormally large	_____.
fingers or toes (digits)	Poly/dactyl/ism means too many *_____.
fingers or toes (digits)	

	5.136
	syn- is a prefix meaning with or together. Syn/dactyl/ism means a joining together of two or more digits. The prefix that means together or with
syn-	is _____.

	5.137
syn/dactyl/ism	A person with two or more fingers joined together has a condition called
sin **dak**′ til izm	_____/_____/_____.

ANSWER COLUMN

5.138

Syn/erg/ism occurs when two or more drugs or organs working together produce an increased effect (**syn-**, join; erg, work; **-ism**, condition or state). Drugs that work together to increase each other's effects are called
____/____/_____ (adjective) drugs.

syn/erg/istic
sin er **jis**′ tik

5.139

Syn/ergetic also means working (erg) together (**syn-**), but usually it refers to muscles that work together. The three muscles in the forearm that work together are ____/____/_____ muscles.

syn/erg/etic
sin er **jet**′ ik

5.140

Tylenol tablets with codeine are frequently more effective for killing pain than Tylenol alone. This is because Tylenol and codeine are
_____ drugs.

synergistic

5.141

Alcohol intake is contraindicated (recommended against) when taking analgesics because the effects can multiply central nervous system depression. This is a dangerous _____ effect.

synergistic

Syndactylism

ANSWER COLUMN

5.142

Analyze synarthrosis.

syn-

arthr

osis

prefix _____

word root (joint) _____

condition _____

5.143

syn/arthr/osis

sin är **thrō'** sis

Syn/arthr/osis indicates an immovable joint. The joined bones are fused together. When bones are fused at a joint so that there is no movement,

_____/_____/_____ occurs.

EXAMPLE: sacrum, pelvis, skull.

5.144

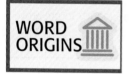

WORD ORIGINS

drom/o comes from the Greek word for run. A hippodrome was an open air stadium built for racing horses or chariots in ancient Greece. Drom/o/mania is an insane impulse to wander or roam. You usually use drom with the prefixes **syn-** and **pro-**.

5.145

syndrome

sin' drōm

A syn/drome is a variety of symptoms occurring (running along) together. The complete picture of a disease is its _____.

Cranial sutures—synarthrotic joints

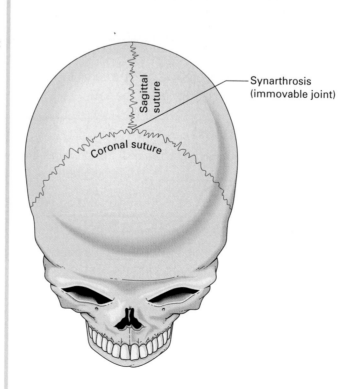

ANSWER COLUMN

INFORMATION FRAME	**5.146** Look up syndrome in your medical dictionary. Read about the syndromes, many of which are named after the scientists who identified them. Korsakoff's syndrome was named after Sergei S. Korsakoff, a Russian neurologist, who described a series of signs and symptoms brought on by alcoholism that pointed to evidence of organic brain damage. Reye's syndrome was named in honor of Ralph Douglas Kenneth Reye, an Australian pathologist, who discovered postinfection encephalopathy in children linked to acute fever, influenza, or chickenpox, which could lead to death from cerebral edema.

Korsakoff's syndrome

syndrome

5.147

A syndrome due to alcoholism is *_____.
Expectant mothers are warned not to drink alcohol during pregnancy to prevent deformities in the newborn, known as fetal alcohol _____ (FAS).

---

syndrome

5.148

Behavior changes and hyperemesis following a viral infection and fever are symptoms occurring together that may indicate Reye's _____.

---

pro/drome
prō′ drōm

5.149

Pro/drome means running before (a disease). A symptom indicating an approaching disease is a _____/_____.

---

prodromes

5.150

The sneezes that come before a common cold are the
_____ (plural) of the cold.

---

pro/drom/al
prō drō′ məl

5.151

Chickenpox has a macular rash that precedes the papules. This is known as a
_____/_____/__ (adjective) rash.

---

dips

5.152

Dipsia is Greek for thirst. Poly/dips/ia means excessive thirst (desire for much fluid). The root word for thirst is _____.

ANSWER COLUMN

5.153

poly- is a prefix meaning too much or too many. Poly/dipsia can be caused by something as simple as eating too much salt. A highly salted meal may cause

poly/dips/ia
pol ē **dip**′ sē ə

_____/_____/__.

5.154

Polydipsia can be caused by something as complex as an upset in pituitary secretion. If the pituitary gland secretes too much of one hormone, salt is retained

polydipsia

in the body, and _____ results.

5.155

High blood sugar levels and lack of insulin in patients with diabetes also cause

polydipsia

_____ (excessive thirst).

5.156

Dips/o/mania is an old term for alcoholism. A person who drinks alcohol excessively and becomes physically and psychologically addicted suffers from

dips/o/man/ia
dip sō **mā**′ nē ə

_____/___/_____/__ or alcoholism.

5.157

Korsakoff's syndrome characterized by nerve inflammation, insomnia, hallucinations, disorientation, and nerve pain is a sequel to

alcohol/ism
al′ kō hol izm

chronic _____/_____.

5.158

TAKE A
CLOSER
LOOK

Alcoholism, a chronic physical and psychological disease, has grave consequences for the individuals who are afflicted as well as for the family members surrounding them. Read more about this disease in your dictionary or encyclopedia. Treatment of alcoholism includes carefully planned withdrawal from alcohol, nutrition, rest, and psychotherapy. Alcoholics Anonymous (AA) offers many support group programs for the alcoholic, spouses (Al- Anon), and children (Ala-Teen). There are even groups (ACOA*) for adults whose parents were alcoholic and who still suffer the effects of being raised in an alcoholic or dysfuntional home.
*Adult Children of Alcoholics

Abbreviation	Meaning
AA	Alcoholics Anonymous
ACOA	Adult Children of Alcoholics
AD	right ear, *auris dextra* (Latin)
AFB	acid-fast bacillus (i.e., TB)
Al-Anon	AA support group for spouses of alcoholics
Ala-Teen	AA support group for children of alcoholics
AS	left ear, *auris sinistra* (Latin)
AU	both ears, auris uterque
C°	Celsius degrees (metric temperature)
C&S	culture and sensitivity (antibiotic susceptibility)
CO_2	carbon dioxide
DM	diabetes mellitus
F°	Fahrenheit degrees
FAS	fetal alcohol syndrome
GB	gallbladder
GNID	gram-negative intracellular diplococcus
HBV	hepatitis B virus
HIV	human immunodeficiency virus
HPV	human papillomavirus
HSV	Herpes simplex virus
LMP	last menstrual period
mcg	microgram(s)*
mg	milligram(s)*
MTD	right eardrum (*membrana tympani dextra*)
MTS	left eardrum (*membrana tympani sinistra*)
NVS	neurologic vital signs
OM	otitis media
O&P	ova and parasites
P	pulse
PAR	perennial allergic rhinitis
R	respiration (rate)
SIDS	sudden infant death syndrome
SOB	short (shortness) of breath
staph	staphylococcus
strep	streptococcus
T, temp	temperature
TB	tuberculosis
VS	vital signs (T, P, R, BP)
°	degree symbol

*We do not pluralize abbreviations. Each stands for singular and plural.

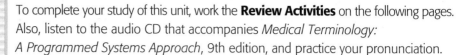

ANSWER COLUMN

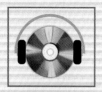

To complete your study of this unit, work the **Review Activities** on the following pages. Also, listen to the audio CD that accompanies *Medical Terminology: A Programmed Systems Approach*, 9th edition, and practice your pronunciation.

Additional practice exercises for this unit are available on the Learner Practice CD-ROM found in the back of the textbook.

REVIEW ACTIVITIES

CIRCLE AND CORRECT

Circle the correct answer for each question. Then check your answers in Appendix A.

1. Sound made by c followed by an o, as in costal
   a. s
   b. k
   c. j
   d. x

2. Sound made by c followed by an i, as in cervicitis
   a. s
   b. k
   c. j
   d. x

3. Plural for round-shaped bacteria
   a. bacilli
   b. bacillus
   c. coccus
   d. cocci

4. Prefix for double
   a. tri-
   b. diplo-
   c. daplo-
   d. ex-

5. Combining form for twisted chains
   a. strep
   b. strepto
   c. stretp
   d. strept

6. Combining form for uvula
   a. staphylo
   b. strepto
   c. vulvo
   d. uvul

7. Suffix for flow or discharge
   a. -itis
   b. -rrhagia
   c. -pnea
   d. -rrhea

8. Combining form for ear
   a. audio
   b. tympano
   c. oto
   d. oculo

9. Suffix for surgical repair
   a. -acopy
   b. -tomy
   c. -ectomy
   d. -plasty

10. Combining form for bile (gall)
    a. chole
    b. calcul
    c. lith
    d. bil

11. Singular for rod-shaped bacteria
    a. bacilla
    b. bacillus
    c. coccus
    d. bacterium

12. Combining form for pus
    a. genic
    b. gen/o
    c. staphyl/o
    d. py/o

13. Word root for nose
    a. ot
    b. rhin
    c. nas/o
    d. lith

14. Suffix meaning infestation (condition)
    a. -iasis
    b. -pathy
    c. -lith
    d. -oid

15. Suffix for breathing
    a. -pne
    b. -pneo
    c. -pnea
    d. -pepsia

16. Combining form for heat
    a. tempero
    b. thermal
    c. thermo
    d. Fahrenheit

REVIEW ACTIVITIES

17. Prefix for small
    a. incro-   b. macro-
    c. micro-   d. hypo-

18. Prefix for large
    a. macro-   b. megaly-
    c. micro-   d. poly-

19. Prefix for join together
    a. inter-   b. intra-
    c. osis-   d. syn-

20. Suffix for thirst
    a. -hydro   b. -dipsia
    c. -mania   d. -poly

21. Word root for finger or toe (digits)
    a. acro   b. dactyl
    c. digit   d. phalang

22. Prefix for many or much
    a. poly-   b. olig-
    c. hyper-   d. sub-

SELECT AND CONSTRUCT

Select the correct word parts (some may be used more than once) from the following list and construct medical terms that represent the given meaning.

a	algia	audio	blast	brady	cardio(a)	cephalus
chole	cysto	cyte	dactylo(ia)	dia	dipso(ia)	drome(al)
dynia	dys	ectomy	ergetic(ergy)	geno(ic) esis	graphy(gram)	hemat
hyper	hypo	ia	iasis	ic	ism	ites
itis	lith(o)	macro	metry	micro	neur	osis
ot(o)(ia)	pepsia	phago(ia)	pnea	poly	pro	pyo
rhino	rrhea	spasm	staphyl	syn	tachy	therapy
therm(o)(al)(y)	tomy	tympan(o)	uvul(o)			

1. slow heart rate   _____

2. fast eating (swallowing) _____

3. inflammation of the uvula _____

4. stones in the gallbladder _____

5. earache   _____

6. process of measuring hearing _____

7. difficulty with digestion _____

8. pus-forming (adjective) _____

9. discharge from the nose _____

10. record of eardrum function _____

11. distended with gas (abdomen) _____

12. x-ray picture of gallbladder _____

13. absence of breathing   _____

14. heat therapy (heating through) _____

15. excessive thirst   _____

REVIEW ACTIVITIES

16. working together   _____

17. abnormally small head   _____

18. very large cell   _____

19. before the onset of illness   _____

20. low body temperature   _____

MIX AND MATCH

Match the organism on the left with its description or disease name on the right.

_____ 1. streptococcus   a. double dot–shaped bacteria

_____ 2. staphylococci   b. HIV is a _____.

_____ 3. diplococcus   c. parasite protozoan with flagella

_____ 4. trichomonas   d. skin bacteria growing in bunches

_____ 5. virus   e. moniliasis

_____ 6. yeast   f. β hemolytic _____ causes throat infection.

_____ 7. filarial worm   g. elephantiasis

_____ 8. giardia   h. giardiasis

DEFINE AND DISSECT

Give a brief definition and dissect each term listed into its word parts in the space provided. Check your answers by referring to the frame listed in parentheses and to your medical dictionary. Then listen to the CD to practice pronunciation.

1. diplococcus (5.10)

_____ / ___ / _____ / _____
        rt   v   rt   suffix

_____
              definition

2. staphylococcus (5.25)

_____ / ___ / _____ / _____
        rt   v   rt   suffix

_____

3. uvulectomy (5.26)

_____ / _____
        rt   suffix

_____

4. pyocele (5.28)

_____ / ___ / _____
        rt   v   suffix

_____

5. otorrhea (5.42)

_____ / ___ / _____
        rt   v   suffix

_____

REVIEW ACTIVITIES

6. tympanotomy (5.50)

_____/____/_____
rt   v   suffix

7. audiogram (5.55)

_____/____/_____
rt   v   suffix

8. rhinolith (5.83)

_____/____/_____
rt   v   rt

9. cholecystitis (5.78)

_____/____/_____/_____
rt   v   rt   suffix

10. trichomoniasis (5.75)

_____/____/____/_____
rt   v   rt   suffix

11. bradyphagia (5.85)

_____/_____/_____
pre   rt   suffix

12. tachypnea (5.96)

_____/_____
pre   suffix

13. dyspepsia (5.115)

_____/_____/_____
pre   rt   suffix

14. cholecystography (5.77)

_____/____/_____/____/_____
rt   v   rt   v   suffix

15. staphyloplasty (5.24)

_____/____/_____
rt   v   suffix

16. gonorrhea (5.10)

_____/____/_____
rt   v   suffix

REVIEW ACTIVITIES

17. diplobacillus (5.17)

_____/____/_____/_____
  rt   v   rt   suffix

18. tympanometry (5.51)

_____/____/_____
  rt   v   suffix

19. audiologist (5.56)

_____/____/_____
  rt   v   suffix

20. aphasia (5.58)

_____/____
  pre   suffix

21. lithotomy (5.70)

_____/____/_____
  rt   v   suffix

22. cholelithiasis (5.74)

_____/____/_____/_____
  rt   v   rt   suffix

23. carcinogenesis (5.108)

_____/____/_____
  rt   v   rt/suffix

24. dyspnea (5.113)

_____/_____
  pre   suffix

25. tympanites (5.52)

_____/_____
  rt   suffix

26. thermometer (5.118)

_____/____/_____
  rt   v   suffix

27. microsurgery (5.127)

_____/_____
  pre   rt/suffix

REVIEW ACTIVITIES

28. macrocephalus (5.130)

_____/_____
     pre   rt/suffix

29. polydactylism (5.134)

_____/_____/_____
    pre   rt   suffix

30. synergistic (5.138)

_____/____/_____
       pre   rt   suffix

31. synarthrosis (5.143)

_____/_____/_____
    pre   rt   suffix

32. syndrome (5.145)

_____/_____
     pre   rt/suffix

33. prodromal (5.151)

_____/_____/_____
    pre   rt   suffix

34. polydipsia (5.153)

_____/_____/_____
    pre   rt   suffix

35. dipsomania (5.156)

_____/____/_____/_____
   rt   v   rt   suffix

36. alcoholism (5.157)

_____/_____
     rt   suffix

37. microgram (5.126)

_____/_____
     pre   suffix

38. hyperthermia (5.123)

_____/_____/____
    pre   rt   suffix

39. syndactylism (5.137)

_____/_____/_____
   pre   rt   suffix

REVIEW ACTIVITIES

40. dactylospasm (5.134)

_____/___/_____
     rt   v   suffix

41. diathermy (5.120)

___/_____/___
  pre   rt   suffix

42. microcyst (5.126)

_____/_____
   pre   rt

43. thermoalgesia (5.119)

_____/___/_____/___
  rt   v   rt   suffix

ABBREVIATIONS MATCHING

Match the following abbreviations with their definition.

_____ 1. AA

_____ 2. T

_____ 3. °F

_____ 4. mcg

_____ 5. SIDS

_____ 6. VS

_____ 7. FAS

_____ 8. GB

_____ 9. MTD

_____10. HPV

_____11. AS

_____12. OM

a. microgram(s)

b. milligram(s)

c. degrees Celsius

d. fetal alcohol syndrome

e. oculomotor

f. degrees Fahrenheit

g. acid-fast bacillus

h. gonorrhea

i. left ear

j. Al-Anon

k. microscopic

l. temperature

m. otitis media

n. right eardrum

o. human papilloma virus

p. vital signs

q. sudden infant death syndrome

r. Alcoholics Anonymous

s. gallbladder

REVIEW ACTIVITIES

CASE STUDY

Write the term next to its meaning given below. Then draw slashes to analyze the word parts. Note the use of medical abbreviations. Look these up in your dictionary or find them in Appendix B. If you have any questions about the answers, refer to your medical dictionary or check with your instructor for the answers in Appendix A.

CASE STUDY 5-1

Operative Report—Cholecystectomy

Pt: Female, age 39, Ht 5'3", Wt 192 lb., BP 130/84, **T 99.6°F**, P 80, R 18

Summary: Ms. Colette Stone is a 39-year-old female who was seen in the office with complaints of repeated pain in the **epigastric** region and **RUQ** of the abdomen. The pain radiates to her shoulder and back. Ms. Stone states that the pain becomes aggravated with consumption of any kind of food, particularly greasy, fatty, or fried food. A complete workup was done, including **ultrasound** of the **gallbladder**. This revealed the presence of a **cholelith**.

Surgical Report Findings: The gallbladder was **edematous** and somewhat thick-walled. There was a stone impacted in the outlet of the gallbladder, measuring about 1 **cm** in diameter. Operative **cholangiograms** showed a small **ductal** system, but there were no filling defects, and there was good emptying of the contrast medium into the duodenum.

1. pertaining to a duct _____

2. swollen _____

3. cholecyst _____

4. gallstone _____

5. x-ray of bile ducts _____

6. centimeter _____

7. upon the stomach _____

8. right upper quadrant _____

9. excision of the gallbladder _____

10. use of high-frequency sound waves _____

11. temperature, 99.6 degrees Fahrenheit _____

REVIEW ACTIVITIES

CROSSWORD PUZZLE

Check your answers by going back through the frames or checking the solution in Appendix C.

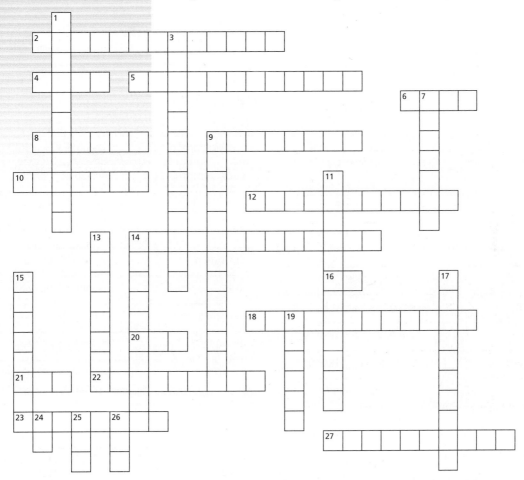

Across

2. inflamed gallbladder
4. suffix for breathing
5. promoting cancer growth
6. prefix for many
8. suffix for paralysis
9. Korsakoff's ____
10. having trouble breathing
12. slow heart rate
14. enlarged fingers
16. tuberculosis (abbreviation)
18. fever
20. culture and sensitivity (abbreviation)
21. human immuno-deficiency virus (abbreviation)
22. large cell
23. failure to develop
27. organism that produces disease

Down

1. surgical repair of the nose
3. round bacteria in twisted chains
7. ear pain
9. excision of the uvula
11. fused joint with no movement
13. eardrum
14. gram-negative intracellular _____
15. purulent discharge
17. runny nose
19. suffix for eating (swallowing)
24. gallbaldder (abbreviation)
25. neurologic vital signs (abbreviation)
26. prefix for joined

REVIEW ACTIVITIES

GLOSSARY

agenesis	lack of development	cholecystotomy	incision into the gallbladder
alcoholism	chronic physical and psychological addiction to alcohol	cholelith	gallstone
		cholelithiasis	infestation with gallstones
amenorrhea	absence of menstruation	coccus	sphere-shaped bacterium
apepsia	cessation of digestion	dactylitis	inflammation of the fingers and/or toes
aphasia	unable to speak	dactylogram	fingerprint
aphonia	no voice, unable to make sounds	dactylospasm	spasm of a digit
apnea	absence of breathing	diplobacillus	double bacillus
audiogram	graphic record of hearing function	diplococci	cocci growing in pairs
		dipsomania	abnormal compulsion to drink
audiologist	hearing specialist	dysmenorrhea	painful menstruation
audiology	science that studies hearing	dyspepsia	poor digestion
audiometer	instrument to test hearing	dysphagia	difficulty swallowing
audiometry	process of testing hearing	dysphasia	difficulty speaking, garbled speech
bacillus	rod-shaped bacterium		
bradycardia	slow heart rate	dysphonia	difficulty making sounds with the voice
bradypepsia	slow digestion	dyspnea	difficulty breathing
bradyphagia	slow eating (swallowing)	hydrocephalus	enlarged head due to fluid accumulation (congenital)
bradypnea	slow breathing		
calculi	small stones	hyperthermia	abnormally high body temperature (synonym fever)
carcinogenesis	formation of cancer		
cholangiogram	x-ray of the bile ducts	hypothermia	abnormally low body temperature
cholecyst	gallbladder	lithometer	instrument to measure stones
cholecystitis	inflammation of the gallbladder	lithotomy	incision for the removal of stones
cholecystogram	x-ray of the gallbladder	macroblast	abnormally large immature cell
cholecystography	process of obtaining x-ray of the gallbladder	macrocephalus	large head size

REVIEW ACTIVITIES

macrocheilia	enlarged lips
macrococcus	large coccus
macrocyte	large cell
macrodactylia	abnormally large digits
macroglossia	enlarged tongue
macrorhinia	enlarged nose
microcardia	abnormally small-sized heart
microcephalus	abnormally small head
microcyst	a small cyst
microcyte	a small cell
microgram	one millionth of a gram
microsurgery	surgery performed using a microscope or other magnifying device
moniliasis	yeast infection
oncogenic	tumor forming
otic	pertaining to the ear
otodynia	earache (synonym otalgia)
otorrhea	discharge from the ear
otoscope	instrument used to look into the ear
paraphasia	abnormal speech
pathogenic	disease producing
peptic	pertaining to digestion
phasology	science that studies speech
phonic	pertaining to the voice
phonology	science that studies the voice sounds

polydactylism	condition of having more than five digits on hands or feet
polydipsia	condition of excessive thirst
prodrome	symptoms before the onset of a disease
pyogenic	pus forming
pyorrhea	flow or discharge of pus
pyothorax	pus in the chest cavity
rhinitis	inflammation of the nose
rhinolith	calculus in the nasal passages
rhinoplasty	surgical repair of the nose
rhinorrhea	runny nose
staphylectomy	excision of the uvula (synonym uvulectomy)
staphylitis	inflammation of the uvula (synonym uvulitis)
staphylococci	bacteria growing in bunches (like grapes)
staphyloplasty	surgical repair of the uvula
streptobacillus	bacillus growing in twisted chains
streptococci	round bacteria growing in twisted chains
synarthrosis	joints that are fused and immovable
syndactylism	fingers or toes that are fused (congenital)
syndrome	symptoms that occur together to characterize a disease
synergistic	works together
tachycardia	fast heart rate

REVIEW ACTIVITIES

tachyphagia	fast eating	thermoplegia	paralysis caused by a person being exposed to too high of a temperature (synonym heat stroke)
tachypnea	fast breathing	trichomoniasis	infestation with *Trichomonas*
thermal	pertaining to heat (synonym thermic)	tympanectomy	excision of the eardrum
thermoesthesia	oversensitivity to heat (synonym thermoalgesia)	tympanic	pertaining to the eardrum
thermogenesis	generation of heat	tympanites	distended with gas (abdomen)
thermophobia	abnormal fear of heat	tympanometry	process of measuring eardrum function
		tympanotomy	incision into the eardrum (synonym myringotomy)

UNIT 6

Urology and Gynecology

Information for Frames 6.1–6.34

Word	Combining Form	New Suffix to Use When Needed
urine	**ur/o**	**-lith** (stone)
kidney	**nephr/o**	**-lysis** (destruction)
	ren/o	**-pexy** (surgical fixation)
renal pelvis	**pyel/o**	**-ptosis** (prolapse)
ureter	**ureter/o**	**-rrhagia** (hemorrhage or "bursting forth" of blood)
bladder	**cyst/o**	**-rrhaphy** (suturing or stitching)
urethra	**urethr/o**	**-uria** (urine, urination)

6.1

Urology is the study of the urinary tract. The urinary tract is responsible for forming urine from waste materials in the blood and eliminating urine from the body. What would you guess to be the combining form for urine? _____.
(See the illustration of a kidney on page 185.)

ur/o

6.2

A ur/o/logist is a physician specialist with expertise in treating disorders of the male and female urinary system and male reproductive system. Men with concerns about infertility or impotence may consult a ____/____/_____.

ur/o/logist
yōō **rol**′ ō jist

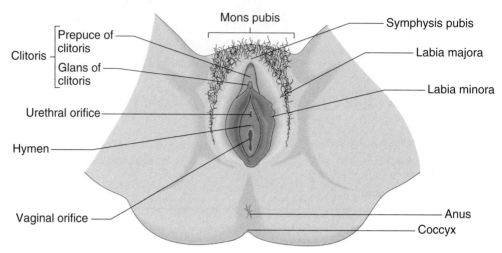

Prepuce of clitoris
Glans of clitoris
Clitoris
Mons pubis
Symphysis pubis
Labia majora
Labia minora
Urethral orifice
Hymen
Vaginal orifice
Anus
Coccyx

External genitalia of the female

ANSWER COLUMN

6.3

Build words meaning
pertaining to urinary tract and genitals
____/____/_____ (genitourinary);

any disease of the urinary tract
____/____/_____.

ur/o/genital
yōō rō **jen**′ i tal

ur/o/pathy
yōō **rop**′ ə thē

CONDITIONS INVOLVING URINATION

Condition	Description
poly/uria	too much (frequent) urination
noct/uria	excessive urination at night
an/uria	suppressed (lack of) urination
olig/uria	abnormally low amounts of urine
hemat/uria	blood in the urine
albumin/uria	protein (albumin) in the urine
glycos/uria	sugar in the urine
keton/uria	ketones in the urine
nocturn/al en/ur/esis	bed wetting
bacter/i/uria	bacteria in the urine

ANSWER COLUMN

6.4

poly/uria
pol ē **yoor**′ ē ə

poly- is a prefix that means many or much. **-uria** is a suffix meaning condition of the urine. Poly/uria means excessive amount of urine. When a person drinks too much water, _____/_____ results.

6.5

noct/uria
nok **tyoor**′ ē ə
poly/uria
pol ē **yoor**′ ē ə
hemat/uria
hem at **yoor**′ ē ə
olig/uria
ō lig **yoor**′ ē ə

Cover the table listing conditions of urination. Build words meaning urinating at night
_____/_____;
frequent urination
_____/_____;
blood in the urine
_____/_____;
low (scant) amount of urine
_____/_____.

6.6

poly/neur/itis
pol ē noo **rī**′ tis

Poly/neur/o/pathy means disease of many nerves. The word for inflammation of many nerves is _____/_____/_____.

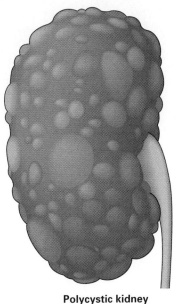

Polycystic kidney

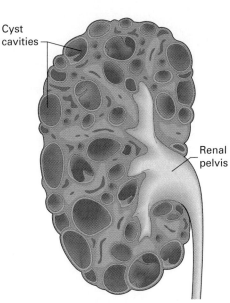

Cyst cavities

Renal pelvis

Section through kidney

6.7

Build words meaning
inflammation of many joints

_____/_____/_____;

pain in many nerves

_____/_____/_____;

state of having too many or more than two ears

_____/_____/_____.

poly/arthr/itis
pol ē är **thrī′** tis
poly/neur/algia
pol ē noo **ral′** jē ə
poly/ot/ia
pol ē **ō′** shē ə

6.8

Define the following terms

poly/cyst/ic *_____;

poly/phagia *_____;

poly/phobia *_____.

having many cysts
eating too much
excessive fear of things
(many phobias)

6.9

ren is one word root for kidney. The combining form for kidney is
_____/_____. Look up all the words that begin with **ren/o** in
your dictionary.

ren/o

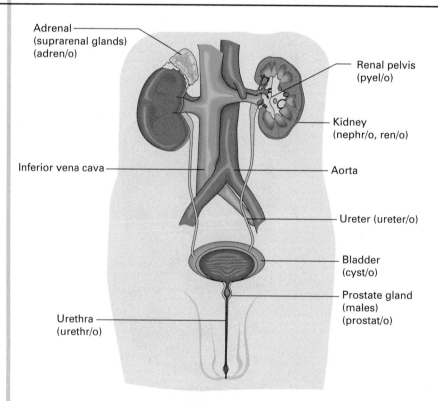

Urinary system

6.10

Build words meaning
pertaining to the kidney
_____/____;
any kidney disease
_____/____/_____;
record from an x-ray of the kidney
_____/____/_____.

NOTE: Ordering a KUB is ordering an x-ray of the kidneys, ureters, and bladder.

ren/al
rē′ nəl
ren/o/pathy
re **nop**′ ə thē
ren/o/gram
rē′ ō gram

6.11

Renointestinal means
* _____.
Renogastric means
* _____.

pertaining to the
  kidney and intestine
pertaining to the
  kidney and stomach

6.12

nephr/o is also used in words to refer to the kidney. A word that means inflammation of the kidney is _____/_____.

nephr/itis
nef **rī**′ tis

6.13

TAKE A CLOSER LOOK

nephr/o comes from Greek, **ren/o** from Latin. Nephrons, the functional units of the kidney, are tiny structures in the renal cortex. They filter blood to remove waste and excess water and form urine. Look up **nephr/o** and **ren/o** in your dictionary. Make a list of terms beginning with each and then compare them.

6.14

-ptosis is a suffix meaning prolapsed. Nephr/o/ptosis can occur from a hard blow or jolt to the kidney. People who ride motorcycles often wear special clothing or
a kidney belt to protect against _____/____/_____.

nephr/o/ptosis
nef′ rop **tō**′ sis

6.15

When nephroptosis occurs, one treament option could be to put the kidney back in place using surgery. Nephr/o/pexy is fixation of a prolapsed kidney. The suffix for fixation is _____.

-pexy

ANSWER COLUMN

nephr/o/pexy **nef′** rō peks ē	**6.16** Nephr/o/plasty is also a repair of the kidney. The specific type of repair to treat nephroptosis is _____/___/_____.

6.17

Recall the suffixes for stone, softening, enlargement, and destruction. Build words meaning
stone in the kidney

nephr/o/lith
nef′ rō lith

_____/___/_____;
softening of kidney tissue

nephr/o/malac/ia
nef rō mə **lā′** shə

_____/___/_____/____;

enlargement of the kidney

nephr/o/megal/y
nef rō **meg′** ə lē

_____/___/_____/____;
destruction of kidney tissue

nephr/o/lysis
nef **rol′** ə sis

_____/___/_____.

6.18

For review build terms that mean
gallstone

chol/e/lith

_____/___/_____;
condition (infestation) of gallstones

chol/e/lith/iasis

_____/__/_____/_____;
nasal stones

rhin/o/lith

_____/___/_____.
Good.

Urinalysis using a reagent strip (dipstick urine)

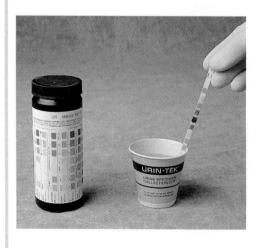

INFORMATION TABLE

Routine urinalysis includes the following tests using a color change reagent strip dipped into the urine sample to determine the following results.

Test	Normal Range
pH	5–8
protein	negative
glucose	negative
ketones	negative
bilirubin	negative
blood	negative
specific gravity	1.001–1.035

6.19

Locate the renal pelvis in the illustration of the kidney. The renal pelvis is formed at the juncture of the calyces. **pyel/o** refers to the

renal pelvis * _____.

6.20

Using what you need from the combining form for renal pelvis, form words meaning

inflammation of the renal pelvis

pyel/itis
pī ə **lī**′ tis
pyel/o/plasty
pī′ e lō plas′ tē

____/_____;

surgical repair of the renal pelvis

____/___/_____.

6.21

condition of renal pelvis and kidney

pyel/o/nephr/itis
pī′ e lō nef **rī**′ tis
pyel/o/gram
pī′ ə lō gram

Pyel/o/nephr/osis means * _____.
Form words that mean
inflammation of the renal pelvis and kidney

____/___/_____/____;

x-ray of the renal pelvis

____/___/____.

NOTE: An IVP is an intravenous pyelogram as shown in the following x-ray illustration.

**X-ray: intravenous
pyelogram (IVP)**

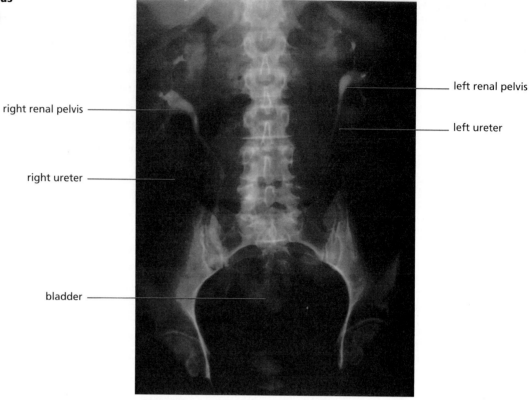

left renal pelvis

right renal pelvis

left ureter

right ureter

bladder

ANSWER COLUMN

6.22

stone or calculus
  in the ureter

ureter/o/cele
yōō **rē**′ tər ō sēl

ureter/o/pathy
yōō rē′ tər **op**′ ə thē

Ureter/o/lith means *_____. Form words that mean
herniation of the ureter

_____/____/_____;

any disease of the ureter

_____/____/_____.

6.23

plastic surgery of the
  ureter and renal pelvis

ureter/o/pyel/itis
yōō rē′ tər ō pī ə **lī**′ tis

Ureter/o/pyel/o/plasty means *_____.

_____.

Form a word meaning inflammation of the ureter and renal pelvis

_____/___/_____/_____.

6.24

ureter/o/cyst/o/stomy
yōō rē′ tə rō sis **tos**′ tə mē

Form words meaning
making a new opening between the ureter and bladder

_____/___/_____/___/_____;

ANSWER COLUMN

ureter/o/py/osis
yōo rē′ tər ō pī **ō**′ sis

a condition of the ureter involving pus

_____ / ___ / ___ / _____.

6.25

Ureter/o/rrhaphy introduces a new word part: **-rrhaphy**. **-rrhaphy** means suturing or stitching. Ureterorrhaphy means

suturing or stitching
of the ureters

*_____.

6.26

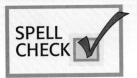

So far you have been introduced to three suffixes with the unique Greek spelling "rrh": **-rrhea**, **-rrhagia**, and **-rrhaphy**. Although the h is silent, don't forget to include it.
-rrhea (runny, flow, or discharge)
-rrhagia (hemorrhage, abnormal bleeding)
-rrhaphy (suturing or wound closure)

6.27

Form the word that means suturing of the ureter:

_____ / ___ / _____.

ureter/o/rrhaphy
yōo rē′ tər **ôr**′ ə fē

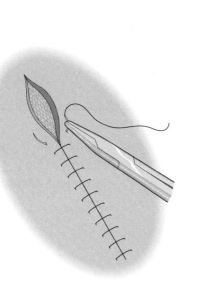
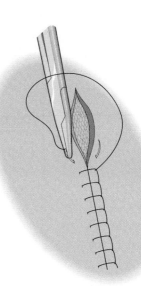

Interrupted (individual) sutures   **Continuous sutures**

6.28

Form words meaning
suturing of a kidney

nephr/o/rrhaphy
nef **rôr**′ ə fē

_____/___/_____;

cyst/o/rrhaphy
sis **tôr**′ ə fē

suturing of the bladder

_____/___/_____.

6.29

Use **neur/o** and **colp/o** to form words meaning
suturing of a nerve

neur/o/rrhaphy
noo **rôr**′ ə fē

_____/___/_____;

colp/o/rrhaphy
kol **pôr**′ ə fē

suturing of the vagina

_____/___/_____.

6.30

SPELL CHECK ✓

Normal anatomy includes two ureters and one urethra. Study these three combining forms. Watch out! Their spellings are very close.

Combining form	Word	Description
urethr/o	urethra	tube from urinary bladder to outside
ureter/o	ureters	tubes from each kidney to the bladder
uter/o	uterus	womb, female reproductive system

6.31

suturing of the urethra

Urethr/o/rrhaphy means *_____.
Form words meaning
incision into the urethra

urethr/o/tomy
yōō rē **throt**′ ə mē

_____/___/_____;

urethr/o/spasm
yōō **rē**′ thrō spaz ə m

spasm of the urethra

_____/___/_____.

6.32

urethra

Urethr/o/rect/al means pertaining to the urethra and rectum.
Urethr/o/vagin/al means pertaining to the _____ and vagina.
Form a word that means inflammation of urethra and bladder:

yōō **rē**′ thrə

urethr/o/cyst/itis
yōō **rē**′ thrō sis tī′ tis

_____/___/_____/_____.

ANSWER COLUMN

INFORMATION
FRAME

6.33

-rrhagia is another complex word part that can be used as a suffix because it follows a word root and ends a word. **-rrhagia** means hemorrhage, or bursting forth of blood.

6.34

hem/o/rrhage
hem′ ôr əg
urethr/o/rrhagia
yōō rē′ thrō **rā′** jē ə
men/o/rrhagia
men′ ō **rā′** jē ə
cyst/o/rrhagia
sis tə **rā′** jē ə
ureter/o/rrhagia
yōō rē′ tər ō **rā′** jē ə

Gastr/o/rrhagia means stomach hemorrhage. Encephal/o/rrhagia means brain
_____/____/_____.
A word that means hemorrhage of the urethra is
_____/____/_____.
Excessive bleeding during menstruation is
_____/____/_____.
hemorrhage of the bladder
_____/____/_____;
hemorrhage of the ureter
_____/____/_____.

6.35

formation of spermatozoa
  or formation of sperm or
  formation of male germ
  cells

Now turn your studies to a new body system. Look at the diagram of the male reproductive system on page 195. Sperma is the Greek word meaning seed. **spermat/o** and **sperm/o(i)** are two combining forms for *spermatozoa* or male germ cells (sperm).
Spermat/o/genesis means *_____
_____.

6.36

sperm/o/lysis or
spûr′ **mol′** ə sis
spermat/o/lysis
spûr mə **tol′** ə sis
spermat/o/blast
or
spûr **mat′** ō blast
sperm/o/blast
spûr′ mō blast

Build words meaning
the destruction of spermatozoa
_____/____/_____;
an immature sperm cell
_____/____/_____.

ANSWER COLUMN

Internal structures of the testes. Spermatogenesis occurs in the seminiferous tubules of the testes; sperm mature in the epididymis and travel to the vas deferens

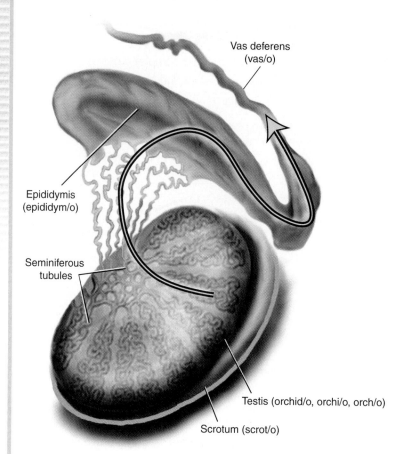

Vas deferens
(vas/o)

Epididymis
(epididym/o)

Seminiferous
tubules

Testis (orchid/o, orchi/o, orch/o)

Scrotum (scrot/o)

6.37

A bladder or sac containing sperm is a
_____/___/_____.

spermat/o/cyst
spûr **mat′** ō sist

A word for resembling sperm is
_____/_____.

spermat/oid
spûr′ mə toid

A word for disease of the sperm is
_____/___/_____.

spermat/o/pathy
spûr′ mə **top′** ə thē

A herniated saclike structure containing sperm is
a _____/_____/_____.

spermat /o/ cele
spûr **mat′** ō sēl

6.38

-cide is a Latin suffix meaning to kill or destroy. Think of suicide or genocide.
An agent used to kill sperm is a _____/___/_____.

sperm/i/cide
spûr′ mə sīd

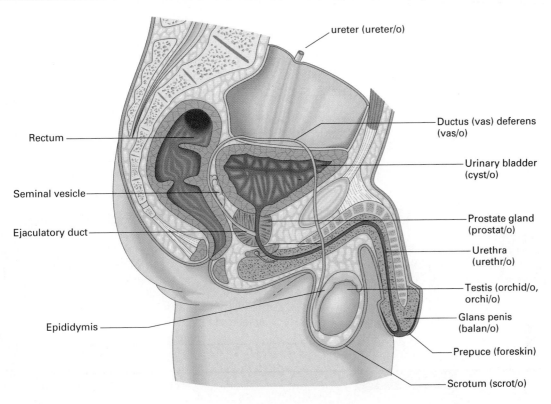

ureter (ureter/o)

Rectum

Ductus (vas) deferens (vas/o)

Urinary bladder (cyst/o)

Seminal vesicle

Ejaculatory duct

Prostate gland (prostat/o)

Urethra (urethr/o)

Testis (orchid/o, orchi/o)

Glans penis (balan/o)

Epididymis

Prepuce (foreskin)

Scrotum (scrot/o)

Male reproductive system

ANSWER COLUMN

6.39

A condom (flexible sheath) placed over the erect penis provides a barrier to sperm. For contraceptive purposes condoms are used with creams and/or

spermicide

foams that contain a _____.

6.40

orchid/o, **orchi/o**, and **orch/o** are all Greek combining forms for testicle. Orchid/ectomy, orchi/ectomy, and orch/ectomy all mean

excision of the testicle

* _____.

NOTE: Look up **orchid/o**, **orchi/o**, and **orch/o** to discover how each is used.

6.41

For this study use only **orchid/o** to build two terms that mean pain in the testes:

orchid/algia
ôr′ kid **al′** gē ə
orchid/o/dynia
ôr′ kid ō **din′** ē ə

_____/_____ and _____/____/_____.

ANSWER COLUMN

6.42

The Latin adjectival form for testicle is testicular. A person with orchidalgia is experiencing _____/_____ pain.

testicul/ar
tes **ti′** kōō lar

6.43

Note that the following terms all refer to the testicles.

TAKE A CLOSER LOOK

test/is	singular noun
test/es	plural noun
test/icle	singular noun
test/icles	plural noun
test/icular	adjectival form

6.44

Cancer of the testes, a very serious condition, occurs more frequently in males between the ages of 18 and 35. Testicular self-exam (TSE) is recommended for early detection of _____ cancer.

testicular

6.45

Around the time of birth, the testicles normally descend from the abdominal cavity into the scrotum. Sometimes this fails to happen (crypt/orchid/ism). Surgical repair may be indicated. The operation is called an _____/____/_____. This operation is also called orchiopexy.

orchid/o/plasty
or′ kid ō plas tē

6.46

Build words meaning
herniation of a testicle
_____/____/_____;
incision into a testicle
_____/____/_____.

orchid/o/cele
ôr′ kid ō sēl
orchid/o/tomy
ôr′ kid **ot′** ə mē

6.47

Crypt/orchid/ism means undescended testicle. crypt means hidden. When a testicle is hidden in the abdominal cavity, the condition is known as _____/_____/_____.

crypt/orchid/ism
krip **tôr′** kid iz əm

ANSWER COLUMN

	6.48
hidden hidden (undescended)	A crypt/ic remark is one with a hidden meaning. A crypt/ic belief is one whose meaning is _____. Cryptorchidism refers to a _____ testicle.
	6.49
prostat/itis pros tā **tī′** tis	**prostat/o** is used for words relating to the prostate gland. Prostat/ic is the adjectival form, as in the condition benign prostatic hyperplasia (BPH, enlargement of the prostate due to increase in number of cells and aging). Build a term meaning inflammation of the prostate gland: _____/_____. See the case study on transurethral resection (TUR) at the end of this unit.
	6.50
semin/al **sem′** i nal semin/al	The normal functioning prostate secretes a fluid that is added to sperm to create semen (**semin/o**). The combination of fluids and sperm is called _____/_____ (adjective) fluid. The _____/_____ vesical secretes fluid to lubricate and nurture sperm.
	6.51
semin/oma se mi **no′** mə	A semin/oma is a malignant neoplasm found most often in young men. It is a growth generated by the spermatoblast cells in a testis. A seminal tissue tumor is called a _____/_____.
	6.52
semen **sē′** men	The seminal vesicles also secrete a fluid that combined with the prostatic fluid and sperm is called _____.
	6.53
prostat/o/rrhea pros′ tā to **rē′** ə	An abnormal flow or discharge from the prostate gland is called _____/____/_____.
	6.54
prostat/algia pros′ tā **tal′** jē ə prostat/ectomy pros′ tāt **ek′** tō mē	Prostatic pain is called _____/_____. Excision of the prostate is _____/_____.

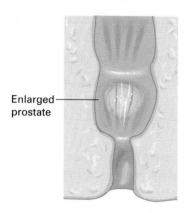

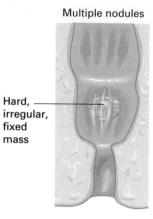

Enlarged prostate

Single nodule — Hard, irregular mass

Multiple nodules — Hard, irregular, fixed mass

Benign prostatic hyperplasia (BPH) rectal view

Cancer of the prostate

ANSWER COLUMN

6.55

balan/o is the combining form for glans penis. Balan/itis is inflammation of the glans penis. Surgical repair of the glans penis is called
_____/___/_____.

balan/o/plasty
bal′ an ō plas tē

6.56

An infection may cause a flow or discharge from the glans penis. This is called
_____/___/_____.

balan/o/rrhea
bal an ō **rē′** ə

6.57

The male external genitalia includes the scrotum and penis. **pen/o** is used to build words about the penis. Pen/ile is the adjectival form. Inflammation of the penis is _____/_____. Scrot/al is the adjective for _____/___.

pen/itis
pē **nī′** tis
scrot/um
skrō′ təm

6.58

Trauma, prostatectomy, or diabetes may cause impotence (the inability to have an erection). A device can be implanted into the penis that is filled with fluid to produce an erection. This is called a _____/_____ prosthesis (implant).

pen/ile
pē′ nil

ANSWER COLUMN

---

scrot/um
skrō′ təm
pen/o/scrot/al
pē′ nō **skrō′** təl

6.59

The saclike structure that contains the testes is the _____/____. Build a term that means pertaining to the penis and scrotum:
_____/___/_____/___.

---

an embryonic egg cell
  (a cell that will become
  an ovum)

6.60

The Greek word for egg is *oon*. In scientific words, **o/o** (pronounce both *o*s) means egg or ovum. An o/o/blast is *_____
_____.

---

o/o/gen/esis
ō ə **jen′** ə sis

6.61

O/o/gen/esis is the formation and development of an ovum. The changes that occur in the cell from ooblast to mature ovum are called
___/___/____/_____.

---

oogenesis

6.62

O/o/gen/esis must be complete for the ovum to be mature. It is impossible for a spermatozoon to fertilize an ovum until _____ is complete.

---

ovary

6.63

The combining form used in words that refer to the ovary is **oophor/o**. (This literally means egg bearing.) When you see oophor in a word, you think of the _____.

---

ovary

6.64

The ovary is the organ that is responsible for maturing and discharging the ovum (ovulation). About every 28 days an ovum (plural ova) is discharged from the _____.

WORD
ORIGINS

6.65

This frame shows the development of the word oophorectomy:
o/o   egg from Greek, *oon*
  phor/o   bear from Greek, *phoros*
    ect/o   out from Greek, *ektos*
      -tomy   cut from Greek, *tomos*
Ovary comes from Latin. An ovarium is a place that holds eggs. Think of aquarium and solarium. Ovarian is the adjective derived from ovarium.

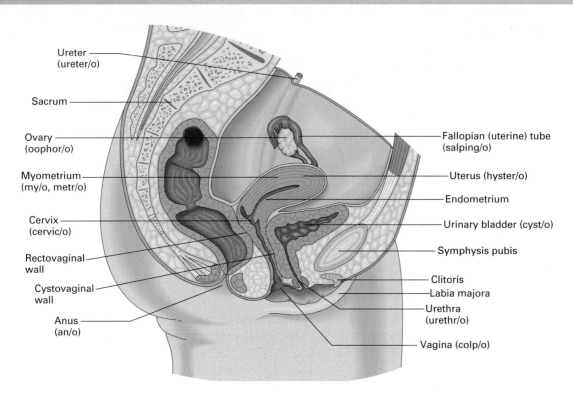

Female reproductive system

ANSWER COLUMN	
	6.66
excision of the ovary	**oophor/o** is used in words to refer to the ovary. Oophorectomy means
	*_____.
	6.67
	Using what you need from **oophor/o**, build words that mean
	inflammation of an ovary
oophor/itis	_____/_____;
ō ə fôr ī′ tis	excision of an ovary
oophor/ectomy	_____/_____;
ō ə fôr **ek**′ tə mē	tumor of an ovary (ovarian tumor)
oophor/oma	_____/_____.
ō ə fôr **ō**′ mə	
	6.68
fixation	Recall that **-pexy** is a suffix meaning fixation. Oophor/o/pexy means fixation of a displaced ovary. **-pexy** is a suffix that means _____. Fixation of a

ANSWER COLUMN

orchi/o/pexy or **ōr′** kē ō peks′ ē orchid/o/pexy **or′** kid ō peks′ ē	displaced testicle is _____/___/_____.

6.69

An oophor/o/pexy is a surgical procedure. When an ovary is displaced,
an _____/___/_____ may be performed.

oophor/o/pexy
ō **of′** ə rō peks′ ē

6.70

TAKE A CLOSER LOOK

If you look up **oophor/o** in your medical dictionary, it will most likely show you
that the correct pronunciation of terms that begin with **oophor/o** is "o of′" or "o".
However, in practice it has become acceptable to use the usual English
pronunciation for oo as an "oo" sound. For example, the term oophorectomy
may be pronounced both as "o͞o fôr **ek′** tō mē" and "ō ôf′ ôr **ek′** tō mē".

6.71

The surgical procedure to fixate a prolapsed (dropped or sagged) ovary is called
an _____.

oophoropexy

6.72

In the male, fixation of a prolapsed or undescended testicle is called
orchid/o/pexy (orchiopexy). The suffix that means fixation is _____.

-pexy

6.73

salping/o, from the Greek word *salpinx,* meaning trumpet (describing the
shape), is used to build words about the fallopian tube(s). A salping/o/scope is an
instrument used to examine the *_____.

fallopian tube(s)

6.74

A new surgical opening made in a fallopian tube is called a
_____/___/_____.

salping/o/stomy
sal pin **gos′** tō mē

6.75

Using what you need of **salping/o**, build words meaning inflammation of a
fallopian tube (or eustachian tubes)
_____/_____;
excision of a fallopian tube (uterine tube)
_____/_____.

salping/itis
sal pin **jī′** tis
salping/ectomy
sal pin **jek′** tə mē

NOTE: **salping/o** is also used to refer to the eustachian tubes in the ears. The
context of the medical report should tell you if it refers to ears or uterine tubes.

ANSWER COLUMN

salping/o-/oophor/itis
sal ping′ gō ō ə fôr ī′ tis

6.76

When you are building compound medical words and use three like vowels between word roots or combining forms, separate them with a hyphen. For a model use salpingo-oophorectomy. Build a word that means inflammation of the fallopian tube and ovary. _____/__-/_____/____

6.77

SPELL CHECK ✓

Do not drop the *o* in **salping/o** when joining it to **oophor/o** because the combining form **o/o** means egg. Remember to use a hyphen: salpingo-oophoritis.

salping/o-/oophor/o/cele
sal ping′ gō ō **of**′ ə rō sēl

6.78

A hernia that encloses the fallopian tube and ovary
is a _____/____-/_____/__/_____.

inflammation of the vagina

6.79

colp/o is used in words about the vagina. Colp/itis means
*_____.

vaginal pain
colp/o/pathy
kol **pop**′ ə thē

6.80

Colp/o/dynia means *_____. Any disease of the vagina
is called _____/____/_____ (vaginopathy).

vaginal spasm
colp/ectomy
kol **pek**′ tə mē

6.81

Colp/o/spasm is a *_____. Excision of a part of the vagina
is a _____/_____ (vaginectomy).

6.82

Build words meaning
fixation of the vagina

colp/o/pexy
kol′ pō peks ē
colp/o/plasty
kol′ pō plast′ ē

_____/____/_____;
surgical repair of the vagina (vaginoplasty)
_____/____/_____.

ANSWER COLUMN

	6.83
	Build words meaning instrument for examining the vagina
colp/o/scope **kol**′ pō skōp colp/o/tomy kol **po**′ tōm ē	_____/_____/_____ ; incision into the vaginal wall _____/_____/_____ .
	6.84
Explanation for next frame	In words built from **laryng/o**, **pharyng/o**, **salping/o**, and **mening/o**, the *g* is pronounced as a hard "g" when followed by o, u, a, or a consonant. The *g* in good, gut, gate, and glad is a hard "g." NOTE: Listen to the CDs that accompany *Medical Terminology: A Programmed Systems Approach,* 9th edition, for assistance with these rules.
	6.85
hard (Pronounce them) pharyng/algia far in **gal**′ jē ə mening/o/cele men **in** gō sēl	In laryng/oscope and salpingocele, the "g" of the word root is pronounced hard, as in goat. In pharyngalgia and meningocele, the "g" is also given a _____ pronunciation.
	6.86
hard	In laryngostomy, pharyngotomy, salpingopexy, and meningomalacia, the "g" is given a _____ sound.
	6.87
o u a consonant	A hard "g" precedes the vowels _____, _____, and _____ or a _____ .
	6.88
Explanation for next frame	In words built from **laryng/o**, **pharyng/o**, **salping/o**, and **mening/o**, the "g" is soft when followed by e, i, or y. The g in germ, giant, and gymnast is soft.

ANSWER COLUMN

6.89

In laryngectomy and salpingitis, the "g" is a soft "g," as in germ. In meningeal and pharyngitis, the g also is given a _____ pronunciation.

soft
mening/eal
men **in'** jē əl
pharyng/itis
far in lī' tis

6.90

In meningitis, salpingectomy, laryngitis, and pharyngectomy, the g is given a _____ sound.

soft
(Pronounce them)

6.91

A soft "g" precedes the vowels _____, _____, and _____.

e
i
y

6.92

"g" is given a hard sound when followed by the vowels _____, _____, and _____.
"g" is given the soft "j" sound when followed by the vowels _____, _____, and _____.

a
o
u
e
i
y

6.93

In compound words a hyphen (-) is used when

* _____

_____.

EXAMPLE: salpingo-oophoritis.

three like vowels join
   word roots or
   combining forms

6.94

INFORMATION FRAME

The spermatozoon is the male germ cell; the ovum is the female egg cell. When they unite in the fallopian tube, fertilization occurs. The fertilized ovum moves to the uterus, implants itself into the endometrium, and grows until birth.

6.95

hyster/o is of Greek origin and is used to build words about the uterus as an organ. A hyster/ectomy is an excision of the _____.

uterus
yōō' ter əs

ANSWER COLUMN

	6.96
uterus uterus	A hyster/o/tomy is an incision into the _____, and a hysterospasm is a spasm of the _____.
	6.97
hyster/o/salping/o/gram his′ tər ō sal **ping**′ ō gram	A hyster/o/gram is an x-ray (picture) of the uterus. A special x-ray (HSG) procedure is performed to determine patency (openness) of the fallopian tubes by injecting a contrast medium. This "picture," an x-ray of the uterus and fallopian tubes, is called a _____/___/_____/___/_____.
	6.98
hyster/o/pathy his′ tər **op**′ ə thē	A general term for any disease of the uterus is _____/___/_____.
	6.99
hyster/o salping/o oophor -ectomy	A hyster/o/salping/o-/oophor/ectomy is the excision of the uterus, fallopian tubes, and ovaries. Analyze this word: _____/___ combining form for uterus _____/___ combining form for fallopian tubes _____ word root for ovary _____ suffix—excision
	6.100
WORD ORIGINS	Dimeter (of the womb) was the goddess of the harvest and the seasons. **metr/o** comes from the Greek word *metra,* meaning womb. The endometrium is the inner layer of tissues of the uterus.
	6.101
hyster/o/scope **his**′ ter ō skōp hyster/o/scopy his′ ter **os**′ kō pē	**hyster/o** is used in words pertaining to the uterus as an organ. In order to view the uterus more closely, an instrument (**-scope**) with a light source is used to see into the uterus. This instrument is called a _____/___/_____. The procedure is called _____/___/_____.

ANSWER COLUMN

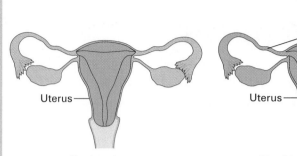

Hysterectomy

**Total hysterectomy—
hysterosalpingo-oophorectomy**

6.102

Uterus (word root uter) comes from a Latin word meaning womb. The adjectival form is uterine. The tubes that attach to the uterus leading to the ovaries are the
_____/_____ (fallopian) tubes.

uter/ine
yōo′ ter in

6.103

There are exceptions to the rule, but in general **hyster/o** means the uterus as an
_____. **metr/o** refers to the uterine _____.

organ
tissues

6.104

Metr/itis means an inflammation of the uterine musculature. Metr/o/paralysis and metr/o/plegia mean paralysis of the
*_____.

uterus or uterine
   musculature

6.105

Using **metr/o** (mē′ trō) and **-rrhea,** build a word meaning abnormal flow or discharge from the uterine tissues:
_____/___/_____.
NOTE: **-metry** and **-meter** are suffixes meaning measure and instrument used to measure. They are pronounced me′ trē and me′ ter, as in audiometry (aw dē om′ et rē) and cytometer (sī tom′ et er).

metr/o/rrhea
mē trō **rē′** ə, or
met rō **rē′** ə

6.106

Build words meaning any uterine disease
_____/___/_____;
herniation of the uterus
_____/___/_____.

metr/o/pathy or
mē **trop′** ə thē
hyster/o/pathy
his′ ter **op′** ə thē

ANSWER COLUMN

metr/o/cele
or
mēt′ rō sēl
hyster/o/cele
his′ ter ō sēl

6.107

The endo/metr/ium is the lining of the uterus.
Build words meaning inflammation of the uterine lining

endo/metr/itis
en dō mē **trī′** tis
metr/o/pathy
mē **trop′** ə thē

_____/_____/_____;
disease of the uterine tissue
_____/___/_____.

6.108

Endo/metr/iosis is a condition in which tissue that looks and acts like endometrial tissue is found in places other than the lining of the uterus. When endometrial-like tissue is found on the outside of the uterus, the ovaries, or bowel, this condition is called _____/_____/_____.

endo/metr/iosis
en′ dō mē trē **ō′** sis

6.109

Build the word that means excision of the uterus, fallopian tubes, and ovaries:
_____/___/_____/___-/_____/_____.

hyster/o/salping/o-/
oophor/ectomy
his′ te rō sal ping′ gō-/
ō′ ə fôr **ek′** tə mē

6.110

INFORMATION FRAME

-ptosis is a suffix meaning prolapse or downward displacement. Ptosis is also a word by itself meaning a condition of displacement. Ptotic is the adjectival form.

6.111

prolapse, falling, or to fall

Hyster/o/ptosis means prolapse of the uterus. *Ptosis* is a Greek word that means *_____.

6.112

hyster/o
ptosis

Hyster/o/ptosis (his ter op tō′ sis) is a compound word constructed from
_____/_____ the combining form for uterus;
_____ a word meaning prolapse.

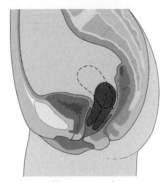

Hysteroptosis

6.113

When prolapse occurs, a fixation is usually done. A hyster/o/pexy would be done to correct or fixate

_____/___/_____.

hyster/o/ptosis
his′ tər op **tō**′ sis

6.114

Many organs can prolapse or sag. When the uterus prolapses, it is called _____.

hysteroptosis

6.115

Build a word meaning prolapse of the vagina:

_____/___/_____.

colp/o/ptosis
kol′ pop **tō**′ sis

6.116

A word meaning surgical fixation of the uterus is

_____/___/_____.

A word meaning uterine hernia is

_____/___/_____.

hyster/o/pexy
his′ tə rō pek sē
hyster/o/cele
his′ tə rō sēl

6.117

Use **cervic/o** to refer to the cervix which is the neck of the uterus. Cervic/o/plasty is a surgical procedure to repair the cervix.
Build a word that means
inflammation of the cervix

_____/_____;

pertaining to the cervix

_____/_____.

cervic/itis
ser vi **sī**′ tis
cervic/al
ser′ vi kal

ANSWER COLUMN

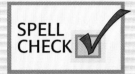

6.118

Cervic/o is also used as a combining form referring to the neck (cervical) area of the spine. The first seven vertebral bones of the neck are the cervical vertebrae. Use the context of your subject and look up terms in the dictionary to know if you are using **cervic/o** correctly in a term when referring to either the neck of the uterus or the neck area of the spine.

6.119

One surgical procedure that may be performed on the cervix is a con/ization. A cone-shaped cut is made in the cervix to remove endo/cervical tissue. This may be done using electr/o/cautery (cautery conization) or a cold knife blade (cold conization).

6.120

con/ization
kō ni **zā**′ shun
endo/cervical
en′ dō **ser**′ vi kal
or
cervic/al

Using what you have just learned, complete the following statement.
A ____/_____ may be performed to remove a cone-shaped sample
of ____/_____ tissue.

6.121

women

gynec/o and **gyn/e** come from the Greek word *gyne,* which means woman. The field of medicine called gynec/o/logy deals with diseases of _____.

Conization

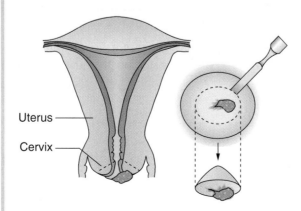

Uterus

Cervix

ANSWER COLUMN

gynec/o/logist gī nə **kol**′ ə jist, or jin ə **kol**′ ə jist gynec/o/log/ic gīn nə kō **lo**′ jik jin ə kō **lo**′ jik	**6.122** Gynec/o/log/ic is the adjectival form of gynecology (GYN). The physician who specializes in female disorders is called a _____/____/_____. This physician may perform a _____/___/_____/____ exam.
gynec/oid **gī**′ nə koid, or **jin**′ ə koid gynec/o/pathy gī′ nə **kop**′ ə thē, or jin ə **kop**′ ə thē gyn/e/phobia gī nə **fō**′ bē ə, or jin ə **fō**′ bē ə	**6.123** Build words meaning resembling woman _____/____; any disease peculiar to women _____/___/_____; abnormal fear of women _____/___/_____.
vessel	**6.124** *Vas* is a Latin word meaning vessel. vas/o is another combining form for blood vessel. Vas/o/dilatation means enlarging the diameter of a _____. Note: Dilatation and dilation are synonyms.
decreasing the size of the diameter of a vessel	**6.125** Vas/o/constriction is the opposite of vas/o/dilatation. Vas/o/constriction means *_____ _____.
vas/o/dilator vas′ ō **dī**′ lā ter	**6.126** Nitroglycerine is a vas/o/dilator. People with angina pectoris experience chest pain due to vas/o/constriction of the blood vessels to the heart. After taking a _____/___/_____, the vessels allow more blood to flow to the heart, and the pain stops.
vessel	**6.127** Vas/o/motor is an adjective that refers to nerves that control the tone of the blood _____ walls.

ANSWER COLUMN

6.128

Using **vas/o**, build words meaning

vas/al
vā′ səl, or **vā**′ zəl
vas/o/spasm
vas′ ō spaz əm, or
vā′ zō spaz əm
vas/o/tripsy
vas′ ō trip sē, or
vā′ zō trip sē

pertaining to a vessel

_____/___;

spasm of a vessel

_____/___/_____;

crushing of a vessel (with forceps to stop hemorrhage)

_____/___/ _tripsy_____.

6.129

INFORMATION FRAME

vas/o can be used to mean many types of vessels. Look at the words used in your dictionary beginning with vas or **vas/o**. They could be confused with **angi/o**. The four words in Frame 6.130 refer to the vas deferens only—no other vessel. The vas deferens is shown in the illustration.

6.130

Build words meaning
incision into the vas deferens

vas/o/tomy
vas **ot**′ ə mē
vas/o/rrhaphy
vas **or**′ ə fē
vas/o/stomy
vas **os**′ tə mē
vas/ectomy
vas **ek**′ tə mē

_____/___/_____;

suture of the vas deferens

_____/___/_____;

making a new opening into the vas deferens

_____/___/_____;

removal of a segment of the vas deferens

_____/_____.

NOTE: Tubal ligation is the excision of the fallopian tubes and is the equivalent of sterilization surgery in women.

Vasectomy

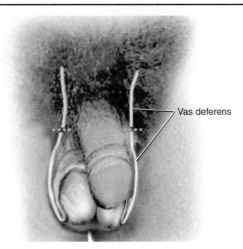

Vas deferens

Abbreviation	Meaning
AID	artificial insemination (donor's sperm)
AIH	artificial insemination (husband's sperm)
BPH	benign prostatic hyperplasia (hypertrophy)
cysto	cystoscopy
ESRD	end-stage renal disease
F, ♀	female
GYN	gynecology (ist)
HSG	hysterosalpingogram
IVP	intravenous pyelogram
KUB	kidney ureter bladder
M, ♂	male
MD	doctor of medicine
Pap	Papanicolaou test (smear)
PID	pelvic inflammatory disease
PSA	prostate specific antigen
RPG	retrograde pyelogram
sp gr, SpG	specific gravity
TAH	total abdominal hysterectomy
TSE	testicular self-exam
TUR (P)	transurethral resection (prostate)
UA	urinalysis
UTI	urinary tract infection

To complete your study of this unit, work the **Review Activities** on the following pages. Also, listen to the audio CDs that accompany *Medical Terminology: A Programmed Systems Approach,* 9th edition, and practice your pronunciation.

Additional practice exercises for this unit are available on the Learner Practice CD-ROM found in the back of the textbook.

REVIEW ACTIVITIES

CIRCLE AND CORRECT

Circle the correct answer for each question. Then check your answers in Appendix A.

1. Sound made by g followed by e
   a. "k"   b. "j"
   c. "s"   d. "g" as in gut

2. Suffix for destruction
   a. -plasty   b. -rrhexis
   c. -lysis   d. -malacia

3. Plural form for sperm
   a. sperms   b. spermat
   c. spermatozoon   d. spermatozoa

4. Word root for penis
   a. penile   b. pen
   c. balan   d. orchid

5. Suffix for prolapse
   a. -ptosis   b. -ectomy
   c. -cele   d. -pexy

6. Suffix for surgical fixation
   a. -ptosis   b. -ectomy
   c. -plasty   d. -pexy

7. Suffix for suturing
   a. -rrhea   b. -rrhaphy
   c. -rrhia   d. -rrhagia

8. Word root for uterus (the organ)
   a. utero   b. hyster
   c. metro   d. meter

9. Adjective for testis
   a. testes   b. orchidic
   c. testicular   d. testicle

10. Suffix for instrument used to make a picture (x-ray)
    a. -graph   b. -scope
    c. -meter   d. -tome

11. Combining form for woman
    a. hystero   b. andro
    c. gyneco   d. femino

12. Adjective for ovary
    a. ovarian   b. ova
    c. oophoral   d. uterine

13. Combining form for kidney
    a. pyelo   b. nephro
    c. oophoro   d. renal

14. Suffix for abnormal bleeding
    a. -rrhea   b. -rrhaphy
    c. -rrhagia   d. -rrhia

15. Suffix for flow or discharge
    a. -clysis   b. -trophy
    c. -rrhea   d. -hydro

16. Adjective for kidney
    a. nephral   b. nephroc
    c. cystic   d. renal

17. Combining form for the tube that leads from the kidneys to the bladder
    a. cysto   b. uretero
    c. urethro   d. pyelo

18. Correct spelling for term meaning bleeding
    a. hemorage   b. hematorrhagia
    c. hyperemia   d. hemorrhage

REVIEW ACTIVITIES
SELECT AND CONSTRUCT

Select the correct word parts from the following list and construct medical terms that represent the given meaning.

algia	ary	balano	centesis	cerviclo(al)	colpo
crypt(o)	cyst(o)	dermato	dynia	ectomy	endo
fibro	genesis	gram	graph	gyneco	hystero
ic	ism	itis	logy(ist)	lysis	metro
nephr/o	oma	oo	oophoro	orchid(o)	osis
ostomy	pathy	pexy	plasty	pneumono	prostato
ptosis	pulmon/o	pyelo	reno(al)	rrhagia	rrhaphy
rrhea	salpingo	scope	scopy	spasm	testiculo
uretero	urethro	uro			

1. inflammation of the renal pelvis and the kidney _____

2. suture of the tube that goes from the kidney to the urinary bladder _____

3. process of examining the urinary bladder by looking through an instrument _____

4. prolapsed kidney _____

5. x-ray of the kidney _____

6. fixation of the urinary bladder _____

7. abnormal bleeding of the urethra _____

8. destruction of kidney tissue _____

9. make a new opening in the urinary bladder _____

10. inflammation of the inner lining of the uterus _____

11. prolapse of the uterus _____

12. undescended testicles _____

13. excision of the prostate gland _____

14. specialist in women's health _____

15. formation of ova _____

16. a discharge from the glans penis _____

17. vaginal pain _____

18. instrument used to look into the uterus _____

19. specialist in men's health _____

20. x-ray of uterus and fallopian tubes _____

21. fixation of a prolapsed testicle _____

22. process of viewing the inside of the vagina with a scope _____

23. inside the cervix _____

REVIEW ACTIVITIES

DEFINE AND DISSECT

Give a brief definition and dissect each term listed into its word parts in the space provided. Check your answers by referring to the frame listed in parentheses and your medical dictionary. Then listen to the audio CD to practice pronunciation.

1. nephropexy (6.16)

_____ / ____ / _____
rt   v   suffix

_____
definition

2. ureterocele (6.22)

_____ / ____ / _____
rt   v   suffix

3. ureteropyelitis (6.23)

_____ / ____ / _____ / _____
rt   v   rt   suffix

4. cystorrhaphy (6.28)

_____ / ____ / _____
rt   v   suffix

5. urethrotomy (6.31)

_____ / ____ / _____
rt   v   suffix

6. nephroptosis (6.14)

_____ / ____ / _____
rt   v   suffix

7. renopathy (6.10)

_____ / ____ / _____
rt   v   suffix

8. nephrolith (6.17)

_____ / ____ / _____
rt   v   rt

9. renal (6.10)

____ / ____
rt suffix

10. ureterocystostomy (6.24)

____ / ____ / _____ / ____ / _____
rt   v   rt   v   suffix

REVIEW ACTIVITIES

11. renogram (6.10)

_____/____/_____
rt   v   suffix

_____

12. spermatozoa (6.36)

_____/____/_____
rt   v   suffix

_____

13. orchidoplasty (6.45)

_____/____/_____
rt   v   suffix

_____

14. testicular (6.42)

_____/____
rt   suffix

_____

15. prostatorrhea (6.53)

_____/____/_____
rt   v   suffix

_____

16. hysterosalpingogram (6.97)

_____/___/_____/___/____
rt   v   rt   v suffix

_____

17. salpingo-oophorocele (6.78)

_____/___/_____/___/_____
rt   v   rt   v   suffix

_____

18. colposcope (6.83)

_____/___/_____
rt   v   suffix

_____

19. endometriosis (6.108)

_____/_____/_____
pre   rt   suffix

_____

20. hysteroptosis (6.113)

_____/___/_____
rt   v   suffix

_____

21. seminal (6.50)

_____/____
rt   suffix

_____

REVIEW ACTIVITIES

22. hysteroscopy (6.101)

_____ / ___ / _____
rt   v   suffix

23. hysterosalpingo-oophorectomy (6.109)

___ / ___ / _____ / ___ / ___ / _____
rt   v   rt   v   rt   suffix

24. orchidalgia (6.41)

_____ / _____
rt   suffix

25. spermicide (6.38)

_____ / ___ / _____
rt   v   suffix

26. gynecologist (6.122)

_____ / ___ / _____
rt   v   suffix

27. vasotripsy (6.128)

_____ / ___ / _____
rt   v   suffix

28. vasectomy (6.130)

_____ / _____
rt   suffix

29. cervicoplasty (6.117)

_____ / ___ / _____
rt   v   suffix

30. vasoconstriction (6.125)

_____ / ___ / _____ / _____
rt   v   rt   suffix

31. conization (6.119)

_____ / _____
rt   suffix

REVIEW ACTIVITIES

ART LABELING

Match the combining forms with the numbered diagram. Write the structure name in the blank.

Combining Form	Name of the Structure
_____ rect/o	_____
_____ cyst/o	_____
_____ urethr/o	_____
_____ balan/o	_____
_____ prostat/o	_____
_____ vas/o	_____
_____ orchid/o	_____
_____ pen/o	_____
_____ ureter/o	_____
_____ scrot/o	_____

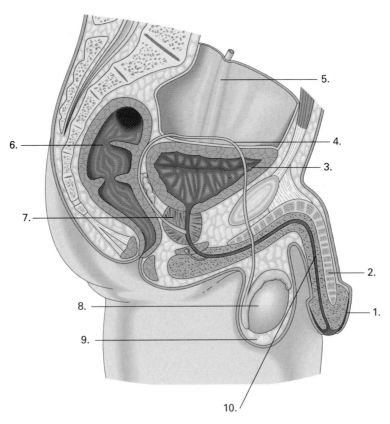

Male reproductive system

REVIEW ACTIVITIES

ART LABELING

Label the structures of the female reproductive system by writing the number in front of the correct word part.

Write the body part indicated.

Combining Form	Body Part
_____ colp/o	_____
_____ hyster/o	_____
_____ oophor/o	_____
_____ metr/o	_____
_____ salping/o	_____
_____ cervic/o	_____
_____ rect/o	_____
_____ clitor/o	_____
_____ labi/o	_____
_____ urethr/o	_____
_____ an/o	_____
_____ ureter/o	_____
_____ cystovagin/o	_____
_____ cyst/o	_____

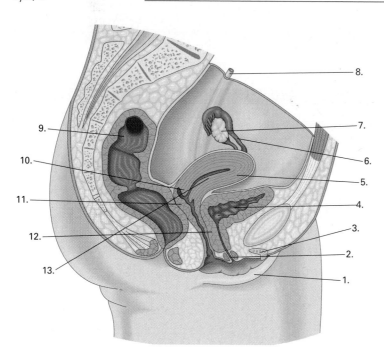

Female Reproductive System

REVIEW ACTIVITIES

ABBREVIATION MATCHING

Match the following abbreviations with their definition.

_____ 1. HSG

_____ 2. cysto

_____ 3. BPH

_____ 4. F, ♀

_____ 5. TUR(P)

_____ 6. M, ♂

_____ 7. GYN

_____ 8. UTI

_____ 9. AID

_____ 10. TSE

_____ 11. RPG

_____ 12. IVP

_____ 13. UA

_____ 14. TAH

a. urinalysis (testing)

b. testicular self-exam

c. transluminal upper restoration

d. hysterectomy (total abdominal)

e. retrograde pyelogram

f. arteriosclerosis

g. benign prostatic hyperplasia (hypertrophy)

h. female

i. transurethral resection of the prostate

j. gynecophobia

k. artificial insemination using husband's sperm

l. intravenous pyelogram

m. male

n. artificial insemination by donor's sperm

o. gynecology (ist)

p. urinary tract infection

q. hysterosalpingogram

r. upper respiratory infection

s. cystoscopy

ABBREVIATION FILL-IN

Fill in the blanks with the correct abbreviation.

15. doctor of medicine _____

16. prostate specific antigen _____

17. kidney, ureter, bladder _____

18. artificial insemination using husband's sperm _____

19. end-stage renal disease _____

20. Papanicolaou test _____

REVIEW ACTIVITIES

CASE STUDY

Write the term next to its meaning given below. Then draw slashes to analyze the word parts. Note the use of medical abbreviations. Look these up in your dictionary or find them in Appendix B. If you have any questions about the answers, refer to your medical dictionary or check with your instructor for the answers in Appendix A.

CASE STUDY 6-1

DISCHARGE SUMMARY—TRANSURETHRAL RESECTION OF THE PROSTATE

Pt: Male, age 72

Dx: Benign prostatic **hyperplasia** with retention and **hydronephrosis**

Mr. Travis Reese was brought to the hospital for a **TUR** for reasons itemized in the **H&P**. He underwent a **transurethral** resection of the trilobar gland on 9/21. On 9/22, **cystoclysis** was clear. He had one degree of temperature and went to straight drainage. On 9/23 his temperature was normal with slight **hematuria**. The **catheter** was removed. On 9/24 he was **afebrile** Urine was light, diluted cherry Kool-Aid color. A **postoperative** instruction sheet was given to Mr. Reese. He read it and had no questions. He was given a prescription for Achromycin 250 **mg qid** and discharged.

Pathology report: 40 g of **benign** tissue with mild focal, acute and **chronic prostatitis**.

1. milligrams four times a day _____

2. noncancerous _____

3. study of disease _____

4. overdevelopment _____

5. inflammation of the prostate _____

6. long-term less severe _____

7. history and physical exam _____

8. urine (water) in the kidney _____

9. transurethral resection _____

10. blood in the urine _____

11. without a fever _____

12. irrigation of the bladder _____

13. tube inserted in the bladder _____

14. after surgery _____

15. across the urethra _____

REVIEW ACTIVITIES

CROSSWORD PUZZLE

Check your answers by going back through the frames or checking the solution in Appendix C.

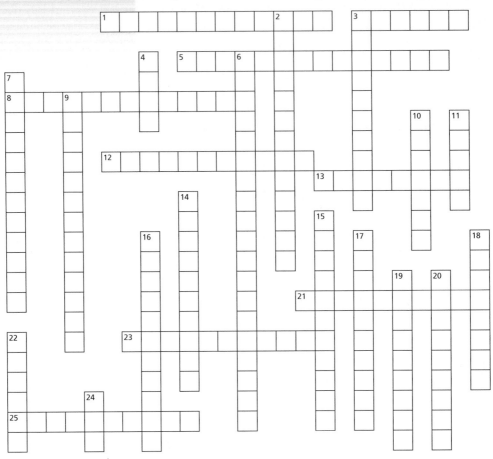

Across

1. suturing of the urinary bladder
3. pertaining to the penis
5. inflammation of the kidney and renal pelvis
8. condition of endometrial tissue on other organs
12. discharge from the glans penis
13. scant amount of urine
21. surgical fixation of orchidoptosis
23. stone in the tube from kidney to bladder
25. pertaining to the testes

Down

2. excision of the prostate gland
3. excessive hunger and eating
4. transurethral resection of the prostate
6. HSG
7. prolapsed kidney
9. surgical repair of testis
10. pertaining to the uterus
11. pertaining to the kidney
14. hysteropathy (synonym)
15. excessive bleeding with menses
16. metrocele (synonym)
17. inflamed ovaries
18. having three ears
19. colpodynia (synonym)
20. blood in the urine
22. combining form for hidden
24. pelvic inflammatory disease (abbreviation)

REVIEW ACTIVITIES

GLOSSARY

antineoplastic	agent that works against tumor growth	gynecology	the science of studying women's health
anuria	unable to produce urine	gynecopathy	any disease peculiar to women
balanoplasty	surgical repair of the glans penis	gynephobia	abnormal fear of women
balanorrhea	discharge from the glans penis	hematuria	blood in urine
cervical	pertaining to the neck and cervix	hemorrhage	bleeding
colpalgia	vaginal pain	hysterectomy	excision of the uterus
colpitis	inflammation of the vagina	hysteropathy	any disease of the uterus
colpopathy	any disease of the vagina (vaginopathy)	hysteropexy	fixation of a prolapsed uterus
colpoptosis	prolapse of the vagina	hysterosalpingogram	x-ray of the uterus and fallopian tubes (uses contrast media)
colposcope	instrument used to examine the vagina and cervix	hysterosalpingo-oophorectomy	total abdominal hysterectomy
colposcopy	the process of using a colposcope to examine tissues of vagina and cervix	hysteroscope	instrument used to examine the inside of the uterus closely
colpotomy	incision into the vaginal wall	hysteroscopy	the process of using a hysteroscope
cryptorchidism	condition of an undescended testis	menorrhagia	abnormally excessive menstruation
cystorrhagia	hemorrhage of the bladder	metrocele	herniation of uterine tissues (hysterocele)
cystorrhaphy	suturing of the urinary bladder	metropathy	any disease of the uterine tissues (hysteropathy)
endocervical	inside the cervix	metrorrhea	discharge from the uterine tissues
endometriosis	condition of endometrial tissue growing outside of the endometrium	nephritis	inflammation of the kidney
endometritis	inflammation of the endometrium	nephrolith	kidney stone
glycosuria	glucose (sugar) in the urine	nephromalacia	softening of kidney tissue
gynecoid	resembling a woman or female structures	nephromegaly	enlargement of a kidney
gynecologist	physician specialist in women's health	nephropexy	surgical fixation of a prolapsed kidney

REVIEW ACTIVITIES

nephroptosis	prolapsed or displaced kidney	polyphagia	excessive hunger and eating
nephrorrhaphy	suturing of kidney tissue	polyphobia	having many fears
neurorrhaphy	suturing of a nerve	polyuria	abnormally excessive urination
nocturia	excessive urination at night	prostatalgia	prostate pain
oliguria	abnormally low amount of urine	prostatectomy	excision of the prostate
oogenesis	formation of ova	prostatitis	inflammation of the prostate gland
oophorectomy	excision of an ovary	pyelitis	inflammation of the renal pelvis
oophoritis	inflammation of an ovary	pyelogram	x-ray of the renal pelvis
oophoroma	tumor of an ovary	pyelonephritis	inflammation of the renal pelvis and the kidney
oophoropexy	surgical fixation of a prolapsed ovary	pyeloplasty	surgical repair of the renal pelvis
oophoroptosis	prolapsed ovary	renal	pertaining to the kidney
orchidalgia	testicular pain (orchidodynia)	renogastric	pertaining to the kidney and stomach
orchidectomy	excision of a testis (orchiectomy, orchectomy)	renogram	x-ray of the kidney (renograph)
orchidocele	herniation of the testes	renointestinal	pertaining to the kidney and intestine
orchidoptosis	prolapsed condition of a testis	renopathy	any disease of the kidney
orchiopexy	fixation of a prolapsed testis (orchidopexy)	salpingectomy	excision of a fallopian tube
orchioplasty	surgical repair of the testes	salpingitis	inflammation of the fallopian tube (or eustachian tube)
orchiotomy	incision into a testis	salpingo-oophoritis	inflammation of the ovary and fallopian tube
penile	pertaining to the penis	salpingo-oophorocele	herniation of the ovary and fallopian tube
penitis	inflammation of the penis	salpingostomy	forming a new opening in the fallopian tube
penoscrotal	pertaining to the penis and scrotum	seminoma	tumor containing sperm
polyarthritis	inflammation of many joints	spermatoblast	immature sperm cell (spermoblast)
polycystic	having many cysts		
polyneuralgia	pain in many nerves		
polyneuritis	inflammation of many nerves		
polyotia	having more than two ears		

REVIEW ACTIVITIES

spermatocele	herniated sac containing sperm		urethrorrhaphy	suturing of the urethra
spermatocyst	saclike structure containing sperm		urethrospasm	spasm of the muscles of the urethra
spermatoid	resembling sperm		urethrotomy	incision into the urethra
spermatolysis	destruction of sperm (spermolysis)		urogenital	pertaining to the urinary tract and genitals
spermatopathy	any disease of the sperm		urologist	physician specialist in disorders of the urinary and male reproductive systems
spermicide	agent that kills sperm			
testicular	pertaining to the testes		urology	the medical specialty that studies the urinary system
ureterocele	herniation of the ureter		uropathy	any disease of the urinary system
ureterocystostomy	procedure to form a new opening between the ureter and the urinary bladder		uterine	pertaining to the uterus
ureterolith	stone in the ureter		vasectomy	excision of the vas deferens (for sterilization)
ureteropathy	any disease involving the ureter		vasoconstriction	decrease in vessel diameter
ureteropyelitis	inflammation of the ureter and the renal pelvis		vasodilation (vasodilatation)	increase in vessel diameter
ureteropyosis	condition of pus in the ureter		vasorrhaphy	suturing of vessel or vas deferens
ureterorrhagia	hemorrhage of the ureter		vasostomy	procedure to make a new opening in the vas deferens
ureterorrhaphy	suturing of the ureter			
urethrocystitis	inflammation of the urethra and urinary bladder		vasotomy	incision into the vas deferens
urethrorrhagia	hemorrhage of the urethra		vasotripsy	surgical crushing of a vessel

UNIT 7

Gastroenterology

Read through the digestive system information in the following table. Locate the organs named by studying the illustration on page 227. Then work Frames 7.1–7.74.

Organ	Combining Form	Suffixes	Examples
mouth	stomat/o	-itis	stomat/itis
teeth	dent/o, odont/o	-ist	dent/ist
tongue	gloss/o, lingu/o	-plegia*	gloss/o/plegia
lips	cheil/o	-plasty	cheil/o/plasty
gums	gingiv/o	-ectomy	gingiv/ectomy
esophagus	esophag/o	-spasm	esophag/o/spasm
stomach	gastr/o	-ectasia*	gastr/ectasia
small intestine	enter/o	-logy	enter/o/logy
duodenum	duoden/o	-ostomy	duoden/ostomy
jejunum	jejun/o	-rrhaphy	jejun/o/rrhaphy
ileum	ile/o	-tomy	ile/o/tomy
large intestine	col/o	-clysis*	col/o/clysis
sigmoid colon	sigmoid/o	-scopy	sigmoid/o/scopy
rectum	rect/o	-cele	rect/o/cele
anus and rectum	proct/o	-scope	proct/o/scope
accessory organs			
liver	hepat/o	-megaly	hepat/o/megaly
gallbladder	cholecyst/o	-gram	cholecyst/o/gram
pancreas	pancreat/o	-lith	pancreat/o/lith

*New suffix.

7.1

Stoma is a Greek word meaning mouth. The combining form for mouth is
_____/____.

stomat/o

ANSWER COLUMN

7.2

inflammation
  of the mouth

Stomat/itis means *_____.

surgical repair of
  the mouth

Stomat/o/plasty means *_____.

7.3

Using the word root for mouth, form words meaning pain in the mouth

stomat/algia
stō mə **tal**′ jē ə

_____/_____;

stomat/o/rrhagia
stō′ mə tō **rā**′ jē ə

hemorrhage of the mouth

_____/____/_____.

7.4

Using the combining form **stomat/o** for mouth, build words meaning condition
of mouth fungus (**myc/o**) _____/____/_____/_____;

stomat/o/myc/osis
stō′ mə tō mī **kō**′ sis

stomat/o/pathy
stō′ mə **top**′ ə thē

any disease of the mouth _____/____/_____.

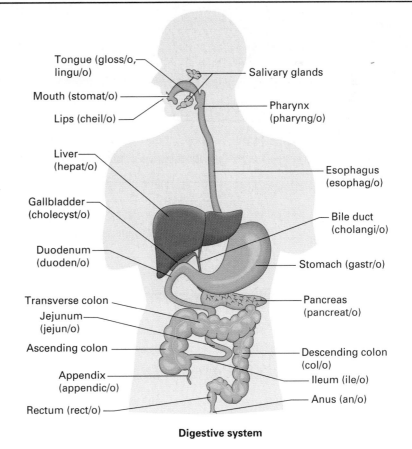

Tongue (gloss/o, lingu/o)

Salivary glands

Mouth (stomat/o)

Pharynx (pharyng/o)

Lips (cheil/o)

Liver (hepat/o)

Esophagus (esophag/o)

Gallbladder (cholecyst/o)

Bile duct (cholangi/o)

Duodenum (duoden/o)

Stomach (gastr/o)

Transverse colon

Pancreas (pancreat/o)

Jejunum (jejun/o)

Ascending colon

Descending colon (col/o)

Appendix (appendic/o)

Ileum (ile/o)

Anus (an/o)

Rectum (rect/o)

Digestive system

ANSWER COLUMN

7.5

Recall that **-scope** is a suffix for an instrument used to examine. A micr/o/scope is an instrument for examining something small. An instrument for examining the mouth is a _____/_____/_____.
The process of examining with this instrument
is _____/_____/_____.

stomat/o/scope
stō **mat**′ ō skōp
stomat/o/scopy
stō mə **tos**′ kə pē

7.6

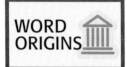

SPELL
CHECK ✓

Be careful to use stomat/o for mouth, not stomach. Remember, **gastr/o** means stomach.

7.7

inflammation of the tongue
excision of the tongue

The Greek combining form for tongue is **gloss/o** (think of a glossary of words). Gloss/itis means *_____.
Gloss/ectomy means *_____.

7.8

gloss/algia
glos **al**′ jē ə
gloss/al
glos′ əl

Using the word root, build words meaning pain in the tongue
_____/_____;

pertaining to the tongue _____/_____.

7.9

under the tongue or
  to the tongue
hypo/gloss/al
hī pō **glos**′ əl   or
sub/lingu/al
sub **lin**′ gwal

hypo- is a prefix meaning below or under. Cranial nerve XII is the hypo/gloss/al nerve. It supplies nerve impulses
*_____

_____.

A medication that is administered under the tongue
is a _____/_____/_____ medication.

7.10

WORD
ORIGINS 🏛

sub- and *lingual* are Latin word parts. **hypo-** and *glossal* are Greek word parts. Generally, original languages are not mixed when forming words. So, sublingual (Latin) and hypoglossal (Greek) are usually used.

ANSWER COLUMN

7.11

lingu/o is a Latin combining form for tongue (think of lingusitics or language). Lingu/al is the adjectival form. **sub-** is a prefix used with **lingu/o**. Build an adjective that means pertaining to under the tongue:

_____/_____/_____.

sub/lingu/al
sub **lin′** gwal

7.12

Nitroglycerin tablets are administered sub/lingual/ly. This means they are placed

under the tongue   * _____.

7.13

Two words that you have learned that mean under the tongue

hypo/gloss/al   are _____/_____/_____ and
sub/lingu/al   _____/_____/_____.

7.14

Using the combining form for tongue, build words meaning prolapse of the tongue

gloss/o/ptosis   _____/_____/_____;
glos op **tō′** sis   examination of the tongue
gloss/o/scopy   _____/_____/_____.
glos **os′** kə pē

7.15

-**plegia** is a suffix meaning paralysis. Build words meaning paralysis of the tongue

gloss/o/plegia   _____/_____/_____ (noun);
glos ō **plē′** jē ə   paralysis of the tongue
gloss/o/plegic   _____/_____/_____ (adjective).
glos ō **plē′** jik

7.16

cheil/o (note: e before i) is a combining form for lips. Cheil/itis means

inflammation of the lips   * _____.
plastic surgery of the lips   Cheil/o/plasty means * _____

_____.

7.17

cheil   The word root for lip is _____.
cheil/o   The combining form for lip is _____/_____.
kī′ lō

The oral cavity

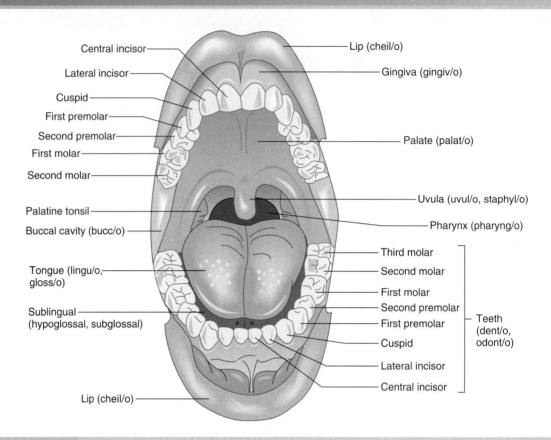

ANSWER COLUMN

7.18

Build words meaning incision of the lips

cheil/o/tomy
kī **lot**′ ə mē

_____/_____/_____;

condition or disorder of the lips

cheil/osis
kī **lō**′ sis

_____/_____.

7.19

A word meaning plastic surgery of the lips and mouth is

cheil/o/stomat/o/plasty
kī′ lō stō **mat**′ ə plas tē

_____/_____/_____/_____/_____.
    lips   mouth   repair

7.20

gingiv/o is the combining form for gums. Gingiv/al means

pertaining to the gums
gingiv/o

*_____.

The combining form for gums is _____/_____.

7.21

Build words meaning inflammation of the gums

gingiv/itis
jin ji **vī**′ tis

_____/_____;

ANSWER COLUMN

gingiv/algia
jin ji **val**′ jē ə

gum pain _____/_____.

7.22

Build words meaning excision of gum tissue

gingiv/ectomy
jin ji **vek**′ tə mē

_____/_____;

gingiv/o/gloss/itis
jin′ ji vō glos **ī**′ tis

inflammation of the gums and tongue

_____/_____/_____/_____;

lingu/o/gingiv/al
lin′ gwō **jin**′ ji vəl

tongue and gums (adjective)

_____/_____/_____/_____.

7.23

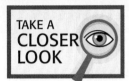

TAKE A CLOSER LOOK

Food is chewed by the teeth (mastica/tion) and mixed with saliva in the mouth. It is then pushed into the pharynx by the tongue and a series of smooth muscle contractions called peristalsis sends it down the esophagus to the stomach (inges/tion). In the stomach, food is mixed with hydrochloric acid (HCl) and enzymes that begin chemical breakdown. Next, it travels to the duodenum. Digestive enzymes are secreted from the duodenal wall and the pancreas, and bile is added from the gallbladder. The enzymes break up starches into glucose, proteins into amino acids, and the bile emulsifies fats (diges/tion). Nutrients including water are absorbed through the small and large intestinal walls into the blood and lymphatic system (absorp/tion). The undigested and unabsorbed food called feces or stool travels through the large intestine to the rectum and is expelled through the anus (defeca/tion).

7.24

From what you have just read, list the words that mean the following:

process of chewing

mastica/tion
ma sti **kā**′ shun

_____/_____;

process of swallowing

inges/tion
in **jest**′ shun

_____/_____;

chemical breakdown of food

diges/tion
dī **jest**′ shun

_____/_____;

movement of nutrients from intestine to the blood

absorp/tion
ab **sorp**′ shun

_____/_____;

expelling solid waste

defeca/tion
de fə **ka**′ shun

_____/_____;

solid waste material

feces
fē sēs

_____ or

stool
stōol

_____.

ANSWER COLUMN

7.25

eso- means in or toward and phag/o means swallow. **esophag/o** is used in words about the esophagus. The adjective is _____/_____.

esophag/eal
ē so fa **jē**′ al

word root   suffix

7.26

sten/osis is a condition of narrowing that may occur in a tube or passageway. Mitral stenosis is a narrowing of the mitral valve opening in the heart. Esophag/o/sten/osis is a narrowing of the _____/_____.

esophag/us
ē **so**′ fə gus

7.27

A person experiencing dysphagia may have a narrowing of the esophagus or _____/_____/_____/_____.

esophag/o/sten/osis
ē so′ fə gō sten **ō**′ sis

7.28

Build an adjective meaning pertaining to the esophagus and stomach:
_____/_____/_____/_____ or
_____/_____/_____/_____.

esophag/o/gastr/ic
gastr/o/esophag/eal
(You pronounce)

7.29

Gastr/o/esophag/eal reflux disease (GERD) causes the gastric and duodenal juices to enter and irritate the esophagus. A person who has chronic heartburn and throat irritation may be suffering from
_____/_____/_____/_____ reflux disease.

gastr/o/esophag/eal
gas′ trō ē sof ə **gē**′ əl

7.30

Not eating just before going to bed, avoiding fatty foods, losing weight, and elevating the head of the bed are all recommendations for people who have GERD or
*_____
_____.

gastroesophageal
   reflux disease

7.31

stomach hemorrhage
inflammation of
   the stomach
pertaining to the stomach

Gastr/o/rrhagia means *_____.
Gastr/itis means *_____.
Gastr/ic means *_____
_____.

ANSWER COLUMN

TAKE A CLOSER LOOK

7.32

An organism called *Helicobacter pylori* (HP) has been found to be a common cause of gastritis in children and adults. It is transmitted through contamination with gastrointestinal substances such as vomit or feces. Symptoms of HP infection include epi/gastr/ic pain, nausea, vomiting, and dys/pepsia. This bacterial infection is treated with antibiotics and H2 antagonists (gastric secretion inhibitors).

7.33

-ectasia (or ectasis) is a suffix meaning stretching or dilatation.
Form words meaning
dilatation (stretching) of the stomach

gastr/ectasia
gas trek **tā**′ shə

_____/_____;

prolapse of the stomach and small intestine

gastr/o/enter/o/ptosis
gas′ trō en′ tər op **tō**′ sis

_____/_____/_____/_____/_____.

7.34

enter/o is used in words about the small intestine or the intestine in general. Tablets that dissolve in the intestine may have an enter/ic coating. Inflammation of the intestine is _____/_____.

enter/itis
en ter **ī**′ tis

7.35

The internal medicine specialty that studies diseases of the stomach and intestine is _____/_____/_____/_____/_____.

gastr/o/enter/o/logy
gas′ trō en′ ter **ol**′ ō gē

7.36

Recall the prefix **dys-**, meaning difficulty or pain. Dys/entery is a disorder of the intestine characterized by inflammation, pain, and dia/rrhea. When caused by an amoeba-type parasite, it is called amoebic _____/_____/_____.

dys/enter/y
dis′ en tair ē

7.37

Form words meaning
pertaining to the stomach and small intestine

gastr/o/enter/ic
gas′ trō en **tair**′ ik

_____/_____/_____/_____;

hemorrhage of the small intestine

enter/o/rrhagia
en tə rō **rā**′ jē ə

_____/_____/_____.

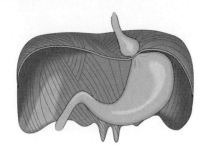

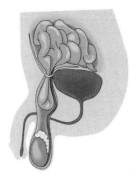

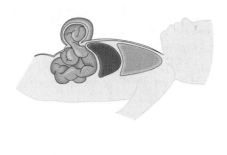

Hiatal hernia **Inguinal hernia** **Umbilical hernia**

ANSWER COLUMN

7.38

Build words meaning
intestinal hernia

enter/o/cele
en′ tə rō sēl
enter/o/clysis
en tə **rok**′ lə sis

_____/_____/_____;

washing or irrigation of the small intestine

_____/_____/_____.

7.39

Build words meaning
paralysis of the small intestine

enter/o/plegia
en tə rō **plē**′ jē ə
enter/ectasia
en tə rek **tā**′ shə

_____/_____/_____;

dilatation of the small intestine

_____/_____.

7.40

prolapse of the
  small intestine
surgical puncture of
  the small intestine

Enter/o/ptosis means *_____.

_____

Enter/o/centesis means *_____

_____.

7.41

col/o is the combining form for colon (large intestine).
Col/ic or colonic means

pertaining to the colon
  or large intestine
surgical puncture
  of the colon

*_____

_____.

Col/o/centesis means *_____

_____.

ANSWER COLUMN

col/o/pexy
kō′ lō pek sē, **kol′** ō pek sē
col/ostomy
ko **los′** tə mē
col/o/ptosis
kōl′ op **tō′** sis

7.42

Build words meaning
surgical fixation of the colon
_____/_____/_____ ;
making a new opening into the colon
_____/_____ ;
prolapse of the colon
_____/_____/_____.

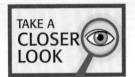

7.43

Constipation, irritable bowel syndrome, and diverticular disease are all disorders associated with slow colonic motility (movement). Although each is treated with different medications, their treatments all include an increase in dietary fiber or a dietary fiber supplement. Chronic lack of moisture and bulk in the feces makes it more difficult for the intestinal muscles to push waste along. The intestine may develop weak walls, pouches, and/or infection.

7.44

Diverticula (singular, diverticulum) are outpouchings or pockets that develop in the colon wall. The presence of diverticula is a condition called diverticul/osis. Food may get trapped in these pockets, putrify, and irritate the tissues causing infection and inflammation of the diverticula. Inflammation of the diverticula is called _____/_____.

diverticul/itis
dī′ ver tik yōō **lī′** tis

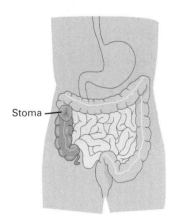

Stoma

Ascending colostomy

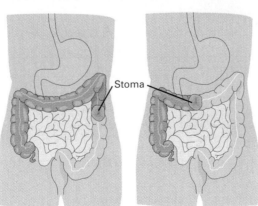

Stoma

Descending colostomy

Transverse colostomy

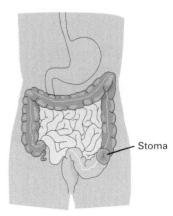

Stoma

Sigmoid colostomy

Colostomy sites

ANSWER COLUMN

7.45

Chronic abdominal pain, cramping, and changes in bowel habits may all
be symptoms of either irritable bowel disease (condition)

diverticul/osis
dī′ ver tik yōō **lō**′ sis

or _____/_____.

7.46

-clysis is a suffix meaning washing or irrigation. Build words meaning washing or
irrigation of the colon

col/o/clysis
kō **lok**′ lə sis
gastr/o/clysis
gas **trok**′ lə sis

_____/_____/_____;

of the stomach

_____/_____/_____.

7.47

Irrigation of the small intestine using contrast media may be done to better view
the small intestine on x-rays. This is called

enter/o/clysis
en′ tr **ok**′ lə sis
enter/o/scope
en′ tə rō skōp

_____/_____/_____.

An instrument to examine the small intestine is the

_____/_____/_____.

7.48

sigmoid/o refers to the sigmoid colon. An instrument used to examine the

sigmoid/o/scope
sig **moid**′ ō skōp
sigmoid/o/scopy
sig moid **ōs**′ kō pē

sigmoid colon is the _____/_____/_____.

The procedure is called _____/_____/_____.

7.49

The combining form for rectum is **rect/o**. Rect/al means

pertaining to the rectum
a rectal hernia or
  herniation of the rectum

* _____.

A rect/o/cele is * _____

_____.

7.50

Build words meaning
washing or irrigation of the rectum

rect/o/clysis
rek **tok**′ lə sis
rect/o/scope
rek′ tə skōp
col/o/rect/al
kō lō **rek**′ təl

_____/_____/_____;

instrument for examining the rectum

_____/_____/_____;

pertaining to the colon and rectum

_____/_____/_____/_____.

ANSWER COLUMN
Diverticulosis

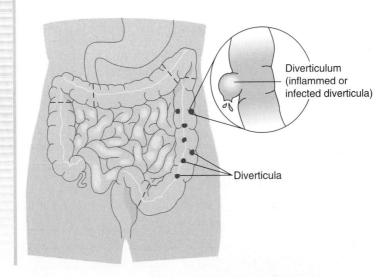

Diverticulum
(inflammed or
infected diverticula)

Diverticula

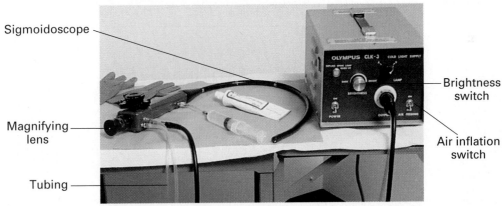

Sigmoidoscope

Brightness
switch

Magnifying
lens

Air inflation
switch

Tubing

Parts of the sigmoidoscope

7.51

rect/o/scopy
rek **tos′** kə pē
rect/ō/scopic
rek tə **skop′** ik

The process of examining the rectum with a rect/o/scope is called
_____/_____/_____. In doing this, the physician
has performed a
_____/_____/_____ examination.
   (adjective)

NOTE: A more common procedure is a sigmoid/o/scopy. This is done using an
endoscope introduced through the anus and rectum to the sigmoid colon.

7.52

rect/o/plasty
rek′ tə plas tē
rect/o/rrhaphy
rek **tōr′** ə fē

Build words meaning
plastic surgery of the rectum
_____/_____/_____;
suturing (stitching) of the rectum
_____/_____/_____.

ANSWER COLUMN

7.53

Build words meaning
pertaining to the rectum and urethra

rect/o/urethr/al
rek tō yoo **rē**′ thrəl
rect/o/cyst/ō/tomy
rek′ tō sis **tot**′ ə mē

_____/_____/_____/_____;
incision of the bladder through the rectum
_____/_____/_____/_____/_____.

    rectum   bladder   incision

7.54

specializes in diseases of
  the anus and rectum
the study of diseases of
  the anus and rectum

proct/o is the combining form for anus and rectum.
A proct/o/logist is one who *_____
_____.

Proct/o/logy is *_____
_____.

7.55

proct/o/clysis
prok **tok**′ lə sis
proct/ō/plegia
prok tə **plē**′ jē ə
proct/o/scope
prok′ tə skōp
proct/o/scopy
prok **tos**′ kə pē

Build words meaning
washing or irrigation of anus and rectum
_____/_____/_____;
paralysis of the anus and rectum
_____/_____/_____.
A proct/o/logist examines the rectum and anus with a
_____/_____/_____.
This examination is called
_____/_____/_____.

7.56

proct/o/rrhaphy
prok **tôr**′ ə fē
proct/ō/pexy
prok′ tō peks ē

Build words meaning
suturing of the rectum and anus
_____/_____/_____;
surgical fixation of the rectum and anus
_____/_____/_____.

7.57

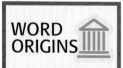
WORD ORIGINS

Catharsis comes from the Greek word *katharsis* meaning purification. A catharsis may be an emotional release from anxiety caused by repressed events. In many ancient Greek plays, the purpose of the story was to produce catharsis for the audience members by acting out their anxieties and giving them an experience of relief. Today, psychoanalysis often works toward this goal by creating an experience of emotional release or catharsis.

ANSWER COLUMN

7.58

Cathartics (laxatives) cause liquification of the stool or relaxation of the bowel to ease defecation producing physical relief. Another name for laxative is
_____/_____.

cathar/tic
ka **thar**′ tik

7.59

Eating a high-fiber diet and increasing water intake may also treat and prevent infrequency of bowel movement (BM) or

constipation
_____.

7.60

Infrequent or small amount of bowel movement is an indication of con/stip/ation. This term comes from Latin word parts meaning to withhold or press together. Slow bowel motility due to anesthesia use, aging, dehydration, or low-fiber intake may be causes of _____.

con/stip/ation
kon sti **pā**′ shun

7.61

The liver has many functions including the production of heparin, which affects the blood-clotting mechanism. It also produces bile. **hepat/o** is the combining form for liver. It comes from the Greek word *hepar,* meaning liver. Hepat/ic

pertaining to the liver
enlargement of the liver
means *_____.
Hepat/o/megaly means *_____
_____.

7.62

Build words meaning
inspection (examination) of the liver

hepat/o/scopy
hep ə **tos**′ kə pē
hepat/ō/pathy
hep ə **top**′ ə thē
_____/_____/_____;
any disease of the liver
_____/_____/_____.

7.63

Build words meaning
incision into the liver

hepat/o/tomy
hep ə **tot**′ ə mē
hepat/ēctomy
hep ə **tek**′ tə mē
_____/_____/_____;
excision of (part of) the liver
_____/_____.

ANSWER COLUMN

7.64

hepat/itis
hep ə **tīt'** is

Hepat/itis is inflammation of the liver. Hepatitis B is a serious condition of the liver caused by a viral infection. Hepatitis B vaccine (Hep B) may be administered as an immunization protection against _____/_____.

7.65

TAKE A
CLOSER
LOOK

According to the National Center for Infectious Diseases, there are five types of viral hepatitis. The three most common forms are Hepatitis A, B, and C.

Hepatitis A (HAV infection) is an acute infection associated with food or water that is contaminated by human waste.

Hepatitis B (HBV infection) is classified as an STD and is transmitted by blood and body fluids.

Hepatitis C (HCV infection) is a chronic condition usually passed through the blood.

7.66

hepat/itis

Using standard precautions to avoid contact with the potentially infections body fluids of others helps to prevent _____/_____ and other viral and bacterial infections.

7.67

pertaining to the pancreas
destruction of
  pancreatic tissue

The pancreas is both a digestive and an endocrine organ. pancreat/o is used in words about the pancreas.
Pancreat/ic means
*_____.
Pancreat/o/lysis means
*_____.

7.68

pancreat/o/lith
pan krē **at'** ō lith
pancreat/o/pathy
pan' krē ə **top'** ə thē

Build words meaning
a stone or calculus in the pancreas
_____/_____/_____;
any pancreatic disease
_____/_____/_____.

7.69

pancreat/ectomy
pan' krē ə **tek'** tə mē

Build words meaning
excision of part or all of the pancreas
_____/_____;

ANSWER COLUMN

pancreat/o/tomy
pan′ krē ə **tot**′ ə mē

incision into the pancreas

_____/_____/_____.

7.70

Recall that cholelithiasis is a condition in which gallstones have formed in the gallbladder. Choleliths can also lodge in the biliary duct blocking bile flow or in the pancreatic ducts causing pancreatitis. An x-ray of the gallbladder is called

chol/e/cyst/o/graph   or
chol/e/cyst/o/gram

_____/_____/_____/_____/_____.

NOTE: -graph originally meant machine, but in practice it has come to mean the x-ray picture (film) itself.

7.71

Build words meaning inflammation of the pancreas

pancreat/itis
pan′ krē ə **tīt**′ is
chol/e/cyst/itis
kōl′ ē sis **tīt**′ is

_____/_____;

gallbladder

_____/_____/_____/_____.

7.72

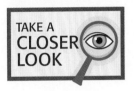

An endoscope can be used to insert a cannula (tube) into the common bile duct or the pancreatic duct. Contrast media is introduced and an x-ray taken. This procedure is known by its abbreviation ERCP, which stands for endoscopic retrograde cholangi/o/pancreat/o/graphy. Look up ERCP in your dictionary or medical text reference and read about it. If a physician is trying to locate a stone that is difficult to see, a

cholangi/o/pancreat/o/-
  graphy
kōl an′ jē ō pan′ krē ə **tog**′
  raf ē

_____/_____/_____/_____/_____

may be ordered.

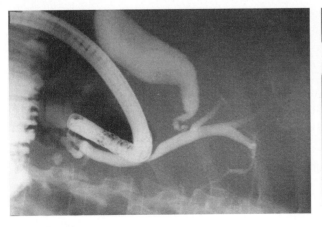

Normal ERCP

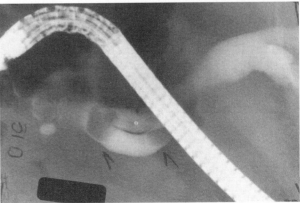

ERCP with stones

ANSWER COLUMN

7.73

Build words meaning
hemorrhage of the liver

_____/_____/_____;

hepat/o/rrhagia
hep ə tō **rā**′ jē ə

suture of a wound of the liver

_____/_____/_____.

hepat/o/rrhaphy
hep ə **tôr**′ ə fē

7.74

Build words meaning
hernia of the liver

_____/_____/_____;

hepat/o/cele
hep **at**′ ō sēl

pain in the liver

_____/_____/_____;

hepat/o/dynia
hep at ō **din**′ ē ə

stone in the liver

_____/_____/_____.

hepat/o/lith
hep **at**′ ō lith

7.75

A/tresia literally means not perforated or not open. Biliary atresia is a condition in which the bile ducts are not open. A congenital condition in which a part of the intestine is closed is intestinal

_____/_____.

a/tresia
a **trē**′ zē ə

7.76

closed
atresia

If a baby is born with esophageal atresia, the esophagus would be _____.
In the heart, congenital closure of the mitral valve is mitral _____.

7.77

atresia

Bile backs up into the liver if the ducts are closed or blocked. Biliary
_____ is a serious condition.

7.78

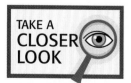

Another debilitating liver disease is cirrh/osis of the liver. In Greek, *kirrhos* means orange-yellow. This disease occurs as a result of malnutrition, alcoholism, poisoning, or a history of hepatitis. Treatment of cirrhosis depends on its cause and may include diet modifications, vitamin supplements, cessation of alcohol use with related support groups, energy conservation, and possibly surgery.

ANSWER COLUMN

7.79

cirrh/osis
si **rō**′ sis

Chronic alcoholism or hepatitis may lead to a dysfunctional liver disease called _____/_____.

7.80

splen/o is used in words about the spleen. Build words meaning

splen/ectomy
spli **nek**′ tə mē
splen/o/megaly
splen ō **meg**′ ə lē
splen/o/ptosis
splen op **tō**′ sis

excision of the spleen

_____/_____;

enlargement of the spleen

_____/_____/_____;

prolapse of the spleen

_____/_____/_____.

7.81

SPELL CHECK ✔

Watch your spelling in words about the spleen. The noun spleen has two *es*, but the combining form has one *e*, i.e., **splen/o**.

7.82

splen/o/pexy
splen′ ō peks ē
splen/o/pathy
splen **op**′ ə thē
splen/ō/rrhaphy
splen **ôr**′ ə fē
splen/ō/rrhagia
splen ō **rā**′ jē ə

Build words meaning
surgical fixation of the spleen

_____/_____/_____;

any disease of the spleen

_____/_____/_____;

suture of the spleen

_____/_____/_____;

hemorrhage from the spleen

_____/_____/_____.

7.83

pain in the spleen

The spleen is one of the blood-forming organs.
Splen/algia means *_____.

7.84

pertaining to the spleen

Splen/ic means *_____.

ANSWER COLUMN

7.85

Recall the suffix **-ostomy**. Anastomosis is a surgical connection between tubular structures. The combining form for esophagus is **esophag/o**. When an entire gastrectomy is performed, a new connection is made between the esophagus and the duodenum. This particular anastomosis can also be called an
_____/____/_____/_____.

esophag/o/duoden/ostomy
i **sof′** ə gō dōō ə də **nos′**-
tə mē

7.86

All of the following operations are types of anastomoses. Using what you have learned about the digestive system, list the body parts indicated in these procedures.
gastr/o/enter/o/col/ostomy

stomach, small intestine,
  and large intestine

*_____

esophag/o/gastr/ostomy

esophagus, stomach

*_____

enter/o/cholecyst/ostomy

small intestine, gallbladder

*_____

7.87

Some medical words get pretty long. Insert the slashes and define the following terms.
jejunoileitis

jejun/o/ile/itis
inflammation of the
  jejunum and ileum

_____
*_____

cholecystoduodenostomy

chole/cyst/o/duoden/-
  ostomy
new opening between the
  duodenum and gallbladder

_____
*_____

esophag/o/gastr/o/-
  duoden/o/scopy
examination of the
  esophagus, stomach,
  and duodenum

esophagogastroduodenoscopy (EGD)

_____
*_____

chol/angi/o/pancreat/o/-
  graphy
x-ray of the biliary and
  pancreatic ducts

cholangiopancreatography

_____
*_____

Good!

ANSWER COLUMN

Abbreviation	Meaning
BM	bowel movement
po	by mouth (Latin: *per os*), orally
NPO, npo	nothing by mouth
EGD	esophagogastroduodenoscopy
ERCP	endoscopic retrograde cholangiopancreatography
GERD	gastroesophageal reflux disease
Hep B	hepatitis B vaccine
HAV	hepatitis A virus
HBV	hepatitis B virus
HCV	hepatitis C virus
HP	*Helicobacter pylori*
GI	gastrointestinal
GB	gallbladder
NG	nasogastric
HCL	hydrochloric acid
BE	Barium enema

To complete your study of this unit, work the **Review Activities** on the following pages. Also, listen to the audio CDs that accompany *Medical Terminology: A Programmed Systems Approach,* 9th edition, and practice your pronunciation.

Additional practice exercises for this unit are available on the Learner Practice CD-ROM found in the back of the textbook.

REVIEW ACTIVITIES

CIRCLE AND CORRECT

Circle the correct answer for each question. Then check your answers in Appendix A.

1. Suffix for dilatation or stretching
   - a. -dilatate
   - b. -clysis
   - c. -ectomy
   - d. -ectasia

2. Prefix for below
   - a. epi-
   - b. inter-
   - c. sub-
   - d. supra-

3. Combining form for small intestine or intestine
   - a. colpo
   - b. entero
   - c. duodeno
   - d. intestino

4. Combining form for liver
   - a. hepat
   - b. hepato
   - c. heparin
   - d. livo

REVIEW ACTIVITIES

5. Suffix for paralysis
   a. -plasia   b. -phagia
   c. -plegia   d. - phasia

6. Prefix for difficult or painful
   a. sub-   b. dynia-
   c. algia-   d. dys-

7. Combining form for spleen
   a. spleno   b. spleeno
   c. spleen   d. splenic

8. Suffix for making a new opening
   a. -tomy   b. -ostomy
   c. -tome   d. -scopy

9. Suffix for irrigation or washing
   a. -colo   b. -ecstasia
   c. -clysis   d. -enema

10. Word root for stomach
    a. stomato   b. stomacho
    c. cheilo   d. gastr

11. Stenosis means
    a. dilation   b. discharge
    c. tubelike   d. narrowing

12. The term for a congenital condition in which a tube is closed is:
    a. stenosis   b. coloclysis
    c. atresia   d. anastomosis

SELECT AND CONSTRUCT

Select the correct word parts from the following list and construct medical terms that represent the given meaning.

al	algia	angi/o	cele	cheilo
chol(e)	clysis	colo	duoden(o)	dys
ectasia	ectomy	entero(ic)	esophago(eal)	gastr(o)(ic)
gingiv(o)(a)	glosso(al)	graphy	hepato(i)c	hypo
ileo	itis	jejuno	linguo(al)	lith
megaly	myc(osis)	ostomy	pancreato	pathy
plasty	pleg(ic)(ia)	procto	ptosis	rect(o)(al)
rrhagia	rrhaphy	rrhea	scope(y)(ic)	sigmoid(o)
sis	spleno	stomato	sub	tomy

1. fungal infection of the mouth   _____

2. below the tongue   _____

3. surgical repair of the lips   _____

4. inflammation of the gums   _____

5. bleeding of the small intestine   _____

6. process of examining the esophagus, stomach, and duodenum by looking with an instrument   _____

7. prolapse of the small intestine   _____

8. irrigation of the rectum   _____

9. paralysis of the anus and rectum   _____

10. stone in the pancreas   _____

REVIEW ACTIVITIES

11. enlargement of the spleen

_____

12. dilatation of the stomach

_____

13. instrument for looking in the sigmoid colon

_____

14. inflammation of the liver

_____

15. herniation of the rectum

_____

16. pertaining to stomach and esophagus

_____

17. x-ray process of biliary and pancreatic ducts

_____

18. pertaining to colon and rectum

_____

DEFINE AND DISSECT

Give a brief definition and dissect each term listed into its word parts in the space provided. Check your answers by referring to the frame listed in parentheses and your medical dictionary. Then listen to the CD to practice pronunciation.

1. cheilostomatoplasty (7.19)

_____/___/_____/___/_____
rt   v   rt   v   suffix

_____
definition

2. gingivoglossitis (7.22)

_____/___/_____/_____
rt   v   rt   suffix

_____

3. gastrorrhagia (7.31)

_____/___/_____
rt   v   suffix

_____

4. esophageal (7.25)

_____/____
rt   suffix

_____

5. enterocentesis (7.40)

_____/___/_____
rt   v   rt/suffix

_____

6. dysentery (7.36)

_____/_____/_____
pre   rt   suffix

_____

7. colopexy (7.42)

_____/___/_____
rt   v   suffix

_____

REVIEW ACTIVITIES

8. rectocele (7.49)

_____/___/_____
rt   v   suffix

9. proctologist (7.54)

_____/___/_____
rt   v   suffix

10. hepatomegaly (7.61)

_____/___/_____
rt   v   suffix

11. pancreatolysis (7.67)

_____/___/_____
rt   v   suffix

12. splenorrhagia (7.82)

_____/___/_____
rt   v   suffix

13. esophagoduodenostomy (7.85)

_____/__/_____/_____
rt   v   rt   suffix

14. diverticulitis (7.44)

_____/_____
rt   suffix

15. cathartic (7.58)

_____/_____
rt   suffix

16. sigmoidoscopy (7.48)

_____/___/_____
rt   v   suffix

17. coloclysis (7.46)

_____/___/_____
rt   v   suffix

18. enterectasia (7.39)

_____/_____
rt   suffix

REVIEW ACTIVITIES

19. glossoplegia (7.15)

_____/____/_____

rt   v   suffix

_____

20. sublingual (7.11)

_____/_____/_____

pre   rt   suffix

_____

21. gastroenterology (7.35)

_____/_____/_____/____/_____

rt   v   rt   v   suffix

_____

22. hepatitis (7.64)

_____/_____

rt   suffix

_____

23. esophagospasm (table page 226)

_____/____/_____

rt   v   suffix

_____

24. gingivectomy (7.22)

_____/_____

rt   suffix

_____

25. stomatomycosis (7.4)

_____/____/_____/____

rt   v   rt   suffix

_____

26. esophagostenosis (7.27)

_____/____/_____/_____

rt   v   rt   suffix

_____

27. cholangiopancreatography (7.72)

_____/____/_____/____/_____

rt   v   rt   v   suffix

_____

28. cirrhosis (7.79)

_____/_____

rt   suffix

_____

REVIEW ACTIVITIES

ART LABELING

Label the diagram of the digestive system by writing the number in the blank.

Write the body part indicated correct word.

_____	hepat/o	_____
_____	gastr/o	_____
_____	col/o	_____
_____	esophag/o	_____
_____	stomat/o	_____
_____	pancreat/o	_____
_____	sigmoid/o	_____
_____	pharyng/o	_____
_____	cholecyst/o	_____
_____	rect/o	_____
_____	duoden/o	_____
_____	appendic/o	_____

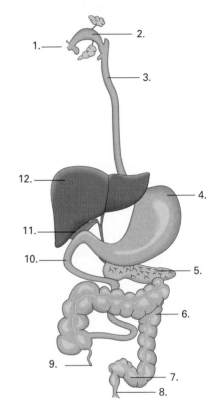

Digestive System

REVIEW ACTIVITIES

ABBREVIATION MATCHING

Match the following abbreviations with their definition.

_____ 1. GB   a. *Helicobacter pylori*

_____ 2. EGD   b. hepatomegaly

_____ 3. GI   c. gums and incisors

_____ 4. po   d. sublingually

_____ 5. npo   e. bowel movement

_____ 6. HBV   f. gallbladder

_____ 7. GERD   g. nothing by mouth

_____ 8. ERCP   h. hepatitis B virus

_____ 9. NG   i. gastrointestinal

_____ 10. BM   j. orally

_____ 11. HP   k. esophagogastroduodenostomy

                          l. esophagogastroduodenoscopy

                          m. AIDS virus

                          n. *Escherichia coli*

                          o. gastroesophageal reflux disease

                          p. after meals

                          q. endoscopic retrograde cholangiopancreatography

                          r. nasogastric (tube)

SUFFIX MATCHING

Match the suffixes on the left with their meanings on the right.

_____ 1. -plegia   a. stretching, dilation

_____ 2. -clysis   b. uncontrolled twitching

_____ 3. -ectasia   c. new permanent opening

_____ 4. -rrhagia   d. suturing

_____ 5. -megaly   e. washing, irrigation

_____ 6. -ostomy   f. hemorrhage

                          g. herniation

                          h. enlarged

                          i. incision into

                          j. paralysis

REVIEW ACTIVITIES

CASE STUDIES

Write the term next to its meaning given below. Then draw slashes to analyze the word parts. Note the use of medical abbreviations. Look these up in your dictionary or find them in Appendix B. If you have any questions about the answers, refer to your medical dictionary or check with your instructor for the answers in Appendix A.

CASE STUDY 7-1

Endoscopy Report

Pt: Female, age 89

Dx: **Gastrointestinal hemorrhage**, duodenal ulcer Tx: **EGD**

Ms. Dena Jitters was admitted through the emergency room because of **vomiting** coffee-grounds material, and passing **melenic** stools. The **nasogastric** tube introduced and showed bright red blood. The patient became **hypotensive** and two units of packed red cells were given. Ms. Jitters became stable with a BP of 120/80. She was lavaged with iced **isotonic** saline and an endoscopy was performed.

REPORT: Premedication: Cetacaine locally. The **endoscope** was easily passed into the esophagus. Numerous amounts of **thrombi** were noted. The scope was introduced into the stomach, which showed increased amounts of bright red blood in the fundus. No **mucosal** lesions could be seen; however, half of the stomach was full of blood. The scope was then passed into the **duodenal** bulb, where clots were also noted. This patient could have a duodenal **ulcer** but because of the amount of blood, it is difficult to delineate an ulcer crater.

A great clot was located on the **anterior** wall. As the scope was withdrawn, the antrum of the stomach could be seen with no lesion noted. It was difficult to clean up all the blood clots and, because of the status of the patient, the procedure was discontinued. Ms. Jitters tolerated the procedure well and did not vomit or **aspirate**.

1. front _____
2. ejecting from the stomach
   through the mouth _____
3. bleed _____
4. pertaining to the nose and stomach _____
5. instrument used to look into _____
6. pertaining to mucosa _____
7. breathe in (suck in) _____
8. having the same concentration _____
9. sore _____
10. pertaining to the stomach and intestine _____
11. black, old blood (adjective) _____
12. low blood pressure (adjective) _____
13. first part of small intestine (adjective) _____
14. clots _____
15. esophagogastroduodenoscopy _____

REVIEW ACTIVITIES

CROSSWORD PUZZLE

Check your answers by going back through the frames or checking the solution in Appendix C.

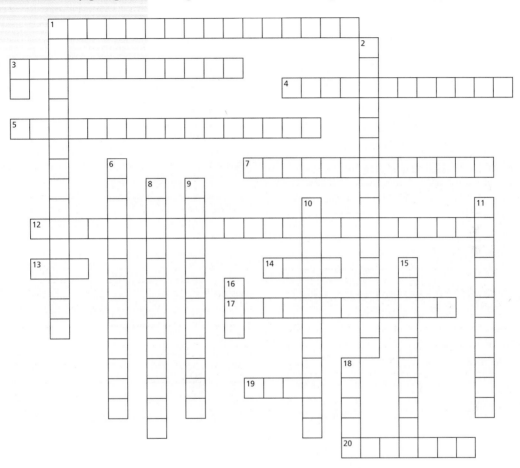

Across

1. specialty in the study of the stomach and the intestine
3. stretching of the stomach
4. enlarged spleen
5. gallbladder x-ray
7. surgical repair of the gums
12. x-ray of the bile ducts (vessels) and pancreatic ducts (process)
13. esophagogastro-duodenoscopy (abbreviation)
14. suffix for stone
17. inflammation of the pancreas
19. endoscopic retrograde cholangiopancreatography (abbreviation)
20. condition of a closed tube or duct (often congenital)

Down

1. pertaining to the stomach and esophagus
2. inflamed gums and tongue
3. gastrointestinal (abbreviation)
6. hemorrhage of the liver
8. instrument used to look into the sigmoid colon
9. irrigation of the anus and rectum
10. suture of the rectum
11. sublingual (synonym)
15. herniation of the intestine
16. nothing by mouth (abbreviation)
18. Greek for mouth

REVIEW ACTIVITIES

GLOSSARY

absorption	movement of nutrients from one layer to another
anastomosis	connecting two tubular structures
atresia	closed ducts or tubes
cathartic	agent that relieves constipation (synonym, laxative)
cheiloplasty	surgical repair of the lips
cheilosis	condition of the lips
cheilostomatoplasty	repair of the lips and mouth
cheilotomy	incision into the lip
cholangio-pancreatography	process of taking X-ray of the biliary and pancreatic ducts using contrast media
cholecystograph (cholecystogram)	X-ray picture of the gallbladder
cirrhosis	chronic liver disease causing loss of liver function and resistance to blood flow through the liver. Etiology may include poor nutrition, alcoholism, previous hepatitis
colic	pertaining to the colon (synonym; colonic)
colocentesis	surgical puncture of the colon to remove fluid
coloclysis	irrigation of the colon
colopexy	surgical fixation of the colon
coloptosis	prolapsed colon
colorectal	pertaining to the colon and rectum
colostomy	making a new opening (stoma) in the colon

constipation	hard stool, infrequent bowel movements
diverticulitis	inflammation of diverticula of the intestine
digestion	breakdown of food
defecation	expelling feces
diverticulosis	condition of having diverticula
dysentery	inflammation of the intestine, pain, diarrhea
enterectasia	stretching of the intestine
enteritis	inflammation of the intestine
enterocele	intestinal hernia
enterocentesis	surgical puncture of the intestine to remove fluid
enteroclysis	irrigation of the intestine
enteroplegia	paralysis of the intestine
enteroptosis	prolapse of the intestine
enterorrhagia	hemorrhage of the intestine
enteroscope	instrument for examining the intestine
esophageal	pertaining to the esophagus
esophagoduodenostomy	anastomosis between the esophagus and duodenum
esophagogastric	pertaining to the esophagus and stomach
esophagostenosis	narrowing of the esophagus
feces	stool, solid waste
gastrectasia	dilatation of the stomach
gastric	pertaining to the stomach
gastritis	inflammation of the stomach

REVIEW ACTIVITIES

gastroclysis	irrigation of the stomach
gastroenteric	pertaining to the stomach and intestine
gastroenterology	the study of diseases of the stomach and intestine
gastroenteroptosis	prolapse of stomach and intestine
gastrorrhagia	hemorrhage of the stomach
gingival	pertaining to the gums
gingivalgia	gum pain
gingivectomy	excision of the gums
gingivoglossitis	inflammation of the gums and tongue
glossal	pertaining to the tongue
glossalgia	tongue pain
glossoplegia	tongue paralysis (adjective, glossoplegic)
glossoptosis	prolapse of the tongue
glossoscopy	examination of the tongue with a scope
hepatectomy	excision of the liver
hepatitis	inflammation of the liver
hepatocele	herniation of the liver
hepatodynia	liver pain (hepatalgia)
hepatolith	liver stone
hepatopathy	any disease of the liver
hepatorrhagia	hemorrhage of the liver
hepatorrhaphy	suture of the liver
hepatoscope	instrument for examining the liver
hepatoscopy	process of using a hepatoscope

hypoglossal	pertaining to below the tongue (synonym, sublingual)
ingestion	swallowing, eating
linguogingival	pertaining to the gums and tongue
mastication	chewing
pancreatectomy	excision of the pancreas
pancreatic	pertaining to the pancreas
pancreatolith	stone in the pancreas
pancreatolysis	destruction of pancreatic tissue
pancreatopathy	any disease of the pancreas
proctoclysis	irrigation of the rectum and anus
proctologist	physician specialist in diseases of the anus and rectum
proctopexy	fixation of a prolapsed anus and rectum (synonyn, rectopexy)
proctoplegia	paralysis of the rectum and anus
proctorrhaphy	suture of the anus and rectum
proctoscope	instrument for examining the anus and rectum
proctoscopy	process of using a proctoscope
rectocele	herniation of the rectum
rectoclysis	irrigation of the rectum
rectocystotomy	incision into the urinary bladder through the rectum
rectoplasty	surgical repair of the rectum
rectorrhaphy	suturing of the rectum
rectoscope	instrument used to examine the rectum

REVIEW ACTIVITIES

rectoscopy	process of using a rectoscope (adjective, rectoscopic)
rectourethral	pertaining to the rectum and urethra
sigmoidoscope	instrument for examining the sigmoid and large colon
splenectomy	excision of the spleen
splenomegaly	enlarged spleen
splenopathy	any disease of the spleen
splenopexy	fixation of a prolapsed spleen
splenoptosis	prolapsed spleen
splenorrhagia	hemorrhage of the spleen
splenorrhaphy	suturing of the spleen
stomatalgia	mouth pain
stomatitis	inflammation of the mouth
stomatomycosis	fungal condition of the mouth
stomatopathy	any disease of the mouth
stomatoplasty	surgical repair of the mouth
stomatorrhagia	hemorrhage of the mouth
stomatoscope	instrument used to examine the mouth
stomatoscopy	process of using a stomatoscope

UNIT 8

Neurology, Psychology, Anesthesiology, and Vascular Terminology

Read through the list of word parts in the following table. Then work the frames in the first part of this unit. Refer back to this list when necessary.

Combining Form	Combining Form	Suffix
neur/o (nerve or neuron)	**blast/o** (germ or embryonic; gives rise to something else)	**-blast** (word itself)
angi/o (vessel)		**-spasm** (word itself)
		-osis (use with **scler/o**)
my/o (muscle)	**spasm/o** (involuntary contraction)	**-lysis** (use with all)
	scler/o (hard)	**-oma** (use with **fibr/o**)
arteri/o (artery)	**lys/o** (breaking down, destruction)	**-pathy**, noun suffix (use with first column)
thromb/o (clot)		**-genesis**, noun suffix (use with **my/o**, **thromb/o**, **neur/o**)
phleb/o (vein)	**fibr/o** (fibrous, fiber)	**-ectasia** (use with **angi/o**, **arteri/o**, **phleb/o**)
hem/o, **hemat/o** (blood)		**-rrhexis** (use with **angi/o**, **arteri/o**, **phleb/o**)
ather/o (fatty or porridgelike)		
ven/i (vein)		

ANSWER COLUMN

8.1

An embryonic (germ) cell from which a muscle cell develops is a my/o/blast. A germ cell from which a nerve cell develops is a

neur/o/blast
noo ō blast

_____/_____/_____.

A germ cell from which vessels develop is an

angi/o/blast
an′ jē o blast

_____/_____/_____.

8.2

A spasm is an involuntary twitching or contraction.
A spasm of a nerve is a neur/o/spasm.
A spasm of a muscle is a

my/o/spasm
mī′ ō spaz əm

_____/_____/_____.

A spasm of a vessel is an

angi/o/spasm
an′ jē ō spaz əm

_____/_____/_____.

8.3

Give the words for
arterial spasm

arteri/o/spasm
är **tir**′ ē ō spaz əm

_____/_____/_____;

gastric spasm

gastr/o/spasm
gas′ trō spaz əm

_____/_____/_____;

softening of the stomach walls

gastr/o/malac/ia
gas′ trō mə **lā**′ shə

_____/_____/_____/_____.

8.4

My/o/pathy means a generalized disease condition of the muscles. Build words meaning
a generalized disease condition of the vessels

angi/o/pathy
an jē **op**′ ath ē

_____/_____/_____;

a generalized disease condition of the nerves

neur/o/pathy
nōōr **op**′ ath ē

_____/_____/_____.

8.5

A (condition of) hardening of nerve tissue is neur/o/scler/osis.
Hardening of a vessel is

angi/o/scler/osis
an′ jē ō sklə **rō**′ sis

_____/_____/_____/_____.

A hardening of muscle tissue is

my/o/scler/osis
mī′ ō sklə **rō**′ sis

_____/_____/_____/_____.

ANSWER COLUMN

8.6

Use **neur/o** plus suffixes you have learned in previous units to build words meaning

a specialist who studies nervous system disorders

neur/o/logist
nōōr **ol**′ ō jist

_____/_____/_____;

the study of the nervous system

neur/o/logy
nōōr **ol**′ ō gē

_____/_____/_____;

inflammation of a nerve

neur/itis
nōōr **ī**′ tis

_____/_____.

TAKE A CLOSER LOOK

8.7

Look up neur/o/logist and neur/o/surgeon in your dictionary and read the definitions and write them below. **_____
_____

8.8

A muscle tumor is a my/oma.
A nerve tumor is a

neur/oma
nōōr **ō**′ mə

_____/_____.

A vessel tumor is an

angi/oma
an jē **ō**′ mə

_____/_____.

A fibrous tumor is a

fibr/oma
f ī **brō**′ mə

_____/_____.

8.9

The destruction of muscle tissue is my/o/lysis.
The destruction of nerve tissue is

neur/o/lysis
nōōr **rol**′ ə sis

_____/_____/_____.

The destruction or breaking down of vessels is

angi/ō/lysis
an′ jē **ol**′ ə sis

_____/_____/_____.

8.10

nerve

nerves

Recall that **neur/o** is used in words that refer to nerves. Neur/algia means pain along the course of a _____.
Neuropathy refers to any disease of the _____.

Afferent and efferent motor pathways of the CNS

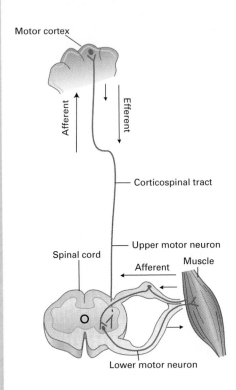

Motor cortex

Afferent

Efferent

Corticospinal tract

Upper motor neuron

Spinal cord

Afferent

Muscle

O

Lower motor neuron

8.11

nerves
joints

Neur/o/arthr/o/pathy is a disease of _____ and _____.

8.12

Neur/o/logy is the medical specialty that deals with the nervous system.
A physician who specializes in diseases of the nervous system is a

neur/o/logist
nōō **rol**′ ə jist

_____/____/_____.

Refer to the illustration of the nerves on page 261.

8.13

Build words meaning
inflammation of a nerve

neur/itis
nōō **ri**′ tis
neur/o/lysis
nōō **rol**′ ə sis
neur/o/plasty
nōō rō plas tē
neur/o/surgeon
nōō′ rō **sur**′ jən

_____/_____;

destruction of nerve tissue

_____/____/_____;

surgical repair of nerves

_____/____/_____;

nervous system surgeon

_____/____/_____.

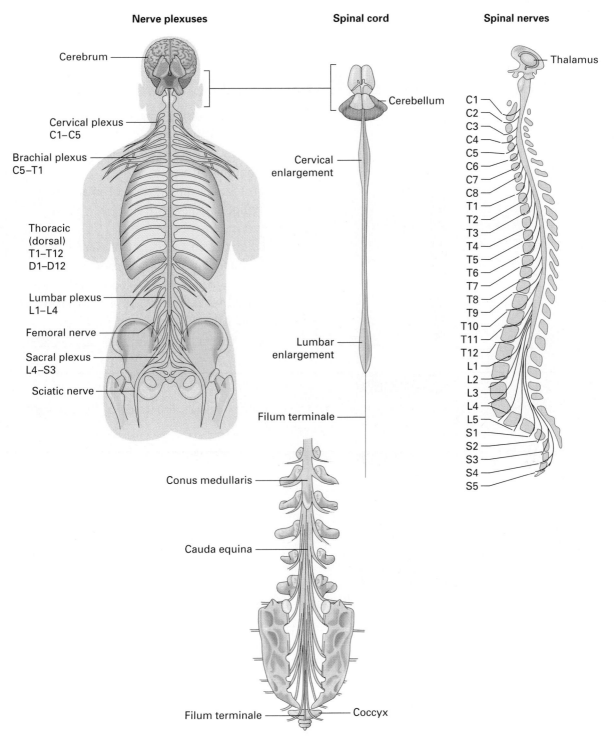

Nerve plexuses

Cerebrum

Cervical plexus
C1–C5

Brachial plexus
C5–T1

Thoracic
(dorsal)
T1–T12
D1–D12

Lumbar plexus
L1–L4

Femoral nerve

Sacral plexus
L4–S3

Sciatic nerve

Spinal cord

Cerebellum

Cervical
enlargement

Lumbar
enlargement

Filum terminale

Conus medullaris

Cauda equina

Filum terminale — Coccyx

Spinal nerves

Thalamus

C1
C2
C3
C4
C5
C6
C7
C8
T1
T2
T3
T4
T5
T6
T7
T8
T9
T10
T11
T12
L1
L2
L3
L4
L5
S1
S2
S3
S4
S5

Spinal cord (myel/o) and spinal nerves

ANSWER COLUMN

This table presents pairs of terms that are often confused in meaning because their spelling is so close. A simple difference between the term beginning with *e* or beginning with *a* makes a big difference in their correct use. Look them up in your dictionary for more information on word origins and use.

afferent	inflowing, *toward a center,* to bring to
efferent	outflowing, *away from a center,* to carry away
affect	to have *influence* upon, i.e. to change mood, thoughts, or actions
effect	the *result* or consequence of an action
accept	include, *bring toward,* embrace
except	exclude, *keep away,* reject
affusion	*pouring upon,* i.e. pouring of water *upon* the body for therapeutic purposes
effusion	the *escaping* of fluid or blood *from* its normal place, i.e. blood from vessels into the lungs or a joint cavity

8.14

trips

Neur/o/tripsy means surgical crushing of a nerve. The word root for crushing (usually by rubbing or grinding) is _____.

8.15

neur/o/tripsy
noo′ rō trip sē

Tripsis, from which we get **-tripsy**, is a Greek word that means rubbing or massage. *Tripsis* can be carried to the point of crushing or grinding. Surgical crushing of a nerve is _____/_____/_____.

8.16

lith/o/tripsy
lith′ ō trip sē

In some cases of lith/iasis, it may be necessary to crush calculi so they may be passed. A word that means surgical crushing of stones, as in the bladder or ureters, is _____/_____/_____.

8.17

lithotripsy

Therapeutic ultrasound (high-frequency sound waves) can be used to fragment stones in the kidney. This is ultrasonic

_____.

ANSWER COLUMN

TAKE A CLOSER LOOK

8.18

Look up myel/itis in your dictionary. From the definition, you conclude that myel is the word root for spinal cord or bone marrow. Write two words for spinal cord and two words for bone marrow using myel.

_____

_____

_____

_____

8.19

Find the word myeloblast in your dictionary and write the meaning.

bone marrow germ cell
myel/o

*_____.

The combining form of myel is _____/_____.

8.20

Find words meaning

myel/o/cyt/ic
mī′ el ō **sit**′ ik
myel/o/cele
mī′ el ō sēl

pertaining to myelocytes

_____/_____/_____/_____;

herniation of the spinal cord

_____/_____/_____.

8.21

-**plasia** means a condition of growth or development. It is used to indicate a change in the form of a structure or an abnormal number of cells. Write the meaning of the following terms.

poor or defective
  development
overgrowth, too
  much growth
lack of development

dys/plasia *_____

hyper/plasia *_____

a/plasia *_____

8.22

myel/o/dys/plasia
mī el ō dis **plā**′ zhə

Build a term that means defective (poor or bad) formation of the spinal cord:

_____/_____/_____/_____

(body part) + (disorder)

8.23

hyper/plasia
hī pər **plā**′ zhə or
hī pər **plā**′ zē ə

A/plasia means failure of an organ to develop properly. A word that means overgrowth or too many cells is

_____/_____.

ANSWER COLUMN

8.24

If growth of too many cells is hyper/plasia, underdevelopment or not enough cells is expressed as _____/_____.

hypo/plasia
hī pō **plā**′ zhə   or
hī pō **plā**′ zē ə

NOTE: Review the text and illustrations in Unit 3 for information on hypertrophy and hypotrophy. The terms hyperplasia and hypoplasia mean something different.

8.25

Using myel/o/dys/plasia as a model, build words meaning defective formation of cartilage

chondr/o/dys/plasia
kon′ drō dis **plā**′ zhə
oste/o/chondr/o/dys/plasia
os′ tē ō kon′ drō-
  dis **plā**′ zhə

_____/_____/_____/_____;

defective formation of bone and cartilage

_____/_____/_____/_____/_____/_____.

NOTE: **-plasia** may also be pronounced **plā**′ zē ə or **plā**′ zhə.

8.26

Form a word meaning inflammation of nerves and spinal cord

neur/o/myel/itis
nōō rō mī′ ə **lī**′ tis

_____/_____/_____/_____.

8.27

SPELL CHECK ✔

psych/o (sī′ kō) refers to the mind. Look up **psych/o** in your dictionary and read the definition. See how many everyday terms begin with the word root psych. Be sure to watch your spelling on this one. The p is silent and the y sound is like an i.

8.28

The study of the mind, mental processes, and human behavior

psych/o/logy
sī **kol**′ ō jē

is _____/_____/_____.

8.29

psych/o/analysis
sī′ kō a **nal**′ ə sis
psych/o/somatic
sī′ kō sō **mat**′ ik
psych/o/sexual
sī′ kō **sex**′ ū əl

Using your dictionary, read and analyze the meanings of
psychoanalysis _____/_____/_____,
**_____;
psychosomatic _____/_____/_____,
**_____;
psychosexual _____/_____/_____,
**_____.

ANSWER COLUMN

	8.30
psych/iatrist sī **kī′** ə trist psych/iatry sī **kī′** ə trē	Psychiatry is the field of medicine that studies and deals with mental and neurotic disorders. The physician who specializes in this field of medicine is called a _____/_____. The treatment of mental disorders by a psychiatrist is called _____/_____.

	8.31
WORD ORIGINS	In Greek mythology Psyche was Cupid's lover. She was the beautiful daughter of a king and the personification of fervent emotion. After many difficult trials, Psyche was made a goddess by Zeus and was united with Cupid on Mount Olympus. *Psyche* in Greek refers to the soul, spirit, or breath that creates life as distinguished from the physical aspects.

	8.32
psych/o/logist sī **kol′** ə jist	Psych/o/logy is the science that studies human behavior. The scientist or therapist who works in this field is called a _____/_____/_____.

	8.33
psych/o/therapy sī′ kō **thair′** ə pē	Psych/o/therapy is a process of healing mental disorders using words, art, drama, or movement to express feelings. A clinical psych/o/logist helps clients with mental disorders by using _____/_____/_____.

	8.34
psych/osis sī **ko′** sis	Psych/o/genesis means the formation of mental characteristics. A severe mental condition marked by loss of contact with reality and having delusions or hallucinations is _____/_____.

	8.35
psych/o/neur/osis sī′ kō nōō **rō′** sis neur/osis nōō **rō′** sis	Psych/o/neurosis (neur/o/sis), an emotional and behavioral disorder, is manifested by anxiety, phobias, and defense mechanisms. A psych/o/neur/o/tic person is one who suffers from a _____/_____/_____/_____ or _____/_____.

ANSWER COLUMN

8.36

The patient suffering from a neurosis knows the real from the unreal but will exaggerate reality. Individuals who will not touch others because they fear contact with germs may suffer from _____.

neurosis

8.37

TAKE A CLOSER LOOK

Obsessive-compulsive disorder (OCD) is a neurosis characterized by repeated distressing thoughts that produce anxiety (obsession) and uncontrollable repeated actions that must be done to relieve the anxiety (compulsion). A person may fear illness and think that they are being constantly exposed to germs. They may refuse to leave the house without wearing gloves and a mask, eat only boiled food, clean their house compulsively, and/or exclude social contact. OCD is a type of _____/_____. Look up OCD and other neuroses in your dictionary.

neuro/sis
no͞o **rō**′ sis

8.38

INFORMATION FRAME

Psych/o/trop/ic (*trope*, Greek for turn) medications may be used to alter emotions or behavior.

8.39

A patient with a psychoneurosis may be given a
_____/_____/_____/_____ medication to lower anxiety.

psych/o/trop/ic
sī′ kō **trō**′ pik

8.40

Use **psych/o** to build words meaning
medication that alters mind and emotions
_____/_____/_____/_____;
severe mental condition (delusional)
_____/_____;
mental processes that cause movement
_____/_____/_____;
mental disorder related to sexual function
_____/_____/_____/_____.

psych/o/trop/ic
sī′ kō **trō**′ pik
psych/osis
sī **kō**′ sis
psych/o/motor
sī′ kō **mō**′ ter
psych/o/sexu/al
sī′ kō **seks**′ yo͞o al

8.41

Psychoneuroses (neuroses, plural) take many forms. Obsessive-compulsive reaction, conversion reaction, and phobias are forms of _____
_____ (plural form).

neuroses   or
psychoneuroses

ANSWER COLUMN

8.42

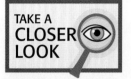

INFORMATION FRAME

In your dictionary read about the psychopath and the psychopathic personality. Also read the definition of psychopathy.

8.43

psych/o/motor
sī′ kō **mō**′ ter

motor is a word root referring to movement. Mental processes that cause movement are _____/_____/_____ functions.

8.44

motor

A neuron that innervates a muscle causes movement. It is called a _____ neuron.

8.45

TAKE A CLOSER LOOK

mental processes
(mental or soul)

Let your eye wander down the columns of psych words in the dictionary. Read about those that interest you. Note the information following the words psychiatric and psychoanalysis. All **psych/o** words refer to

*_____.

8.46

psych/o/pharmac/o/logy
sī′ kō fär ma **kol**′ ō jē

pharmac/o (as in pharmacy) means drugs or medicine. Neur/o/pharmacology is the study of drugs that affect the nervous system. The study of drugs that act on the mind and emotions is

_____/_____/_____/_____/_____.

8.47

INFORMATION FRAME

Psych/o/pharmac/o/logy includes the study of using medications to treat mental illness. The following are examples of psychotropic medications: antidepressants (Prozac), tranquilizers (Thorazine), neuroleptics, sedatives, and anticonvulsants (Dilantin).

8.48

pharmac/o/logy
fär′ ma **kol**′ ō jē

A pharmac/ist is licensed to dispense prescription and nonprescription medications from a pharmacy. To become a pharmacist, a person must study _____/_____/_____.

PROFESSIONAL PROFILES

A **registered pharmacist** (R.Ph) is licensed by each state to prepare and dispense all types of medications as well as medical supplies related to medication administration. They may practice in hospitals and clinics or own and operate and/or be employed in private pharmacies. The minimum training for a pharmacist is a five-year Baccalaureate Degree, and some pharmacists pursue a Doctor of Pharmacy Degree (Pharm D) offered by major universities around the United States. **Pharmacy technicians** assist the pharmacist with preparation and administration of medications as well as with reception and billing duties. Professional certification of pharmacy technicians varies from state to state and is administered by state pharmacy associations.

Pharmacy technicians preparing medications (Courtesy of the Michigan Pharmacists Association and the Michigan Society of Pharmacy Technicians)

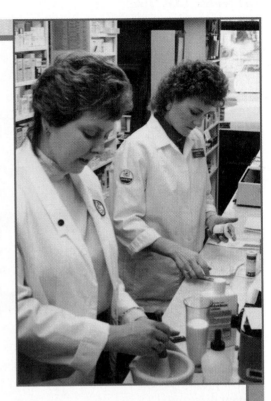

ANSWER COLUMN

8.49

narc/o is the combining form for sleep. A narc/o/tic is a drug that produces sleep. Opium produces stuporous sleep. Opium is a

_____/_____/_____.

narc/o/tic
när **kot'** ik

8.50

A narcotic produces pain relief as well as numbness or stuporous sleep. A narcotic should be used only on the advise of a physician. Codeine produces pain relief and sleep. Codeine is a _____.

narcotic

8.51

WORD ORIGINS

Morpheus was the Greek god of dreams. Morphine is a narcotic derived from opium poppies and produces a dreamlike state as well as analgesia.

ANSWER COLUMN

	8.52
narcotic	Morphine (MS-morphine sulfate) is used as a pain reliever (analgesic) and is also a _____.
	8.53
narcotics	Because narcotics can cause addiction, a physician must have a narcotic license to either dispense or write orders for _____ (plural).
	8.54
narc/osis när **kō**′ sis	The condition induced by narcotics is called _____/_____.
	8.55
TAKE A CLOSER LOOK epilepsy **ep**′ i lep sē	*Epilepsia* is a Greek word meaning to seize upon. In the past epilepsy has been classified by types of seizures described as petit mal and grand mal. Today epilepsy is described by the area of the brain involved, and it is divided into two categories including partial and general. Medical and surgical therapies are used in treatment of seizure disorders called _____.
	8.56
narc/o/lepsy **när**′ kō lep sē	**-lepsy** is used in words to mean seizure. Narc/o/lepsy means seizure or attacks of sleep. A person who is absolutely unable to stay awake suffers from _____/_____/_____.
	8.57
narcolepsy	Narcolepsy is a type of sleep disorder. A person may fall sound asleep standing at a bus stop. This is _____.
	8.58
narcolepsy	Cerebroma, cerebral arteriosclerosis, and paresis are some causes of sleep seizures, which are called _____.
	8.59
sleep, stupor, or stuporous sleep	You may get "tired" of hearing this, but **narc/o** any place in a word should make you think of *_____ _____.

8.60

Build words meaning
destruction (breakdown) of fat (lipids)

_____/_____/_____;

destruction (breakdown) of cells

_____/_____/_____.

lip/o/lysis
li **pol′** ə sis
cyt/ō/lysis
sī **tol′** ə sis

8.61

arteri/o is used in words about the arteries. Arteries are blood vessels that carry blood away from the heart. A word meaning hardening of the arteries

is _____/_____/_____/_____ (AS).

arteri/o/scler/osis
är tir′ ē ō sklə **rō′** sis

8.62

Arteri/o/scler/osis means hardening of the arteries.
Build words meaning
a fibrous condition of the arteries

_____/_____/_____/_____;

a softening of the arteries

_____/_____/_____.

arteri/o/fibr/osis
är tir′ ē ō fī **brō′** sis
arteri/o/malacia
är tir′ ē ō mə **lā′** shə

8.63

Refer to the diagram of atherosclerosis. Recall that **ather/o** means fatty or porridgelike. Hardening of the blood vessels (arteries) caused by a fatty substance (atheroma) is a condition called _____/_____/_____/_____.

ather/o/scler/osis
a′ ther ō skler **ō′** sis

8.64

Atherosclerosis occurs primarily in medium to large blood vessels and can decrease vascular supply causing ischemia and necrosis. This leads to myocardial infarction (heart attack) or cerebral infarction (stroke). Fatty streaks inside the carotid arteries are an indication

of _____/_____/_____/_____.

NOTE: Look up ischemia and necrosis in your dictionary.

ather/o/scler/osis
a′ ther ō skler **ō′** sis

8.65

If a large ather/oma develops from the fatty streak, an ather/ectomy may be performed. Excision of an ather/oma is called _____/_____

or _____/_____/_____. This procedure is most commonly performed on the carotid artery.

ather/ectomy
a′ ther **ek′** tō mē
end/arter/ectomy
end är′ ter **ek′** tō mē

Major arteries and vascular conditions associated with atherosclerosis

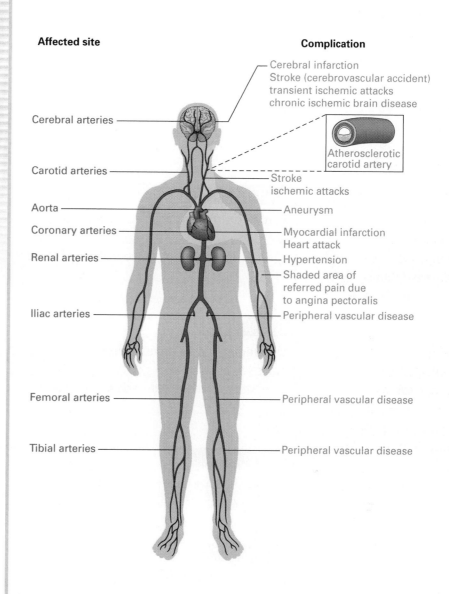

Affected site

Cerebral arteries

Carotid arteries

Aorta

Coronary arteries

Renal arteries

Iliac arteries

Femoral arteries

Tibial arteries

Complication

Cerebral infarction
Stroke (cerebrovascular accident)
transient ischemic attacks
chronic ischemic brain disease

Atherosclerotic
carotid artery

Stroke
ischemic attacks

Aneurysm

Myocardial infarction
Heart attack

Hypertension

Shaded area of
referred pain due
to angina pectoralis

Peripheral vascular disease

Peripheral vascular disease

Peripheral vascular disease

8.66

Nonsurgical treatment of atherosclerosis includes bringing cholesterol to normal levels, increasing the high-density lipoproteins (HDL), decreasing the low-density lipoproteins (LDL), and stopping smoking. Diet, exercise, and lifestyle changes can help reduce the risk of death from _____.

atherosclerosis

8.67

Ather/o/scler/o/tic coronary artery disease is the most common cause of angina pectoris. If the oxygen demand is higher than that supplied to the heart muscle, * _____ can occur.

NOTE: Look up angina pectoris in your dictionary.

angina pectoris
an **jī**′ na pek **tor**′ is   or
an′ ji na pek **tor**′ is

ANSWER COLUMN

8.68

hem/o refers to blood. A benign tumor of a blood vessel is a hem/angi/oma. (Note that the o is dropped.) An embryonic blood vessel cell is a

hem/angi/o/blast
hēm **an**′ gē ō blast

_____/_____/____/_____.

A condition of blood in a joint is

hem/arthr/osis
hēm är **thrō**′ sis

_____/_____/_____.

8.69

hemat/o also refers to blood. Another word for destruction of blood cells

hemat/o/lysis
hēm ə **tol**′ ə sis

is _____/____/_____.

-phobia means fear. An abnormal fear of blood is

hemat/ō/phobia
hēm′ ə tō **fō**′ bē ə

_____/____/_____.

8.70

blood
hemat/o/logy
hēm ə **tol**′ ə jē
hemat/ō/log/ist
hēm ə **tol**′ ə jist

Use **hemat/o** once more to mean _____.
The study of blood is _____/____/_____.
One who specializes in the science of blood is a

_____/____/_____/_____.

8.71

blood clot

thromb/o is the combining form that means blood clot.
Thromb/o/angi/itis means inflammation of a vessel with formation
of a *_____.

8.72

excision of a
   thrombus (clot)

Thromb/ectomy means *_____

_____.

8.73

thrombus
throm′ bus
thrombi
throm′ bī

The medical name for blood clot is thrombus.
A synonym for clot is _____.

The plural form is _____.

8.74

inflammation of a lymph
   vessel with formation
   of a thrombus (clot)

Recall **lymph/o** means lymphatic tissue. Thromb/o/lymph/ang/itis means
*_____

_____.

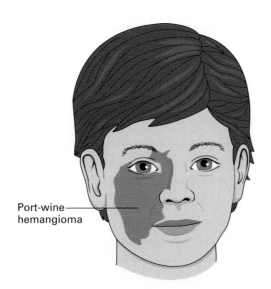

Port-wine hemangioma

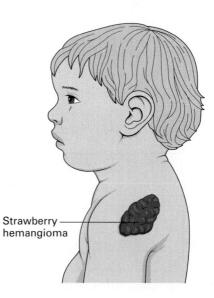

Strawberry hemangioma

ANSWER COLUMN

8.75

phleb/o is a combining form for vein. Thromb/o/phleb/itis means

inflammation of a vein with thrombus formation

*_____

_____.

8.76

See, you are great at figuring out meanings. Now, using
thromb/o, build words meaning
a condition of forming a thrombus

thromb/osis
throm **bō′** sis

_____/_____;

a cell that aids clotting

thromb/o/cyte
throm′ bō sit

_____/_____/_____;

resembling a thrombus

thromb/oid
throm′ boid

_____/_____.

8.77

Build words meaning
pertaining to the formation of a thrombus

thromb/o/gen/ic
throm′ bō **jen′** ik

_____/_____/_____/_____;

destruction of a thrombus

thromb/o/lysis
throm **bol′** ə sis

_____/_____/_____;

lack of cells that aid in clotting (platelets)

thromb/o/cyt/o/penia
throm′ bō sī′ tō **pē′** nē ə

_____/_____/_____/_____/_____.

Great! You are good at word building, too.

ANSWER COLUMN

INFORMATION FRAME

8.78

A thrombus may block or "occlude" a vessel. This occlusion may cause ischemia, stopping blood supply to the tissues and producing an infarct (necrosis of tissue). If this happens in the heart muscle, the condition is called myocardial infarction (MI).

TAKE A CLOSER LOOK

8.79

Look up the following terms in your medical dictionary and write their definitions.
occlusion *_____
_____;
infarct *_____
_____;
myocardial *_____
_____.

---

occlusion
ō **klōō**′ shun

8.80

A thrombus or piece of a thrombus may move through blood vessels to another part of the body. This moving thrombus is called an embolus. An embolus may cause a block in a vessel called an _____/___.

---

my/o/cardi/al in/farct/ion
mī ō **kär**′ dē əl
in **fark**′ shun

8.81

If an artery of the heart muscle is occluded and an area of tissue has no blood supply, a *____/____/_____/____ ____/_____/_____ (MI) may occur.

---

cerebr/al in/farct/ion
se **rē**′ bral in **fark**′ shun

8.82

If an artery supplying the cerebrum (brain) is occluded,
a *_____/____ ____/_____/_____
(cerebrovascular accident [CVA] stroke) could occur.

---

heart

8.83

Recall that arteries (**arteri/o**) are vessels that carry blood away from the heart. Veins (**phleb/o**) are vessels that carry blood back to the _____.

---

arteries
phleb/o/scler/osis
fleb′ ō sklə **rō**′ sis

8.84

One combining form for vein is **phleb/o**. Arteriosclerosis is hardening of the _____. Hardening of veins is called _____/____/_____/_____.

8.85

Build words meaning
excision of a vein

phleb/ectomy
fli **bek**′ tə mē   _____ / _____ ;

phleb/o/pexy   surgical fixation of a vein
fleb′ ō pek sē   _____ / _____ / _____ .

8.86

Dilation and dilatation are synonyms for stretching or increase in diameter. **-ectasia**
is used as a suffix for dilatation.
Build words meaning
venous dilatation (stretching)

phleb/ectasia   _____ / _____ ;
fleb′ ek **tā**′ shə   arterial dilatation

arteri/ectasia   _____ / _____ ;
är tir′ ē ek **tā**′ shə   vessel dilatation

angi/ectasia   _____ / _____ .
an′ jē ek **tā**′ shə

8.87

Phleb/o/plasty means

surgical repair of a vein   * _____ .
incision into a vein or   Phleb/o/tomy means
    venipuncture   * _____ .
vēn′ i punk tyo͞or

Venipuncture

8.88

ven/o and **ven/i** are also combining forms for vein. To obtain a ven/ous
ven/i/puncture   blood sample, a _____ / _____ / _____ is performed.
vēn′ i punk tyo͞or

ANSWER COLUMN

ven/ous **vēn′** us ven/ous	**8.89** Venous blood is the dark blood in the veins. Blood flow through the veins back to the heart is called _____/_____ return. Administering medication within a vein is an intra/_____/_____ injection.
rupture of the uterus	**8.90** **-rrhexis** is a suffix meaning rupture. Hyster/o/rrhexis means * _____.
suffixes	**8.91** With **-rrhexis** you learn the last of the Greek "rrh" forms. **-rrhea**, **-rrhagia**, **-rrhaphy**, and **-rrhexis** are _____.
rupture of the bladder rupture of the small intestine	**8.92** Cyst/o/rrhexis means * _____. Enter/o/rrhexis means * _____.
-rrhea, discharge or flow -rrhagia, hemorrhage -rrhaphy, suture -rrhexis, rupture	**8.93** To summarize, the four "rrh" suffixes you have learned are _____, meaning _____ _____, meaning _____ _____, meaning _____ _____, meaning _____
cardi/o/rrhexis kär′ dē ō **rek′** sis angi/o/rrhexis an′ jē ō **rek′** sis	**8.94** Build words meaning rupture of the heart _____/____/_____; rupture of a vessel _____/____/_____.
arteri/o/rrhexis är tir′ ē ō **rek′** sis phleb/o/rrhexis fleb′ ō **rek′** sis	**8.95** Build words meaning rupture of an artery _____/____/_____; rupture of a vein _____/____/_____.

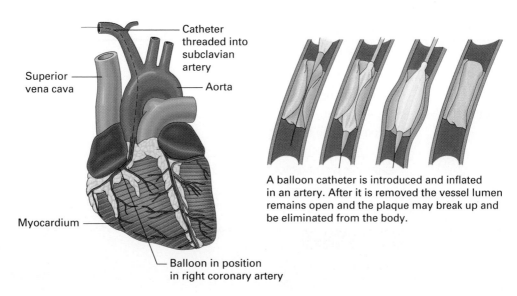

Superior vena cava
Catheter threaded into subclavian artery
Aorta
Myocardium
Balloon in position in right coronary artery

A balloon catheter is introduced and inflated in an artery. After it is removed the vessel lumen remains open and the plaque may break up and be eliminated from the body.

Balloon angioplasty

ANSWER COLUMN	
	8.96
	Build terms that mean repair of a vessel
angi/o/plasty **an′** jē ō plas tē	_____/_____/_____;
angi/o/graphy an jē **og′** raf ē	process of obtaining an x-ray of a vessel _____/_____/_____;
angi/o/scopy an jē **os′** kō pē	process of using a looking device to examine a vessel _____/_____/_____;
angi/o/gram **an′** jē ō gram	image of a vessel. _____/_____/_____.
	8.97
	Give the meaning of the following terms phleb/o/plasty
repair of a vein	*_____;
process of obtaining an x-ray of a vein	phleb/o/graphy (ven/o/graphy) *_____ _____.
	8.98
	Rupture of the tissues of the uterus is called either
metr/o/rrhexis or mē trō **rek′** sis hyster/o/rrhexis his′ ter ō **rek′** sis	_____/_____/_____ or _____/_____/_____.

ANSWER COLUMN

8.99

Build words meaning
rupture of the liver

hepat/o/rrhexis
hep at ōr **eks**′ is

_____/_____/_____;

hepat/o/rrhaphy
hep at **ōr**′ a fē

suturing of the liver (wound)

_____/_____/_____;

hepat/o/rrhea
hep at ō **rē**′ ə

excessive discharge of bile from the liver

_____/_____/_____.

8.100

Build words meaning
rupture of the bladder

cyst/o/rrhexis
sis′ tō **reks**′ is

_____/_____/_____;

cyst/o/rrhagia
sis′ tō **rā**′ jē ə

hemorrhage from the bladder

_____/_____/_____;

cyst/o/rrhea
sis tō **rē**′ ə

discharge from the bladder

_____/_____/_____;

cyst/o/rrhaphy
sis **tōr**′ a fē

suturing of the bladder

_____/_____/_____.

Good!

8.101

INFORMATION FRAME

Esthesia is a word meaning feeling or sensation. Think of the English word aesthetics, meaning that which we perceive or sense. **an-** is a form of the prefix **a-**. **an-** means without (e.g., anemia, lack of blood; anorexia, lack of appetite).

8.102

Recall that **a-** and **an-** are prefixes meaning without or lack of. Analyze the following words by dividing them into their word parts. Look up the meanings in your dictionary.

esthesiometer

esthesi/o/meter
es thēs′ ē **om**′ ə ter

_____/_____/_____

anesthesia

an/esthesi/a
an es **thēs**′ ē ə

_____/_____/_____

anesthesiology

an/esthesi/o/logy
an es thēs′ ē **ol**′ o jē

_____/_____/_____/_____

anesthetist

an/esthet/ist
an **es**′ the tist

_____/_____/_____

ANSWER COLUMN

8.103

Build words that mean
without or lack of sensation

anesthesia

_____;

a person who administers anesthetic agents

anesthetist

_____;

a physician specialist in anesthesia

anesthesiologist

_____.

8.104

Novocaine is used to remove sensation in a specific area. It is a local

an/esthet/ic
an es **the**′ tik

_____/_____/_____.

8.105

Think of the meaning as you analyze the following words.
dysesthesia

dys/esthesi/a
dis es **thēs**′ ē ə
hypo/esthesi/a
hī′ pō es **thēs**′ ē ə

_____/_____/_____

hypoesthesia

_____/_____/_____

8.106

Algesia is a noun meaning oversensitivity to pain. Hyper/esthesi/a is a synonym
for algesia. Algesia means

oversensitivity to pain
 or hyperesthesia

*_____

_____.

8.107

Use the word root alges to build words meaning
instrument used to measure pain

alges/i/meter
al jē **səm**′ et er
alges/ic
al **jēs**′ ik
an/ alges/ia
an al **jēs**′ ē ə

_____/_____/_____;

pertaining to pain (adjective)

_____/_____;

condition without pain (noun)

_____/_____/_____.

ANSWER COLUMN

DICTIONARY EXERCISE A-Z

without pain

abnormal pain

abnormal pain

paralysis of the lower body

8.108

Look up the following words in your medical dictionary and write their meanings below.

analgesia
*_____

paralgesia
*_____

paralgia
*_____

paraplegia
*_____

---

inflammation near
 the kidney
inflammation near
 the liver
works beside a physician
 assisting in rescue
 operation—EMT with
 advanced training

8.109

para- is a Greek prefix that means beside, beyond, near, abnormal.
Para/nephr/itis means
*_____.

Para/hepat/itis means
*_____.

Para/medic means
*_____
_____.

---

para/nephr/itis
par′ ə nef rī′ tis
para/salping/itis
par′ ə sal pin jī′ tis
para/hepat/itis
par′ ə hep at ī′ tis
para/oste/o/arthr/o/pathy
par′ ə os′ tē ō är **throp′-**
 ə thē

8.110

Using the prefix **para-**, build terms that mean
inflammation near the kidney
_____/_____/_____;
inflammation near the fallopian tubes
_____/_____/_____;
inflammation near the liver
_____/_____/_____;
disease near a bone and joint
_____/_____/_____/_____/_____/_____.

---

para/lysis
par **al′** ə sis

8.111

Paralysis is a loss of muscle function and sensation. Para/plegia
is _____/_____ of the lower body.

ANSWER COLUMN

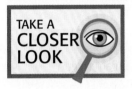

DICTIONARY EXERCISE A-Z

partially paralyzed
   (lower body)
delusions of persecution
part of the autonomic
   nervous system
abnormal touch sensation

8.112

Look up the following terms that begin with **par/a-** and write their meaning below.

para/plegia _____

para/noid _____
para/sympathetic _____

par/esthesia _____

TAKE A CLOSER LOOK

8.113

The autonomic nervous system (ANS) is the functional organization of the nervous system that responds during stress. The sym/path/etic nerves send signals to prepare the body for fight or flight when danger is either near or perceived. The para/sym/path/etic nerves return the body to its normal resting state.

8.114

Imagine that a person is driving and the car begins to slide out of control after hitting an ice patch. The person's eyes dilate, the heart and respiration rates increase, and epinephrine is released from the adrenal glands. This response to danger is brought on by the

sym/path/etic
sim pa **the**′ tik
para/sym/path/etic
par′ ə sim pa **the**′ tic

_____/_____/_____ nerves of the autonomic nervous system.
After the danger has passed, the
_____/_____/_____/_____ nerves return the
body to a resting state.

INFORMATION FRAME

8.115

Paroxysmos is a Greek word meaning an irritation. A symptom that comes upon someone suddenly, for example difficulty breathing in the middle of the night, is called a paroxysm. Paroxysmal nocturnal dyspnea (PND) is the sudden onset of shortness of breath (SOB) at night.

8.116

Waking in the middle of the night with difficulty breathing is called

paroxysm/al
par oks **iz**′ mal

_____/_____ nocturnal dyspnea.

Use the following combining forms and suffixes in Frames 8.117–8.124.

Combining Form	Meaning	Suffix
my/o	muscle	-graph (instrument for recording)
		-gram (record, picture)
		-algia (pain)
		-logy (study of)
kinesi/o	movement	-oma (tumor)
rhabd/o	rod shaped	-pathy (disease)
lip/o	fat	
fibr/o	fibrous	

8.117

Myon is a Greek word meaning muscle. Myocarditis means inflammation of the heart muscle. **my/o** is used in words referring to the _____.

muscles

INFORMATION FRAME

8.118

There are three main types of muscle found throughout the body. Study the table on page 283 to discover each type, its location, and main function.

8.119

The words my/o/gram, my/o/graph, and my/o/graphy mean

myogram   _____ the tracing
myograph   _____ the instrument
myography   _____ the process

8.120

muscles

My/asthenia gravis is a condition of the _____.

8.121

Using **my/o**, **fibr/o**, and **-oma**, build a term meaning a fibrous muscle tumor:

my/o/fibr/oma   _____/_____/_____/_____. This is also called a leiomy/oma uteri
mī ō fib rō′ mə   or fibroid tumor of the uterine _____ or my/o/metr/ium.
muscle

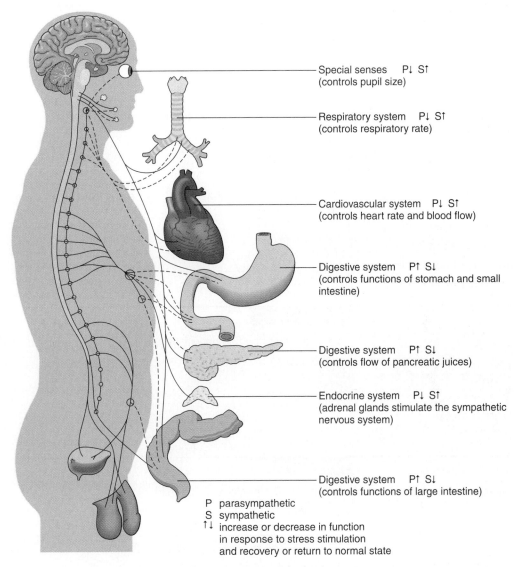

Special senses   P↓ S↑
(controls pupil size)

Respiratory system   P↓ S↑
(controls respiratory rate)

Cardiovascular system   P↓ S↑
(controls heart rate and blood flow)

Digestive system   P↑ S↓
(controls functions of stomach and small intestine)

Digestive system   P↑ S↓
(controls flow of pancreatic juices)

Endocrine system   P↓ S↑
(adrenal glands stimulate the sympathetic nervous system)

Digestive system   P↑ S↓
(controls functions of large intestine)

P parasympathetic
S sympathetic
↑↓ increase or decrease in function
in response to stress stimulation
and recovery or return to normal state

The autonomic nervous system controls the involuntary actions of the body

Muscle Type	Location	Function
striated (skeletal, voluntary) **rhabd/o/my/o**	covers skeleton Example: rhabdomyosarcoma	skeletal movement
smooth (visceral, involuntary) **leiomy/o**	organs, vessels Example: leiomyofibroma	movement of liquids, gases, and solids
cardiac **myocardi/o**	heart Example: myocardiopathy	maintain heartbeat

ANSWER COLUMN

8.122

Build words meaning
resembling muscle
____/_____;

my/oid
mī′ oid

muscle tumor containing fatty elements
____/____/_____/_____;

my/o/lip/oma
mī ō lip **ō′** mə

muscle disease
____/____/_____;

my/o/pathy
mī **op′** ath ē

heart muscle disease

cardi/o/my/o/pathy   or
kär′ dē ō mi **op′** ə thē

my/o/cardi/o/pathy
mī′ ō kär dē **op′** ə thē

_____/____/____/____/_____.

8.123

TAKE A
CLOSER
LOOK

Look up words beginning with **my/o** in your dictionary. Count how many of the words you know. Write the number here:

more than 60

* _____

8.124

muscles

When you see **my/o**, you will think of _____.
When you see **leiomy/o**, you will think of

smooth muscle

* _____.
When you see **myocardi/o**, you will think of

heart muscle

* _____.

8.125

The main function of muscles is movement. **kinesi/o** is used in words to mean movement or motion. Brady/kinesia means

slowness of movement

* _____.

8.126

pain on movement or
  movement pain

Kinesi/algia means * _____
_____.

8.127

Kinesi/algia occurs when you have to move any sore or injured part of the body.
Moving a broken arm causes

kinesi/algia
ki nē′ sē **al′** jē ə

_____/_____.

ANSWER COLUMN

Types of muscle tissue:
(A) skeletal muscle;
(B) smooth muscle;
(C) cardiac muscle

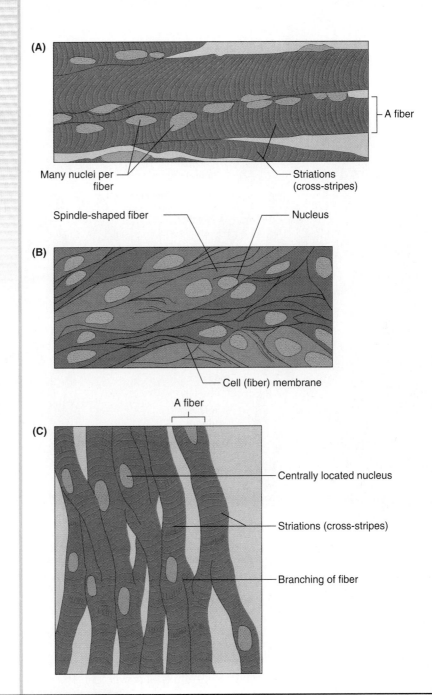

8.128

After one's first ride on horseback, almost any movement causes

kinesialgia _____.

8.129

-logy is used like a suffix to mean study of. (Remember **-logist**?) The study of muscular body movements is

kinesi/o/logy
ki nē′ sē **ol**′ ə jē _____/_____/_____.

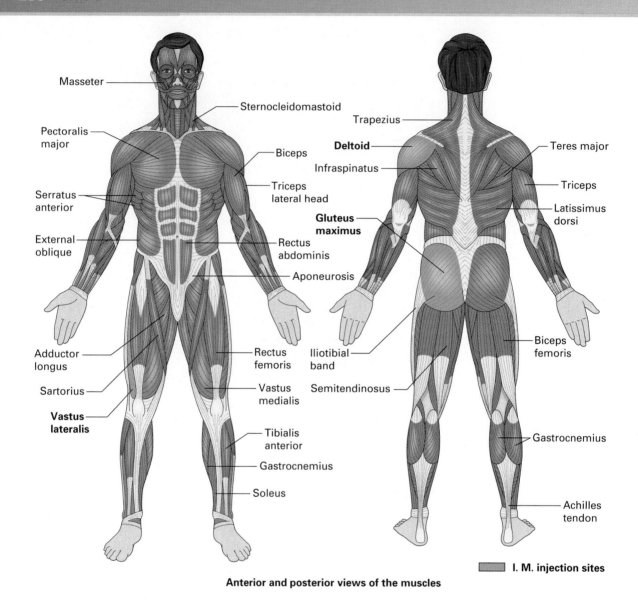

Anterior and posterior views of the muscles

▭	**I. M. injection sites**

ANSWER COLUMN

8.130

Kinesi/o/logy is the study of movement. The study of muscular movement during exercise would be done in the field of

_____.

kinesiology

PROFESSIONAL PROFILES

Physical therapists (PTs) assess, prevent, and treat movement dysfunction and physical disabilities by using technological interventions as well as personal contact. In addition to patient care, the physical therapist may consult, supervise, administer, research, and provide community service through private practice or employment within an inpatient facility or clinic. **Physical therapy assistants** are supervised by the physical therapist and may administer physical therapy treatments as well as help with record keeping, billing, and reception. There are several professional organizations involved with education and credentialing of physical therapists. They include the American Association of Rehabilitation Therapy (AART), the American Physical Therapy Association (APTA), and the American Congress of Physical Medicine and Rehabilitation (ACPMR).

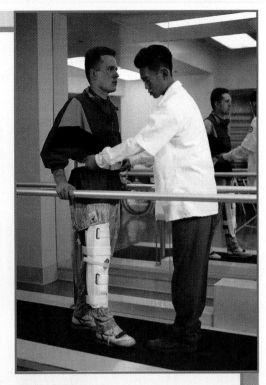

Physical therapist

ANSWER COLUMN

	8.131
	An exercise physiologist studies the science of how the body moves, called
kinesiology	_____.

	8.132
	Recall **brady-** is the prefix for slow. Slowness of movement is called
brady/kinesia brād′ i ki **nē**′ sē ə or brād′ ē ki **nē**′ sē ə	_____/_____.

Abbreviation	Meaning
AANA	American Association of Nurse Anesthetists
AART	American Association of Rehabilitation Therapy
ACPMR	American Congress of Physical Medicine and Rehabilitation
ADL	activities of daily living
AE	above the elbow
AK	above the knee
AOD	arterial occlusive disease
ANS	autonomic nervous system
APTA	American Physical Therapy Association
AS	arteriosclerosis, left ear
ASCVD	arteriosclerotic cardiovascular disease
ASHD	arteriosclerotic heart disease
BE	below the elbow, barium enema
BK	below the knee
C1–C8	cervical spinal nerve pairs
CABG	coronary artery bypass graft
CAD	coronary artery disease
CNS	central nervous system
CRNA	Certified Registered Nurse Anesthetist
C-section	cesarean section
EMG	electromyogram
HA	headache, hearing aid
HDL	high-density lipoproteins
IV	intravenous
L1–L5	lumbar spinal nerve pairs
MD	muscular dystrophy, medical doctor
MFT	muscle function test
MI	myocardial infarction
MS	multiple sclerosis, morphine sulfate
NVS	neurologic vital signs
OCD	obsessive-compulsive disorder
PND	paroxysmal nocturnal dyspnea, postnasal drip
PNS	peripheral nervous system
pro time, pt	prothrombin time
PT	physical therapy (therapist)

ANSWER COLUMN

Abbreviation	Meaning
RPh	Registered Pharmacist
ROM	range of motion
S1–S5	sacral spinal nerve pairs
SOB	shortness (short) of breath
T1–T12 (D1–D12)	thoracic spinal nerve pairs same as dorsal spinal nerve pairs
TENS	transcutaneous electric nerve stimulation

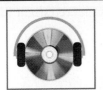

To complete your study of this unit, work the **Review Activities** on the following pages. Also, listen to the audio CDs that accompany *Medical Terminology: A Programmed Systems Approach*, 9th Edition, and practice your pronunciation.

Additional practice exercises for this unit are available on the Learner Practice CD-ROM found in the back of the textbook.

REVIEW ACTIVITIES

CIRCLE AND CORRECT

Circle the correct answer for each question. Then, check your answers in Appendix A.

1. Suffix for surgical fixation
   a. -ptosis
   b. -plasty
   c. -pexy
   d. -ectasia

2. Combining form for vein
   a. phlebo
   b. ven
   c. venous
   d. thrombo

3. Suffix for rupture
   a. -ptosis
   b. -ectasis
   c. -rrhaphy
   d. -rrhexis

4. Suffix for most x-ray procedures
   a. -graphy
   b. -electric
   c. -Roentgen
   d. -graph

5. Prefix for without
   a. not-
   b. inter-
   c. an-
   d. dys-

6. Word root for oversensitivity to pain
   a. alges
   b. analgia
   c. esthesia
   d. algia

7. Prefix for abnormal, near, or beyond
   a. meta-
   b. para-
   c. ultra-
   d. ab-

8. Word root for movement
   a. my
   b. esthesi
   c. kinesi
   d. motor

REVIEW ACTIVITIES

9. Suffix for tumor
   a. -algia
   b. -itis
   c. -genic
   d. -oma

10. Combining form for hard
    a. cranio
    b. skullo
    c. osteo
    d. sclero

11. Word root for vessel
    a. arterio
    b. arter
    c. angi
    d. vesic

12. Suffix for destruction
    a. -plasty
    b. -rrhexis
    c. -lysis
    d. -malacia

13. Word root for blood clot
    a. thromb
    b. hem
    c. hemat
    d. embolism

14. Combining form for blood
    a. hemato
    b. penia
    c. emia
    d. thrombo

SELECT AND CONSTRUCT

Select the correct word parts from the following list and construct medical terms that represent the given meaning.

a	algeso(ic)	algia(esic)	an	analg
angio	arterio	ather/o	brady	cardio
dynia	dys	echo	ectasia	entero
esthesi/o(a)	fibr/o	gram	graph(y)	hepato
ist	itis	kinesi/o(a)	logist	logy
ma	meter	myo	neur/o	osis
para	pathy	psych/o	pharm/o	phlebo
plasty	plegia(ic)	rrhexis(ia)	sclero	scopy
spasm	tachy	thromb/o	tropic	veno

1. hardening of an artery _____

2. dilation of a vein _____

3. rupture of the intestine _____

4. x-ray of a vessel _____

5. instrument for measuring touch _____

6. physician specialist who prepares patients for painless surgery _____

7. pain-relieving medication (adjective) _____

8. inflammation near the liver _____

9. mental condition characterized by anxiety, phobias _____

10. instrument for measuring muscle function _____

11. difficult or painful movement _____

12. specialist in drug therapy _____

REVIEW ACTIVITIES

13. drugs that affect mental processes   _____

14. paralysis of the lower body   _____

15. fibrous and muscle tumor   _____

16. large vessel hardening due to fatty streaks   _____

17. repair of a vessel   _____

18. condition of blood clots   _____

19. abnormal muscle contraction   _____

20. tumor of fiber and nerve   _____

21. inflammation of vein caused by clots   _____

22. specialist in nerve disorders   _____

23. heart muscle disease   _____

24. pertaining to heart muscle   _____

DEFINE AND DISSECT

Give a brief definition and dissect each term listed into its word parts in the space provided. Check your answers by referring to the frame listed in parentheses and your medical dictionary. Then listen to the CDs to practice pronunciation.

1. neuroblast (8.1)

    _____/____/_____
      rt   v   rt

    _____
              definition

2. myelocele (8.20)

    ____/____/_____
     rt   v   suffix

    _____

3. arteriofibrosis (8.62)

    _____/___/_____/_____
       rt   v   rt   suffix

    _____

4. hematolysis (8.69)

    _____/___/_____
        rt   v   suffix

    _____

5. thrombogenic (8.77)

    _____/___/_____/____
        rt   v   rt   suffix

    _____

6. occlusion (8.80)

    _____/_____
        rt   suffix

    _____

REVIEW ACTIVITIES

7. neurologist (8.6)

_____/___/_____
rt   v   suffix

8. myocardial (8.81)

___/___/_____/___
rt   v   rt   suffix

9. hemangioma (8.68)

_____/_____/_____
rt   rt   suffix

10. phlebosclerosis (8.84)

_____/___/_____/_____
rt   v   rt   suffix

11. arteriectasia (8.86)

_____/_____
rt   suffix

12. narcolepsy (8.56)

_____/___/_____
rt   v   suffix

13. angioplasty (8.96)

_____/___/_____
rt   v   suffix

14. phlebography (8.97)

_____/___/_____
rt   v   suffix

15. anesthetist (8.103)

___/_____/_____
pre   rt   suffix

16. dysesthesia (8.105)

_____/_____/___
pre   rt   suffix

17. analgesia (8.107)

___/_____/___
pre   rt   suffix

18. paranephritis (8.109)

_____/_____/_____
pre   rt   suffix

REVIEW ACTIVITIES

19. paranoid (8.112)

                                      _____ / ___

                                        pre   suffix

20. sympathetic (8.114)

_____ / _____ / _____

pre   rt   suffix

21. cardiomyopathy (8.122)

_____ / __ / ____ / __ / _____

rt   v   rt   v   suffix

22. myography (8.119)

__ / __ / _____

rt   v   suffix

23. thrombophlebitis (8.75)

_____ / ___ / _____ / _____

rt   v   rt   suffix

24. kinesiology (8.129)

_____ / ___ / _____

rt   v   suffix

25. bradykinesia (8.125)

_____ / _____ / ___

pre   rt   suffix

26. phlebotomy (8.87)

_____ / ___ / _____

rt   v   suffix

27. anesthesiologist (8.103)

__ / _____ / ___ / _____

pre   rt   v   suffix

28. angioscopy (8.96)

_____ / ___ / _____

rt   v   suffix

29. myofibroma (8.121)

_____ / __ / __ / _____

rt   v rt suffix

30. paralysis (8.111)

_____ / _____

pre   suffix

REVIEW ACTIVITIES

31. chondrodysplasia (8.25)

_____/___/___/_____
   rt   v   pre   suffix

_____

32. neurosurgeon (8.13)

_____/___/_____/___
   rt   v   rt   suffix

_____

33. paraplegia (8.112)

_____/_____
   pre   suffix

_____

34. endarterectony (8.65)

_____/_____/_____
  pre   rt   suffix

_____

35. ischemia (8.78)

_____/___
        rt   suffix

_____

36. infarction (8.81)

___/_____/_____
  pre   rt   suffix

_____

37. paroxysmal (8.116)

_____/____
              rt   suffix

_____

REVIEW ACTIVITIES

ABBREVIATION MATCHING

Match the following abbreviations with their definition.

_____ 1. CNS   a. muscular dystrophy

_____ 2. MS   b. milliamperes

_____ 3. EMG   c. arteriosclerotic heart disease

_____ 4. HA   d. range of motion

_____ 5. AANA   e. arteriosclerotic cardiovascular disease

_____ 6. ASHD   f. multiple fracture test

_____ 7. R.Ph   g. American Association of Nurse Anesthetists

_____ 8. MFT   h. electroencephalogram

_____ 9. ROM   i. American Association of Naturopaths

_____10. ADL   j. hearing aid

         k. central nervous system

         l. electromyogram

         m. heartache

         n. muscle function test

         o. ad lib

         p. Registered Pharmacist

         q. above the elbow

         r. activities of daily living

         s. below the elbow, barium enema

         t. multiple sclerosis

ABBREVIATION FILL-IN

Fill in the blanks with the correct abbreviations.

11. high-density lipoproteins _____

12. myocardial infarction _____

13. prothrombin time _____

14. coronary artery bypass graft _____

15. intravenous _____

16. below the knee _____

17. muscular dystrophy _____

18. transcutaneous electrical nerve stimulation _____

19. paroxysmal nocturnal dyspnea _____

20. obsessive-compulsive disorder _____

REVIEW ACTIVITIES

CASE STUDIES

Write the term next to its meaning given below. Then draw slashes to analyze the word parts. Note the use of medical abbreviations. Look these up in your dictionary or find them in Appendix B. If you have any questions about the answers, refer to your medical dictionary or check with your instructor for the answers in Appendix A.

CASE STUDY 8-1

Summary

Pt: 83-year-old woman, Ht 5'2", Wt 110, **BP** 104/60, **T** 98.9, **R** 20

Dx: 1. **Obsessive-compulsive disorder**

2. **Hypothyroidism**

3. **Incontinence**

This 83-year-old, single woman presented to the emergency room with complaints of anxiety, fear of impending death, panic, fatigue, and **diarrhea**. She has a history of hospitalization for obsessive-compulsive disorder between the ages of 35 and 55 when she was treated with **EST**, psychotropic medication, and **psychotherapy**. She was released to an adult foster care home where she lived for approximately 10 years, moving from home to home with difficulty conforming to house rules about bathroom privileges and having **paranoia**. She is currently living in an apartment. Although fully aware of her condition and advised of new treatments for **OCD**, she has refused medication and continues her daily routine of hand washing for as long as 30 minutes at a time several times a day. She explains that she is afraid people have entered her apartment and touched her bag of soaps and towels and that she had to throw it all away. She also states that the women in her building have tried to have her evicted because she looks so young for her age. She does not go out at night for fear of being raped. **Psychiatric** referral and 50 mg Melaril tid is recommended.

Physical examination reveals no significant abnormality, and she appears in remarkably good cardiovascular health. She states that she walks the equivalent of two miles a day from her apartment to the store or restaurant. The skin on her hands is thin, pink, and dry from hand washing. She does feel fatigued and has a history of hypothyroidism. She has taken no medication for several weeks since her prescription ran out. Rx 200 mcg Synthroid is recommended after lab results called. She has occasional accidents from incontinence and diarrhea. She was advised on the use of incontinence garments and will be assessed for **UTI**. Lab order: T3, T4, CBC, **Ua with C&S** if necessary, occult blood (OB) stool. Psychiatric consult ordered.

1. abnormally slow-acting thyroid _____

2. uncontrolled bowel movement or urination _____

3. pertaining to psychiatry _____

4. neurosis characterized by anxiety and ritual behavior _____

5. urinary tract infection _____

6. electroshock therapy _____

7. watery stool _____

8. blood pressure, temperature, respiration _____

9. urinalysis with culture and sensitivity _____

10. delusions of persecution and grandeur _____

REVIEW ACTIVITIES

CROSSWORD PUZZLE

Check your answers by going back through the frames or checking the solution in Appendix C.

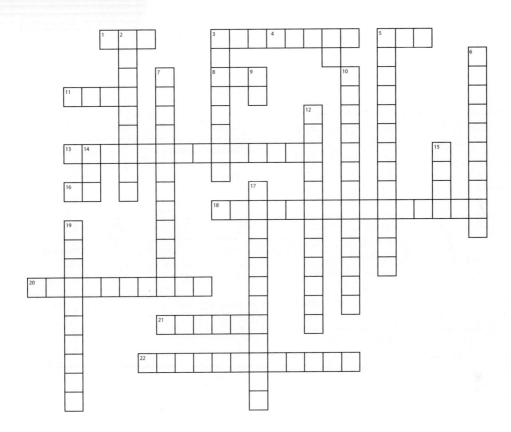

Across

1. obsessive-compulsive disorder
3. anxiety and phobia, nervous condition
5. high density lipoproteins (abbr.)
8. range of motion (abbr.)
11. combining form for vessel
13. study of producing loss of sensation for surgery
16. multiple sclerosis
18. condition; fatty deposits in large vessels, hardening
20. medication; produces loss of sensation
21. combining form for vein
22. pertaining to producing blood clots

Down

2. destruction of cells
3. medication; sleep-producing analgesic
4. intravenous
5. oversensitivity to touch
6. seizures of sleep
7. physician; treats mental disorders
9. myocardial infarction (abbr.)
10. dilation of an artery
12. medication; affects mental processes
14. neurologic vital signs
15. transcutaneous electric nerve stimulation (abbr.)
17. study of drugs
19. synonym for venipuncture

REVIEW ACTIVITIES

GLOSSARY

algesia	condition of pain sensitivity
algesic	pertaining to algesia
algesimeter	instrument for measuring level of pain
analgesia	condition without pain
anesthesia	condition of no sensation
anesthesiology	science of studying the administration of anesthetics
anesthetic	agent that produces loss of sensation
angiectasia	dilation of a vessel
angioblast	immature vessel cell
angiogram	x-ray of a vessel
angiolysis	vessel destruction
angioma	vessel tumor
angiopathy	vessel disease
angioplasty	surgical repair of a vessel
angiorrhexis	rupture of a blood vessel
angiosclerosis	hardening of a vessel
angioscopy	process of looking into a vessel using a scope
angiospasm	vessel spasm
arteriectasia	dilation of an artery
arteriofibrosis	condition of fibrous growth in the arteries
arteriomalacia	softening of the arteries
arteriorrhexis	rupture of an artery
arteriosclerosis	hardening of the arteries
arteriospasm	spasm of an artery

atherectomy	excision of an atheroma
atheroma	fatty tissue tumor inside a large vessel
atherosclerosis	fatty deposits on medium to large vessels, causing hardening
autonomic	self-controlling, stress response center of the nervous system
cardiorrhexis	rupture of the heart
chondrodysplasia	defective development of cartilage
cystorrhexis	rupture of the bladder
cytolysis	cell destruction
dysesthesia	difficult or painful sensation
enterorrhexis	rupture of the small intestine
esthesiometer	instrument used to measure the amount of sensation
fibroma	fibrous tumor
gastromalacia	softening of the stomach
gastrospasm	stomach spasm
hemangioblast	immature blood vessel cell
hemarthrosis	blood in a joint
hematologist	physician specialist in blood disorders
hematology	specialty of studying the blood
hematolysis	destruction of blood (hemolysis)
hematophobia	abnormal fear of blood
hepatorrhexis	rupture of the liver

REVIEW ACTIVITIES

hyperesthesia	oversensitivity to touch (may be painful)
hyperplasia	abnormal over growth of cells
hypoesthesia	below normal ability to feel (touch)
hysterorrhexis	rupture of the uterus
infarction	necrosis of tissue due to ischemia
ischemia	condition of stopping blood supply
lipolysis	lipid destruction
metrorrhexis	rupture of uterine tissues
myelocele	spinal cord herniation
myelocyte	bone marrow or spinal cord cell
myoblast	immature muscle cell
myocardial	pertaining to the heart muscle (myocardium)
myocarditis	inflammation of the myocardium
myofibroma	fibrous muscle tumor
myograph	instrument used to make a picture of muscle function
myography	the process of using a myograph to make a myogram
myolysis	muscle tissue destruction
myoma	muscle tumor
myopathy	muscle disease
myosclerosis	hardening of a muscle
myospasm	muscle spasm
narcolepsy	seizures of uncontrolled sleep

narcosis	condition of being affected by narcotics
narcotic	analgesic and sleep-producing drug
neuroblast	immature nerve cell
neurologist	physician specialist in nervous system disorders
neurolysis	nerve destruction
neuroma	nerve tumor
neuropathy	nerve disease
neurosis	nerve condition characterized by anxiety and phobias
neurospasm	nerve spasm
neurosurgeon	physician specialist who performs surgery on the brain and nerves
neurotripsy	surgical crushing of a nerve
parahepatitis	inflammation near the liver
paralgesia	pain in the lower body
paralgia	abnormal pain
paralysis	loss of muscle function and sensation
paramedic	emergency medical technician with advanced training
paranephritis	inflammation near the kidney
paraosteoarthropathy	disease near the bone and joint
paraplegia	paralysis in the lower body
parasympathetic	nerves that return the body to normal following stress
paroxysmal	pertaining to the sudden onset of an attack, symptoms, or emotion

REVIEW ACTIVITIES

pharmacist	specialist in drug therapy and dispensing drugs	psychotherapy	therapy for mental disorders
pharmacology	study of drug therapy	psychotropic	agent that affects mental processes
phlebectasia	dilation of a vein	thrombectomy	excision of a clot
phlebectomy	excision of a vein	thromboangiitis	blood clot in a vessel causing inflammation
phlebography	process of taking an x-ray of a vein	thrombocyte	blood clotting cell (platelet)
phlebopexy	fixation of a prolapsed vein	thrombocytopenia	lack of platelets
phleboplasty	surgical repair of a vein	thrombogenic	pertaining to producing clots
phleborrhexis	rupture of a vein	thromboid	resembling a clot
phlebosclerosis	hardening of a vein	thrombolymphangitis	inflammation of a lymph vessel caused by a clot
phlebotomy	venipuncture	thrombolysis	clot destruction
psychiatrist	physician specialist in treatment of mental disorders	thrombophlebitis	inflammation of a vein caused by a clot (thrombus)
psychoanalysis	analysis of mental and emotional state for treatment	thrombosis	condition of forming clots
psychology	study of the mind and mental processes	venipuncture	incision into a vein with a needle to remove a venous blood sample (synonym, phlebotomy)
psychomotor	mental processes that control movement		
psychosexual	mental processes related to sexuality	venous	pertaining to veins

UNIT 9

Anatomic Terms

9.1

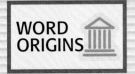

WORD ORIGINS

Ana/tomy comes from the Greek word *anatome* meaning cutting apart. Galen (A.D. 129–199), one of the earliest respected anatomists of the Western world, relied on animal experiments and dissecting corpses to identify and name body parts. As did many scholars of his day, he spoke and wrote in Greek and Latin. Those who followed him continued the creation of the anatomic and medical language that was later converted to English. You will notice that many anatomic terms have both Greek and Latin forms. The study of naming body structures is

_____/_____.

ana/tomy
ə **na**′ tō mē

9.2

Study the following table of new anatomic word parts. These will be used to build terms throughout this unit.

Directional Word	Combining Form	Meaning
dorsal	**dors/o**	near or on the back
ventral	**ventr/o**	near or on the belly side of the body
anterior (ant)	**anter/o**	toward the front or in front of
posterior (post)	**poster/o**	following or located behind
cephalic	**cephal/o**	upward, toward the head
caudal, caudad	**caud/o**	downward, toward the tail
medial	**medi/o**	toward the midline

(continues)

301

Directional Word	Combining Form	Meaning
lateral	**later/o**	toward the side, away from the midline
superior	**super-**	above
inferior	**sub-** or **infra-**	below
proximal	**proxim/o**	near the point of origin
distal	**dist/o**	away from the point of origin
sagittal	**sagitt/o**	vertical, anteroposterior direction or plane dividing into left and right
coronal	**coron/o**	resembling a crown or encircling

9.3

The combining forms for anterior and posterior do not include the i. They are **anter/o** and **poster/o**. Using the information about directional terms in the table, build terms that mean pertaining to the

front and side

anter/o/later/al
an ter ō **lat**′ er al

_____/____/_____/____;

front and middle

anter/o/medi/al
an ter ō **mēd**′ ē al

_____/____/_____/____;

front and top

anter/o/super/ior
an ter ō sup **ēr**′ ē or

_____/____/_____/_____.

9.4

Build terms that mean pertaining to the

back and side

poster/o/later/al
pōst′ er ō **lat**′ er al

_____/____/_____/____;

back and outside of the body

poster/o/extern/al
pōst′ er ō eks **tern**′ al

_____/____/_____/____;

back and inside of the body

poster/o/intern/al
pōst er ō in **tern**′ al

_____/____/_____/____.

9.5

Build terms that mean pertaining to the

front and back (from front to back)

anter/o/poster/ior or
an′ ter ō pōst **ēr**′ ē

_____/____/_____/_____ (AP)

or

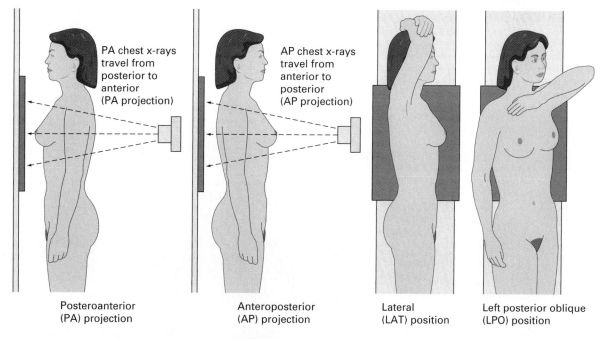

Posteroanterior (PA) projection	Anteroposterior (AP) projection	Lateral (LAT) position	Left posterior oblique (LPO) position

Radiographic projection positions

ANSWER COLUMN

ventr/o/dorsal vent rō **dor**′ sal dors/o/cephal/ad dor sō **sef**′ əl ad ventr/ad (ventral) or **vent**′ rad (**ven**′ trəl) anter/ior an **tēr**′ ē or	_____/_____/_____ ; toward the back of the head _____/_____/_____/____ ; toward the front _____/_____ or _____/_____ . Note: **-ad** as a suffix means toward.

9.6

Proximal (**proxim/o**) means closer to a designated point (like the origin of a muscle or limb), and distal (**dist/o**) means further from a designated point. Because the elbow is closer to the shoulder than the hand is, the elbow is _____/_____ to the shoulder. Because the ankle is further from the hip than the knee, the ankle is _____/_____ to the hip.

proxim/al
proks′ i mal
dist/al
dis′ tal

9.7

A fracture in the upper part (closer to the hip) of the femur (thigh bone) is a fracture of the _____ end of the femur. A fracture in the lower part of the femur is a fracture of the _____ end.

proximal
distal

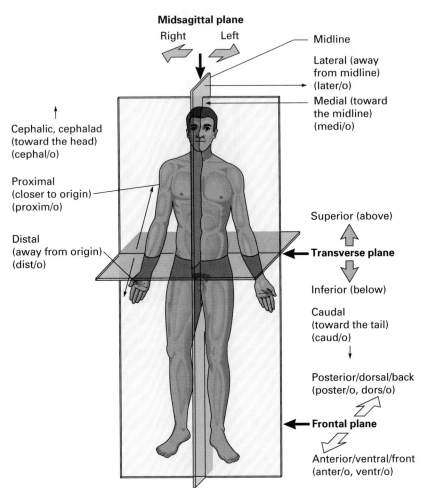

Directions and planes of the body in anatomic position

9.8

distal

The bone in the tip of a finger (phalanx) is the _____ phalanx, because it is farther from the origin of the finger.

proximal

The phalanx close to the palm is the _____ phalanx.

9.9

After studying the table on pages 301 and 302 provide the meaning for the following terms

middle and side
above and to the side
head to tail

medi/o/later/al *_____;
super/o/later/al *_____;
cephal/o/caud/al *_____.

9.10

It is often necessary to look at anatomy by taking views of planes or slices of the body. This happens when using tomography and sonography. A sagittal cut is

ANSWER COLUMN

mid/sagitt/al
mid **saj**′ i tal

made in a vertical, anteroposterior direction. Such a cut made at the midline to divide the body into equal right and left halves is called the
_____/_____/_____ plane.

9.11

sagitt/al
saj′ i tal

Any vertical slice from front to back is a _____/_____ view.

9.12

WORD ORIGINS

In Latin *sagittalis* means arrowlike. The constellation and astrological sign Sagittarius is the shape of a mythological character, a Centaur, that is half man, half horse drawing a bow with a star for its arrow point. It is as if to say if struck with an arrow, a person would be cut into halves.

9.13

crown
circle (encircle)

The coron/al suture line of the skull sits at the crown of the skull. Coron/al comes from a Greek word root meaning crown or circle. The corona dentis is the _____ of a tooth. The coron/ary arteries _____ the heart to supply the muscle with blood.

9.14

coron/ary
kor′ ən air ē
coron/ary

The arteries encircling the heart are the _____/_____ arteries.
The veins encircling the heart are the _____/_____ veins.

9.15

INFORMATION FRAME

To find a word root for navel, look up navel in the dictionary. A synonym for navel is the Latin word *umbilicus.* The Greek combining form **omphal/o** comes from *omphalos.*

9.16

omphal/itis
om fəl **ī**′ tis

Inflammation of the umbilicus is _____/_____.

9.17

omphal/o

In the dictionary, turn to words beginning with **omphal/o**. The combining form for navel is _____/_____.

ANSWER COLUMN

9.18

Using **omphal/o**, build words meaning
pertaining to the navel

omphal/ic
_____/_____ ;

om **fal**′ ik
excision of the umbilicus

omphal/ectomy
_____/_____ ;

om fə **lek**′ tə mē
herniation of the navel (umbilical hernia)

omphal/o/cele   or
_____/_____/_____ or

om′ fə lō sēl, om **fal**′ ō sēl

umbilic/o/cele
_____/___/_____

um bil′ **i kō** sēl

9.19

Build words meaning
umbilical hemorrhage

omphal/o/rrhagia
_____/_____/_____ ;

om′ fâ lō **rāj**′ ē ə
discharge flowing from the navel

omphal/o/rrhea
_____/_____/_____ ;

om′ fâ lō **rē**′ ə
rupture of the navel

omphal/o/rrhexis
_____/_____/_____ .

om′ fəl ō **reks**′ is

9.20

navel
Words containing **omphal/o** refer to the _____, which is also called

umbilicus
the _____ .

9.21

ad- is used as a suffix meaning toward. Build words meaning
toward the head

cephal/ad
_____/_____ and

sef′ al ad
toward the tail (lower spine)

caud/ad
_____/_____ .

kaw′ dad

9.22

Human development is usually in a head-to-body (tail) direction. (The structures
of the head develop first.) This is called

cephal/o/caud/al
_____/_____/_____/_____ development.

sef′ al ō **kaw**′ dal

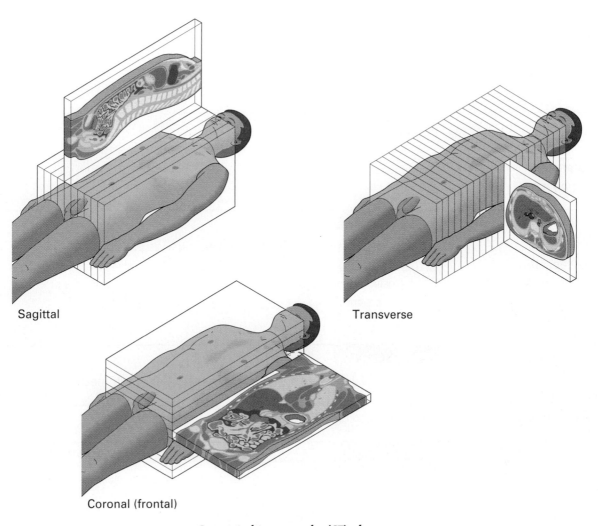

Sagittal

Transverse

Coronal (frontal)

Computed tomography (CT) planes

INFORMATION
FRAME

9.23

In your dictionary look at the words beginning with gnos. They come from the Greek word meaning knowledge.

9.24

The words gnosia and gnosis are medical words built from the Greek word meaning _____.

knowledge

ANSWER COLUMN

	9.25
	pro- is a prefix meaning in front of; pro/gnos/is (P$_x$) means foreknowledge or predicting the outcome of a disease. The prefix that means before or in front of
pro	is _____ .
	9.26
	Leukemia is a serious disease associated with leukocytes. The
pro/gnos/is	_____ / _____ / _____ of acute leukemia is grave.
prog **nō′** sis	
	9.27
	Procephalic means in the front of the head. Analyze procephalic
pro/cephal/ic	_____ / _____ / _____ .
prō sə **fal′** ik	Prognostic means giving an indication concerning the outcome of a disease.
pro/gnos/tic	Analyze prognostic: _____ / _____ / _____ .
prog **nos′** tik	
	9.28
	dia- means through or complete. Dia/gnos/is (D$_x$) literally means
knowing through or	* _____
know through	(identification of a disease through signs and symptoms).
	9.29
	Dia/gnos/tic is the adjectival form of diagnosis and dia/gnos/e is the verb.
dia/gnos/tic	When the results of the _____ / _____ / _____
dī ag **nos′** tik	(adjective) tests are complete, the physician will
dia/gnos/e	_____ / _____ / _____ (verb) the condition of the patient.
dī′ ag nōs	
	9.30
	A diagnosis (identification of a disease) is made by studying through its symptoms. When a patient tells of having chills, hot spells, and a runny nose, the physician
dia/gnos/is	may make the _____ / _____ / _____ of viral syndrome.
dī əg **nō′** sis	
	9.31
	Nurses observe patients for signs and symptoms of conditions that require treatment. After careful observation, a nurse will summarize these findings
dia/gnos/is	by writing a nursing _____ . The patient may have several
dia/gnos/es	_____ / _____ .
dī əg **nō′** sēs	

ANSWER COLUMN

9.32

The literal meaning of dia/rrhea (watery stool) is

flowing through

*_____.

INFORMATION
FRAME

9.33

Dia/lysis is the separation of substances in a solution.
Hem/o/dia/lysis removes waste from the blood by using an artificial kidney machine.

9.34

Dialysis is a process of destroying waste products in the blood by diffusion through a membrane. People with kidney failure (ESRD, end-stage renal disease)

dia/lysis
dī al′ i sis

may need _____/_____ to remove waste from their blood.

9.35

dialysis

Peritoneal dialysis and hemodialysis are two types of _____.

9.36

A dia/scope is placed on the skin, and the skin is looked at *through* the instrument to see superficial surface lesions and other things. The word part for

dia

through is _____ .

9.37

aer/o is used in words to mean air. You undoubtedly know the words aer/ial and

air

aer/ialist. **aer/o** always makes you think of _____ .

9.38

Using what you need of **aer/o**, build words meaning
abnormal fear of air

aer/o/phobia
air′ ō **fō**′ bē ə
_____/_____/_____ ;
treatment with air

aer/o/therapy
air′ ō **ther**′ ə pē
_____/_____/_____ ;
herniation containing air

aer/o/cele
air′ ō sēl
_____/_____/_____ .

9.39

Bios is the Greek word for life. Bi/o/chemistry is the study of chemical changes in living things. The science (study of) living things is

bi/o/logy
bī o′ lə jē
_____/_____/_____ .

Peritoneal dialysis

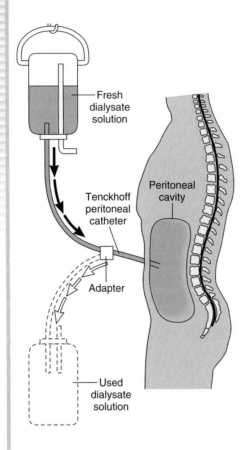

Fresh dialysate solution

Tenckhoff peritoneal catheter

Peritoneal cavity

Adapter

Used dialysate solution

Hemodialysis

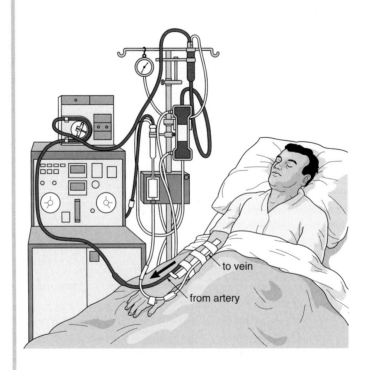

to vein

from artery

ANSWER COLUMN

9.40

living things or life

A bi/o/logist is one who studies
*_____.

living things

Bi/o/genesis is the formation of
*_____.

9.41

An an/aer/o/bic plant or animal cannot live in the presence of air (**an-**—without).
Analyze anaerobic:

an

prefix (without) _____ ;

aer/o

combining form (air) _____/_____ ;

bic

suffix (life) _____ .

9.42

If anaerobic means existing without air (oxygen), build a word that means
needing air (oxygen) to live (adjective);

aer/o/bic

_____/_____/_____ .

air ō′ bik

9.43

Use aerobic or anaerobic in Frames 9.43–9.45.
The bacterium that causes pneumonia requires air to live. These bacteria are

aerobic

considered _____ bacteria.

9.44

The tetanus bacillus causes lockjaw. Lockjaw can develop only in closed wounds
where air does not penetrate (e.g., stepping on an old nail). The tetanus bacillus

an/aer/o/bic

is an _____/_____/_____/_____ bacterium. Read about

an ə rō′ bik

tetanus in your medical dictionary.

9.45

Botulism is a serious type of food poisoning. It occurs from eating improperly
canned meats and vegetables. Cans do not admit air. The bacillus that causes

anaerobic

botulism is _____ .

9.46

A bi/o/psy is an excision of tissue for examination of

living or live

*_____ tissue.

9.47

A combining form that means color is **chrom/o**. The Greek word for a color is
chroma. There are English words chroma and chrome. **chrom/o** makes you

color

think of _____ .

ANSWER COLUMN

Neisseria gonorrhoeae **in synovial fluid** *(gram-negative intracellular diplococci)*

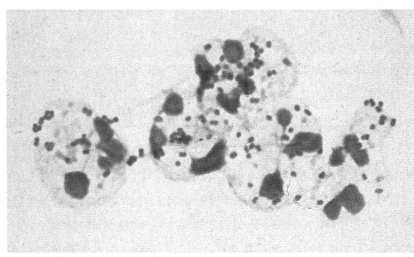

---

chrom/o/blast
krō′ mō blast

9.48

A chrom/o/cyte is any colored cell. An embryonic color (pigment) cell is called a _____/_____/_____.

---

chrom/o/lysis
krō **mol′** ə sis
chrom/o/gen/esis
krō′ mō **jen′** ə sis
chrom/o/meter
krō **mom′** ə ter

9.49

Build words meaning
destruction of color (in a cell)
_____/_____/_____;
formation of pigment (color)
_____/_____/_____/_____;
instrument for measuring amount of color in a substance
_____/_____/_____.
(chromat/o/graph)

---

chrom/o/philic
krō′ mō **fil′** ik

9.50

phil is a word root meaning attracted to or loves. A chrom/o/philic cell is one that takes a stain easily (attracts stain). Some leukocytes stain deeper than others. They are more _____/_____/_____ than the less easily stained leukocytes.

---

chromophilic

9.51

Some cells are chrom/o/phobic and will not stain at all. They are not _____.

EXAMPLE: Gram-negative bacteria will not attract color from the Gram stain.

ANSWER COLUMN

	9.52
staining easily	Chromophilic means *_____.
	The word that means something does not (without) stain easily is
a/chrom/o/philic	_____/_____/_____/_____.
ā′ krō mō **fil**′ ik	

	9.53
abnormal, bad, painful, or	**dys-** means *_____.
difficult	The opposite of **dys-** is **eu-**, which means
well or easy	*_____.

	9.54
	Form the word that means the opposite of
	dys/pepsia
eu/pepsia	_____/_____ ;
yōo **pep**′ sē ə	dys/peptic
eu/peptic	_____/_____ ;
yōo **pep**′ tik	dys/pnea
eu/pnea	_____/_____.
yōop **nē**′ ə or	
yōop′ nē ə	

	9.55
	Form the opposite of
	dys/kines/ia
eu/kinesi/a	_____/_____/_____ ;
yōo ki **nē**′ zhə	dys/esthes/ia
eu/esthesi/a	_____/_____/_____ ;
yōo es **thē**′ zhə	dys/phor/ia
eu/phor/ia	_____/_____/_____.
yōo **fôr**′ ē ə	

	9.56
	-tocia is a suffix meaning labor. Dys/tocia (dis tō′ shə) means difficult labor.
	Eu/tocia (ū tō′ shə) means
easy or normal labor	*_____.
and childbirth	

	9.57
	If you work a frame and have forgotten what the word root means, look it up
	in your medical dictionary. Use this frame to take a breath and _____.

ANSWER COLUMN

9.58

Thanatos is a Greek word meaning death. The word root for death is than. When someone has an easy or peaceful death, it is called

eu/than/asia
yōō than ā′ zhə
euthanasia

_____/_____/_____ .

Many ethical medical questions surround the subject of _____.
If this interests you, you may want to learn about active and passive euthanasia.

9.59

Another area of ethics is the study of eu/gen/ics (good development).
Researchers are working on ways to improve humans through genetic engineering. Look up eugenic in your dictionary and analyze the word parts

good
form or produce
adjective ending

eu- _____ ;
gen *_____ ;
-ic *_____ .

9.60

Eugenic sterilization is selective sterilization of individuals that society says have undesirable traits or would be unable to be good parents. One controversial topic of bi/o/ethics is whether severely mentally impaired adult patients may be

eu/gen/ic
yōō **jen**′ ik

selected for _____/_____/_____ sterilization.

9.61

INFORMATION FRAME

Bi/o/ethics and medical ethics are topics that deal with decisions about life and medical treatments that concern right and wrong as seen by both society and individuals.

9.62

Euthanasia and eugenics are both controversial topics concerning

bi/o/ethics
bī ō **eth**′ iks

_____/_____/_____ .

9.63

Recall that **enter/o** is the combining form for intestine. Infections of the intestine can be viral, bacterial, or parasitic and cause pain and diarrhea. This painful or difficult condition of the small intestine is called _____/_____/___.

dys/entery
dis′ en tair ē

NOTE: **enter/o** is used more with words about the small intestine, and **col/o** is used for the large intestine.

ANSWER COLUMN

9.64

dysentery

Travelers are cautioned not to drink water in countries with poor sanitation systems to avoid contracting amebic _____.

9.65

men/o is used in words referring to the menses. In Latin *mensis* means month. Men/ses is another way of saying men/struation, which occurs in monthly cycles. **men/o** in any word should make you think of _____ / _____.

men/ses   or
men′ sis
men/struation
men strōō **ā′** shun

9.66

SPELL
CHECK ✓

Watch the spelling and pronunciation of menstruation. There is "a u" after the "str", and it is pronounced with a long "u" sound.

9.67

Men/arche (men ar′ kē) comes from the Greek words *men* for month and *arche* for beginning. Menarche refers to a female's first menstrual period. Build words meaning flow of menses

men/o/rrhea
men ə **rē′** ə
dys/men/o/rrhea
dis′ men ə **rē′** ə

_____ / _____ / _____ ;
painful (bad or difficult) menstrual flow
_____ / _____ / _____ / _____ .

9.68

Men/o/pause (men′ ō paws) means permanent cessation of

menstruation or menses

* _____.
Men/o/rrhagia (men ō rā′ jē ə) means

excessive menstruation   or
menstrual hemorrhage

* _____
_____.

9.69

Build words meaning
absence (without) menstrual flow

a/men/o/rrhea
ā men ə **rē′** ə
men/o/stasis
mə **nos′** te sis

_____ / _____ / _____ / _____ ;
stopping menstrual flow
_____ / _____ / stasis _____ .

ANSWER COLUMN

9.70

-**stasis** means the act or condition of stopping or controlling.

act of controlling
blood flow

Hem/o/stasis means *_____.

A word meaning control of blood flow in veins is

phleb/o/stasis or
fli **bos**′ tə sis
ven/o/stasis
vē **nos**′ tə sis

_____/_____/_____.

9.71

Build words meaning
control of flow in arteries

arteri/o/stasis
är tir′ ē **os**′ tə sis
lymph/o/stasis
lim **fos**′ tə sis

_____/_____/_____;

control of lymph flow

_____/_____/_____.

PRONUNCIATION NOTE

Medical terms ending in -**stasis** are formally pronounced as indicated in Frames 9.70 and 9.71. In practice and transcription you will probably hear the following instead

phlebostasis—flē bō **stā**′ sis
venostasis—vē nō **stā**′ sis
arteriostasis—är tir ē ō **stā**′ sis
hemostasis—hē mō **stā**′ sis

9.72

syphil/o

Syphilis is a sexually transmitted disease (STD). Read about the disease in your dictionary. Note the origin of the word. Look at the words beginning with syphil. The combining form used in words referring to this disease is _____/_____.

9.73

Using syphil, build terms that mean
mental condition caused by syphilis

syphil/o/psych/osis
sif′ il ō sī **kō**′ sis
syphil/o/phobia
sif′ il ō **fōb**′ ē ə
syphil/o/therapy
sif′ il ō **ther**′ a pē

_____/_____/_____/_____;

fear of contracting syphilis

_____/_____/_____;

therapy for syphilis

_____/_____/_____.

Syphilitic chancre

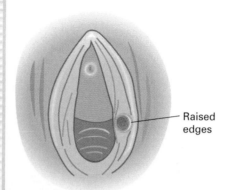

Raised
edges

9.74

Build words meaning
a syphilitic tumor

syphil/oma
sif il **ō**′ mə

_____/_____ ;

any syphilitic disease

syphil/o/pathy
sif il **op**′ ə thē

_____/_____/_____ .

9.75

-cyesis comes from the Greek word *kyesis* meaning pregnancy. **pseudo-** means false. A pseud/o/cyesis (sōō dō sī ē′ sis) or pseud/o/pregnancy is a false pregnancy. A pseud/o/science is a

false science

* _____ .

9.76

Pseud/o/mania is a psychosis in which patients have a false or pretended mental disorder. Pseud/o/paralysis means

false paralysis
(paralysis not due
  to nerve damage)

* _____ .

9.77

Build words meaning
a false cyst

pseud/o/cyst
sōō′ dō sist

_____/_____/_____ ;

false edema

pseud/o/edema
sōō′ ə **dē**′ mə

_____/_____/_____ ;

false or imaginary sensation

pseud/o/esthesi/a
sōō′ dō es **thē**′ zhə

_____/_____/_____/_____ .

Look up and learn the meaning of edema.

ANSWER COLUMN

9.78

Build words meaning
false hypertrophy

pseud/o/hyper/trophy   _____/_____/_____/_____ ;

false tuberculosis (TB)

pseud/o/tubercul/osis   _____/_____/_____/_____ ;

false nerve tumor

pseud/o/neur/oma   _____/_____/_____/_____ .
(You pronounce)

9.79

SPELL CHECK ✓

Words built with **pseud/o** often give students spelling and pronunciation problems. Remember, the *p* is silent and the *eu* has a long *u* sound.

9.80

viscer/o

The viscera (singular viscus) are the internal organs of the body. Viscer/ad means toward the viscera. Viscer/o/genic means development of organs. The combining form for viscera is _____/_____ .

9.81

organs (internal)

In the words viscer/o/motor, viscer/o/pariet/al, and viscer/o/pleur/al, **viscer/o** refers to _____ .

9.82

periton/eum
per i tō **nē**′ um

Locate the peritoneum on page 319. The membrane that lines the abdominal cavity is the _____/_____ .

9.83

pleur/al
plōor′ əl

Locate the pleura on page 319. The membrane that covers the lungs is the visceral _____/_____ membrane.

9.84

INFORMATION FRAME 💡

pariet/o is the combining form for wall. Uses of visceral (vis′ er əl) and parietal (pa rī′ ə təl) include

visceral pleura   (membrane on the surface of the lung)
parietal pleura   (membrane on chest cavity wall)
visceral peritoneum (membrane on the surface of the organs of the
                            abdominal cavity)
parietal peritoneum (membrane on the abdominal cavity wall)

ANSWER COLUMN

Ventral cavity membranes

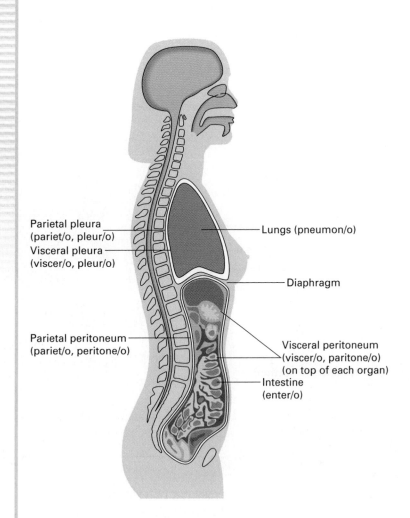

Parietal pleura
(pariet/o, pleur/o)

Visceral pleura
(viscer/o, pleur/o)

Lungs (pneumon/o)

Diaphragm

Parietal peritoneum
(pariet/o, peritone/o)

Visceral peritoneum
(viscer/o, paritone/o)
(on top of each organ)

Intestine
(enter/o)

9.85

Name the membrane that
covers the surface of the lungs

viscer/al

vis′ er əl

pariet/al

pa **rī**′ ə təl

_____/_____ pleura;

is on the thoracic cavity wall

_____/_____ pleura.

9.86

Build words meaning
prolapse of organs

viscer/o/ptosis

vis′ ər op **tō**′ sis

viscer/algia

vis′ ər al′ jē ə

viscer/al

vis′ ər əl

_____/_____/_____ ;

pain in organs

_____/_____ ;

pertaining to organs

_____/_____ .

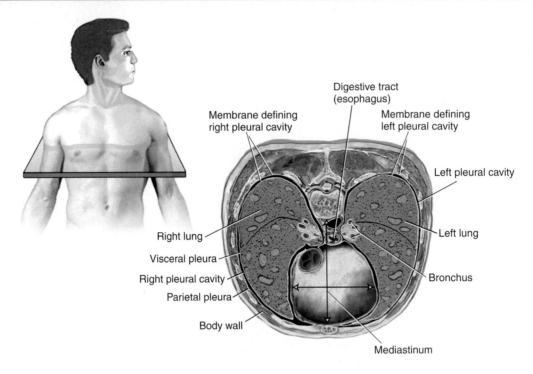

Thorax (transverse section)

ANSWER COLUMN

9.87

Build words beginning with **viscer/o** that mean

sensory function of organs

viscer/o/sensor/y
vis′ er ō **sens**′ ôr ē

_____/____/_____/____ ;

pertaining to organs and the skeleton

viscer/o/skelet/al
vis′ er ō **skel**′ e tal

_____/____/_____/_____ ;

pertaining to the development of organs

viscer/o/gen/ic
vis′ er ō **jen**′ ik

_____/____/_____/_____ .

The following table is for use in building words for Frames 9.88-9.120.

Prefix of Location	Meaning
ecto-	outer-outside
endo-	inner-inside
meso-	middle
retro-	backward-behind
para-	near

ANSWER COLUMN

9.88

The blast/o/derm is an embryonic disk of cells that gives rise to the three main layers of tissue in humans. The outer germ layer is called the ecto/derm. The inner germ layer is called the _____/_____ .

endo/derm
en′ dō dûrm

9.89

Between the ectoderm and endoderm is a middle germ layer called the _____/_____ .

meso/derm
mez′ ō dûrm

9.90

The ectoderm forms the skin. The nervous system arises from the same layer as the skin. This layer is the _____/_____ .

ecto/derm
ek′ tō dûrm

9.91

Sense organs and some glands are also formed from the _____ .

ectoderm

9.92

The endo/derm forms organs inside the body. The stomach and small intestine arise from the _____ .

endoderm

9.93

The mesoderm forms the organs that arise between the ectoderm and endoderm. Muscles are formed by the _____ .

mesoderm

9.94

The blastoderm gives rise to the three germ layers. They are

outer   _____ ;
middle _____ ;
inner   _____ .

ectoderm
mesoderm
endoderm

9.95

ecto- is a Latin prefix for outside. **exo-** is a Greek prefix for outside. Something produced within an organism is said to be endo/gen/ous. Something produced outside an organism is _____/_____
or
_____/_____ .

ecto/genous
ek **toj′** ə nəs
exo/genous
eks **oj′** ə nəs

ANSWER COLUMN

9.96

ectogenous or exogenous

Type 1 diabetics produce very little endogenous insulin. Therefore, they must take _____ (from an outside source) insulin.

9.97

poly/ur/ia
poly/dips/ia
poly/phag/ia

People with type 1 diabetes have hyperglycemia and no insulin to carry the glucose into the cells. Therefore they exhibit the three *P*s as classic symptoms. Recall the prefix **poly-** and build words that represent these symptoms:
excessive urination _____/_____/_____;
excessive thirst _____/_____/_____;
excessive hunger _____/_____/_____.

9.98

endo/cyst/ic
en′ dō **sis**′ tik

Ecto/cyt/ic is an adjective meaning outside a cell. An adjective meaning inside a bladder is _____/_____/_____.

9.99

ecto/plasm
endo/plasm   or
cyt/o/plasm
(You pronounce)

-plasm is used as a suffix in words about the substance of cells (cyt/o/plasm). **proto-** means first. Think of prot/o/type. Prot/o/plasm is the substance of life. The protoplasm that forms the outer membrane of the cell is called _____/_____. The protoplasm within the cell is called _____/_____/_____.

9.100

endo/chondr/al
en′ dō **kon**′ drəl

Endo/crani/al is an adjective meaning within the cranium. An adjective meaning within cartilage is _____/_____/_____.

9.101

endo/cardial   or
endo/cardiac
endo/colitis
(You pronounce)

Endo/enter/itis means inflammation of the lining of the small intestine. Build words meaning
pertaining to the lining of the heart (adjective)
_____/_____;
inflammation of the lining of the colon
_____/_____.

9.102

An endo/scope is an instrument used to look into a hollow organ or cavity of the body, as in viewing the stomach. The process of viewing the stomach through an instrument is called _____/_____

endo/scopy
en' **dos**' kō pē
gastr/o/scopy
gas **tros**' kō pē

or

_____/_____/_____.

9.103

endoscopy

Esophag/o/gastr/o/duoden/o/scopy (EGD) is one type of _____.

WORD BUILDING
■ ■ ■ ■ ■

ESOPHAG/O	+	GASTR/O	+	DUODEN/O	+	SCOPY
combining form		combining form		combining form		suffix

9.104

Using what you know about **endo-**, **arter**, and **-ectomy**, complete the definition of this term

end/arter/ectomy—removal of a substance (usually an atheroma) from the

inside

_____ of an artery.

9.105

INFORMATION
FRAME

Note the involved development of the word ectopic (out of place)
ect/o—outside
top/os—place (Greek word)
-ic—adjectival suffix

9.106

An ectopic pregnancy occurs outside of the uterus (usually in a fallopian tube). A salpingectomy may be required after the rupture of an

ec/topic
ek **top**' ik

_____/_____ pregnancy.

9.107

ectopic

If endometrial tissue occurs in the fallopian tubes, a fertilized egg can lodge in it, thus causing pregnancy. This is an _____ pregnancy.

9.108

ectopic

An embryo's development in the abdominal cavity is another example of an

_____ pregnancy.

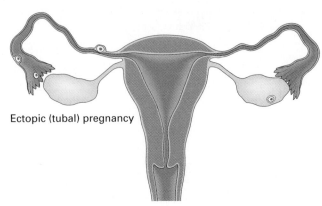

Ectopic (tubal) pregnancy

9.109

mes/entery
mez′ en tair ē
meso/colon
mez′ ō **kol′** in
meso/dont/ic
mez′ ō **don′** tik

meso- is a prefix for middle. Build words meaning peritoneum attaching intestine to the abdominal wall (literally: middle intestine)

_____/_____ ;

peritoneum attaching large intestine to the abdominal wall (mesentery of the colon)

_____/_____ ;

pertaining to middle-sized teeth

_____/_____/_____ .

9.110

retro/colic
ret′ rō **kol′** ik
retro/mammary
ret′ rō **mam′** ə rē
retro/stern/al
ret′ rō **stûr′** nəl

retro- is a prefix meaning behind. Build adjectives meaning

behind the colon

_____/_____ ;

behind the breast (mammary glands)

_____/_____ ;

behind the stern/um

_____/_____/_____ .

9.111

retro/version
ret′ rō vûr zhən

Ante/version means turning forward. The word for turning backward

is _____/_____ .

9.112

behind

retro/periton/itis
ret′ rō per′ i tə **nī′** tis

The retro/periton/eum is the space _____ the peritoneum. An inflammation of this space is called

_____/_____/_____ .

ANSWER COLUMN

9.113

Recall that ERCP is an x-ray procedure in which an endo/scope is used to inject a contrast medium into the ducts of the pancreas and gallbladder so that any obstructions can be viewed. Using what you know about the word parts you have already learned, draw the slashes for the ERCP terms:

endo/scop/ic
retro/grade

endoscopic _____;
retrograde _____;
cholangiopancreatography

chol/angi/o/pancreat/o/
 -graphy

_____.

Refer to the illustration near frame 7.72

9.114

Flex/ion is bending or shortening of a body part (usually at a joint). **ante-** is the prefix for front or forward. Therefore, the word ante/flexion means

bending forward

*_____.

9.115

retro- means behind (or backward). Build a term meaning bending backward:

retro/flexion
re′ trō flek shən

_____/_____.

9.116

Retro/flexion of the uterus means that the uterus is

bending backward

*_____.

Uterine Positions

Anteversion   Marked retroversion   Retroflexion

9.117

para- as a prefix means near, beside, or around.

near the center or
 around the center
inflammation around
 the appendix

Para/centr/al means *_____

_____.

Para-/appendic/itis means *_____

_____.

ANSWER COLUMN

9.118

Build words meaning
inflammation around (near) the bladder
_____/_____/_____ ;
inflammation of tissues around (near) the vagina
_____/_____/_____ .

para/cyst/itis
par′ ə sis **tī**′ tis
para/colp/itis
par′ ə kol **pī**′ tis

9.119

Build words meaning inflammation of tissues
near the liver
_____/_____/_____ ;
near the kidney
_____/_____/_____ .

para/hepat/itis

para/nephr/itis
(You pronounce)

9.120

outer
inner
middle
around (near)
behind

ecto- means _____.
endo- means _____.
meso- means _____.
para- means _____.
retro- means _____.

Abbreviation	Meaning
ā	before
AD	right ear (*auris dextra*)
AP	anterior to posterior, anteroposterior
AS	left ear (*auris sinstra*)
AU	both ears (*auris uterque*)
Bx	biopsy
CT	computed tomography
DRG	diagnostic-related group
Dx	diagnosis, diagnoses
ESRD	end-stage renal disease
Hx	history
LAT	lateral
LMP	last menstrual period
LOA	left occiput anterior

ANSWER COLUMN

Abbreviation	Meaning
LPO	left posterior oblique
OD	right eye (*ocula dextra*)
OS	left eye (*ocula sinistra*)
OT	occupational therapy
OU	both eyes (*ocula uterque*), each eye
PA	posterior to anterior
p̄	after
Px	prognosis, prognoses
ROP	right occiput posterior
RPO	right posterior oblique
RPR, VDRL	syphilis test (blood test)
STD, STI	sexually transmitted disease (infection)
TB	tuberculosis
VD	venereal disease (old use STD)

To complete your study of this unit, work the **Review Activities** on the following pages. Also, listen to the audio CDs that accompany *Medical Terminology: A Programmed Systems Approach,* 9th edition, and practice your pronunciation.

Additional practice exercises for this unit are available on the Learner Practice CD-ROM found in the back of the textbook.

REVIEW ACTIVITIES

CIRCLE AND CORRECT

Circle the correct answer for each question. Then check your answers in Appendix A.

1. Prefix for in front of
   a. sub-   b. pro-
   c. post-   d. an-

2. Prefix for through
   a. gnosis-   b. pre-
   c. pro-   d. dia-

3. Suffix for substance that affects
   a. -pathic   b. -tropic
   c. -trophic   d. -phobic

4. Word root for front
   a. frontal   b. post
   c. ante   d. anter

REVIEW ACTIVITIES

5. Combining form for back
   a. posto
   b. posterio
   c. ventr
   d. postero

6. Adjectival form for side
   a. anterial
   b. dorsal
   c. lateral
   d. laterial

7. Combining form for umbilicus
   a. omphalo
   b. onycho
   c. umbilical
   d. omphalic

8. Combining form for without air
   a. pneumo
   b. apnea
   c. anaero
   d. aerobic

9. Suffix for attraction to
   a. -philic
   b. -phobic
   c. -phagic
   d. -appeal

10. Prefix for false
    a. fraud-
    b. psycho-
    c. pseudo-
    d. mal-

11. Prefix for easy or good
    a. a-
    b. eu-
    c. dys-
    d. eas-

12. Prefix or suffix for toward
    a. rrhexis
    b. al
    c. ad
    d. to

13. Word root for color
    a. chrom
    b. chlor
    c. xanth
    d. philic

14. Combining form for menstruation
    a. metro
    b. metrio
    c. orrhea
    d. meno

15. Suffix for controlling or stopping
    a. -rrhagia
    b. -centesis
    c. -stasis
    d. -dilation

16. Combining form for wall
    a. peritoneo
    b. parieto
    c. viscero
    d. septum

SELECT AND CONSTRUCT

Select the correct word parts from the following list and construct medical terms that represent the given meaning.

a/an	aero	anter/o/ior	bio/bic	caud/al
cephal/o/ic	chrom/o	cyesis	derm	dia
dist/o	dys	ecto	edema	endo
eu	gen/ous	gnosis	gustr/o	hemo
hyper	itis	later/o/al	log/y/ist	lysis
medi/o	men/o	meso	omphal/o	omphal/o/ic
osis	pariet/o/al	pepsia	periton/eam/a/	philia/ic
phobia	phoria	pleur/o/al	poster/o/ior	pro
proxim/o/al	pseud/o	retro	rrhea	scopy
stasis	syphil/o/is	thanas/o/ia	topic	tropic
ventr/o	viscer/o/al			

1. looking into the stomach with a scope   _____

2. behind the peritoneum (adjective)   _____

3. filtering blood through a membrane (artificial kidney)   _____

REVIEW ACTIVITIES

4. inner germ layer that gives rise to muscle _____

5. outside of the normal location (i.e., pregnancy) _____

6. pertaining to direction from back to front _____

7. pertaining to in front of the head _____

8. identification of a disease through signs and symptoms _____

9. inflammation of the umbilicus (navel) _____

10. pertaining to the side and front _____

11. pertaining to a direction from head to tail _____

12. lack of digestion _____

13. false pregnancy _____

14. feeling of well-being (good) _____

15. easy (peaceful) death _____

16. difficult (painful) menstruation _____

17. membrane attached to the lung _____

18. control of blood flow _____

19. uses air to live (metabolism with oxygen) _____

20. absorbs stain easily _____

21. membrane that lines the abdominal wall _____

22. discharge from the navel _____

23. fear of contracting syphilis _____

24. pertaining to the middle and the side _____

25. formed outside of the body (from another source) _____

DEFINE AND DISSECT

Give a brief definition and dissect each term listed into its word parts in the space provided. Check your answers by referring to the frame listed in parentheses and your medical dictionary. Then listen to the CD to practice pronunciation.

1. diagnostic (9.29)

_____/_____/_____
    pre   rt   suffix

_____
              definition

2. dialysis (9.34)

_____/_____
    pre   suffix

_____

REVIEW ACTIVITIES

3. ectoderm (9.90)

_____/_____

pre   rt

4. exogenous (9.95)

_____/_____/_____

pre   rt   suffix

5. polyphagia (9.97)

_____/_____

pre   suffix

6. endoscopy (9.102)

_____/_____

pre   suffix

7. mesentery (9.109)

_____/_____/____

pre   rt   suffix

8. retroversion (9.111)

_____/_____/____

pre   rt   suffix

9. prognosis (9.26)

_____/____/____

pre   rt   suffix

10. hemodialysis (9.33)

_____/___/____/_____

rt   v   pre   suffix

11. cholangiopancreatography (9.113)

_____/_____/___/_____/___/_____

rt   rt   v   rt   v   suffix

12. para-appendicitis (9.117)

_____-/_____/_____

pre   rt   suffix

13. paranephritis (9.119)

_____/___/_____

pre   rt   suffix

14. proximal (9.6)

_____/___

rt   suffix

REVIEW ACTIVITIES

15. dorsocephalad (9.5)

_____ / ___ / _____ / ___
rt   v   rt   suffix

16. posterolateral (9.4)

_____ / ___ / _____ / ___
rt   v   rt   suffix

17. omphalocele (9.18)

_____ / ___ / _____
rt   v   suffix

18. dysentery (9.63)

___ / ___ / _____
rt   v   rt/suffix

19. anaerobic (9.44)

___ / _____ / ___ / _____
pre   rt   v   suffix

20. biopsy (9.46)

___ / ___ / _____
rt   v   suffix

21. chromolysis (9.49)

_____ / ___ / _____
rt   v   suffix

22. eukinesia (9.55)

___ / _____ / ___
pre   rt   suffix

23. euthanasia (9.58)

___ / _____ / _____
pre   rt   suffix

24. menorrhea (9.67)

_____ / _____ / _____
rt   v   suffix

25. syphilopsychosis (9.73)

_____ / ___ / _____ / _____
rt   v   rt   suffix

26. pseudoesthesia (9.77)

_____ / ___ / _____ / ___
rt   v   rt   suffix

REVIEW ACTIVITIES

27. pseudoneuroma (9.78)

_____/___/_____/_____
rt   v   rt   suffix

_____

28. visceroptosis (9.86)

_____/__/_____
rt   v   suffix

_____

29. visceropleural (9.81)

_____/__/_____/_____
rt   v   rt   suffix

_____

30. distal (9.6)

_____/_____
rt   suffix

_____

31. mediolateral (9.9)

_____/__/_____/_____
rt   v   rt   suffix

_____

32. omphalorrhagia (9.19)

_____/__/_____
rt   v   suffix

_____

33. dyspnea (9.54)

_____/_____
pre   suffix

_____

34. cephalocaudal (9.22)

_____/__/_____/_____
rt   v   rt   suffix

_____

35. achromophilic (9.52)

__/_____/__/_____
pre   rt   v   suffix

_____

36. phlebostasis (9.70)

_____/__/_____
rt   v   suffix

_____

37. visceromotor (9.81)

_____/__/_____
rt   v   rt/suffix

_____

38. chromoblast (9.48)

_____/__/_____
rt   v   suffix

_____

REVIEW ACTIVITIES

DIAGRAM LABELS

From what you have learned about directional terms, complete the diagram below by labeling the blanks with the proper direction term or word part.

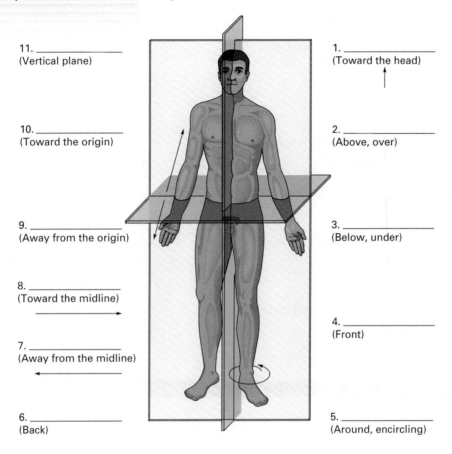

11. _____
(Vertical plane)

10. _____
(Toward the origin)

9. _____
(Away from the origin)

8. _____
(Toward the midline)

7. _____
(Away from the midline)

6. _____
(Back)

1. _____
(Toward the head)

2. _____
(Above, over)

3. _____
(Below, under)

4. _____
(Front)

5. _____
(Around, encircling)

REVIEW ACTIVITIES

ABBREVIATION MATCHING

Match the following abbreviations with their definition.

_____ 1. Dx   a. treatment

_____ 2. Bx   b. prescribe

_____ 3. Hx   c. diagnosis-related group

_____ 4. OD   d. anterior

_____ 5. Px   e. prognosis

_____ 6. ESRD   f. last menstrual period

_____ 7. AP   g. certified pharmacy technician

_____ 8. LMP   h. diagnosis

_____ 9. DRG   i. esophagogastric disease

_____10. ANT   j. physician's assistant

                                                                 k. history

                                                                  l. biopsy

                                                              m. right eye

                                                             n. end-stage renal disease

                                                              o. both eyes

                                                              p. anterior to posterior

ABBREVIATION FILL-INS

Fill in the blanks with the correct abbreviations.

11. left occiput anterior _____

12. sexually transmitted disease _____

13. syphilis test _____

14. lateral _____

15. last menstrual period _____

16. posterior to anterior _____

17. occupational therapy _____

18. tuberculosis _____

CASE STUDIES

Write the term next to its meaning given on page 335. Then draw slashes to analyze the word parts. Note the use of medical abbreviations. Look these up in your dictionary or find them in Appendix B. If you have any questions about the answers, refer to your medical dictionary or check with your instructor for the answers in Appendix A.

REVIEW ACTIVITIES

CASE STUDY 9-1

Consultation Note

Pt: Female, age 34

Dx: 1. Obesity **hypoventilation syndrome**

2. Diabetes mellitus type 1

Ms. Betty Sweet presented with a history of morbid obesity and a previous admission for respiratory insufficiency. She entered the emergency room complaining of progressive fatigue, sleepiness, **cephalalgia, narcolepsy,** general weakness, and **dyspnea.** She admits to a dry nonproductive cough without congestion, **URI symptoms,** recent fevers, sweats, and chills. For her headache she had been taking an occasional nonprescription **analgesic** amounting to 2 aspirins/week and she denied any other drug use. Ms. Sweet has a history of type 1 diabetes and had been maintained on 25 **U** of insulin until August 11 when she was increased to 40 U. A urinary tract infection was an incidental finding. She has done no blood sugar checks at home. No **hypoglycemic** reactions have been recorded. Ms. Sweet has progressive, increasing lethargy and feels unrested. Past history is also significant for a hospitalization in 1988 for which she required **ventilatory** support for obstructive **apnea.** She was discharged home on nasal **CPAP** and was able to lose 20–30 pounds with marked improvement in her symptoms. She has gained the weight back over the last 6 months and is dieting again. Of note at that time was Swan-Ganz **catheterization,** which revealed elevated pulmonary artery pressures.

1. introduction of a tube to evacuate or irrigate a body cavity _____
2. cessation of breathing _____
3. type one diabetes mellitus _____
4. upper respiratory infection _____
5. sleep seizures _____
6. continuous positive air pressure _____
7. reduced depth of breaths _____
8. symptoms that run together _____
9. how the patient feels _____
10. units _____
11. low blood sugar (adjective) _____
12. pain reliever _____
13. headache _____
14. difficulty breathing _____
15. getting air in lungs (adjective) _____

REVIEW ACTIVITIES

CROSSWORD PUZZLE

Check your answers by going back through the frames or checking the solution in Appendix C.

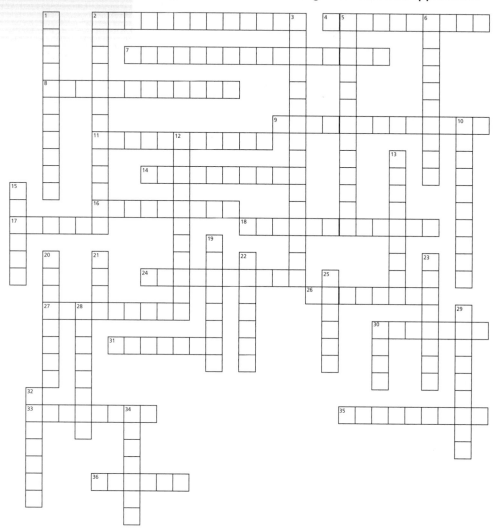

Across

2. does not absorb stain
4. partial paralysis (lower body)
7. inflammation behind the peritoneum
8. twisting backward
9. pertaining to the back and head
11. bending forward
14. formed outside the body
16. grows without air
17. synonym for posterior
18. inflammation near the bladder
24. below normal amount of growth
26. filtration of blood with artificial kidney
27. examination by looking into the body
30. pregnancy outside of the uterus
31. difficulty breathing
33. choosing good genetic traits only
35. cessation of reproductive cycle
36. synonym for menorrhea

Down

1. hemorrhage during menstruation
2. pertaining to the front and side
3. defective cartilage development
5. control of blood flow in the arteries
6. easy death
10. absence of menstruation
12. crushing of a stone
13. opinions of good and bad choices for living things
15. middle
19. toward the head
20. below
21. outer-prefix
22. side
23. difficult labor
25. away from the point of origin
28. flowing of watery stool
29. identifying a disease
30. inner-prefix
32. synonym for anterior
34. pertaining to the crown

REVIEW ACTIVITIES

GLOSSARY

achromophilic	resisting color (stain)	coronary	pertaining to the crown or encircling (reference to around the heart)
aerobic	requiring air to live		
aerocele	herniation containing air	diagnosis	identifying a disease
aerophobia	abnormal fear of air	dialysis	separating of substances in a solution (filtration)
aerotherapy	treatment using air (respiratory therapy)		
		diarrhea	abnormally loose watery bowel movement
amenorrhea	cessation of menstruation		
anaerobic	able to live without air	distal	away from a point of origin or designated point
anterolateral	front and side		
anteromedial	front and middle	dorsal	back (posterior)
anteroposterior	from front to back	dorsocephalad	from back toward the head
anterosuperior	front and top	dysentery	inflammation of the intestine
arteriostasis	control of flow through arteries	dysmenorrhea	difficult or painful menstruation
bioethics	study of what is good and bad for living things	dyspepsia	poor digestion
		dyspnea	difficulty breathing
biology	science studying living things	dystocia	difficulty in labor
blastoderm	embryonic disk that gives rise to the endoderm, mesoderm, ectoderm	ectocytic	outside the cell (extracellular, adjective)
		ectoderm	outer embryonic (germ) layer
caudad	toward the tail (sacrum)	ectogenous	formed outside the body (from another source, adjective)
cephalad	toward the head		
cephalocaudal	from head to tail		
chondrodysplasia	defective development of cartilage	ectopic	outside of the normal location (adjective)
chromogenesis	formation of color	ectoplasm	outer membrane of the cell
chromolysis	destruction of color	endocardium	inner membrane layer of the heart
chromometer	measuring color		
chromophilic	attracting color (stain)	endochondral	within the cartilage (adjective)
coronal	pertaining to the crown or encircling	endocolitis	inflammation of the lining of the colon

REVIEW ACTIVITIES

endocystic	inside the urinary bladder or inside a cyst (adjective)
endoderm	inner embryonic (germ) layer
endoenteritis	inflammation of the lining of the small intestine
endogenous	made by one's own body (adjective)
endoscopy	process of using a scope to look into the body
eugenics	choosing good genetic trait to propagate
eupepsia	good digestion
eupnea	easy breathing
euthanasia	easy death
eutocia	easy labor
hyperplasia	overdevelopment (too many cells)
hypoplasia	underdevelopment (too few cells)
inferior	below
lateral	side
lithotripsy	surgical crushing of a stone
lymphostasis	control of lymph flow
medial	middle
menopause	cessation of menstruation, ovulation, and atrophy of female reproductive system
menorrhagia	hemorrhage during menstruation
menses	menstruation (menorrhea), plural: menses
midsagittal	the plane dividing the body into equal right and left halves
neurotripsy	surgical crushing of a nerve

omphalectomy	excision of the umbilicus
omphalic	pertaining to the umbilicus
omphalitis	inflammation of the umbilicus
omphalocele	umbilical hernia (umbilicocele)
omphalorrhagia	hemorrhage of the umbilicus
omphalorrhea	discharge from the umbilicus
omphalorrhexis	rupture of the umbilicus
osteochondrodysplasia	defective development of bone and cartilage
para-appendicitis	inflammation of near the appendix
paracentral	pertaining to near the center (adjective)
paracolpitis	inflammation near the vagina
paracystitis	inflammation near the urinary bladder
parahepatitis	inflammation near the liver
paranephritis	inflammation near the kidney
parietal	pertaining to the wall
peritoneum	membrane of the abdomen
phlebostasis	control of flow through a vein (venostasis)
pleura	membrane of the lungs
posteroanterior	from back to front
posteroexternal	back and outside
posterointernal	back and inside
posterolateral	back and side
procephalic	in front of the head
prognosis	predicting the outcome of a disease
prognostic	pertaining to a prognosis

REVIEW ACTIVITIES

proximal	near the point of origin or a designated point		retroperitonitis	inflammation of the area behind the peritoneum
pseudocyesis	false pregnancy (pseudopregnancy)		retrosternal	behind the sternum (adjective)
pseudocyst	false cyst		retroversion	twisting (turning) backward
pseudoedema	false swelling		sagittal	vertical in an anteroposterior direction or plane
pseudoesthesia	false sensation (i.e., phantom limb)		superior	above
retrocolic	behind the colon (adjective)		syphilophobia	abnormal fear of syphilis
retroflexion	bending (flexing) backward		syphilopsychosis	severe mental condition caused by untreated syphilis
retroperitoneum	behind the peritoneum		syphilotherapy	treatment for syphilis

UNIT 10

Surgery, Diabetes, Immunology, Lesions, and Prefixes of Numbers and Direction

ANSWER COLUMN

	10.1
abdominal wall	**lapar/o** means abdominal wall. A laparectomy is an excision of part of the * _____.
	10.2
lapar/o/scopy lap ə **ros**′ kō pē	The process of examining the abdominal cavity with an end/o/scope is called _____/_____/_____.
INFORMATION FRAME	**10.3** A lapar/o/scope is a special instrument that allows a physician to view the inside of the abdominal cavity and its organs. Surgery can also be performed while using a laparoscope (usually attached to a video screen). See the illustration on page 341.
	10.4
lapar/o/scope **lap**′ är ō skōp	Lapar/o/scop/ically assisted vaginal hyster/ectomy (LAVH) is actually the removal of the uterus through the vagina assisted by looking through the _____/_____/_____ from within the abdominal cavity.
	10.5
lapar/o/scop/ic lap′ är ō **skō**′ pik	Chole/cyst/ectomy can also be performed with the assistance of the laparoscope. This would be called _____/_____/_____/_____ cholecystectomy.

ANSWER COLUMN

---

lapar/o/tomy lap′ ə **rot**′ ə mē lapar/o/rrhaphy lap′ ə **rôr**′ ə fē	**10.6** An incision into the abdominal wall is a _____/____/_____. Suturing of the abdominal wall is _____/____/_____.

10.7

Give the meaning for the following words about the abdomen (use your dictionary if needed)

laparohepatotomy (lap′ ə rō hep′ ə **tot**′ ō mē)

*_____;

laparocolostomy (lap′ ə rō cō **los**′ tō mē)

*_____;

laparogastrotomy (lap′ ə rō gas **trot**′ ō mē)

*_____.

incision into the liver
  through the abdomen
new opening in the colon
  through the abdomen
incision into the stomach
  through the abdomen

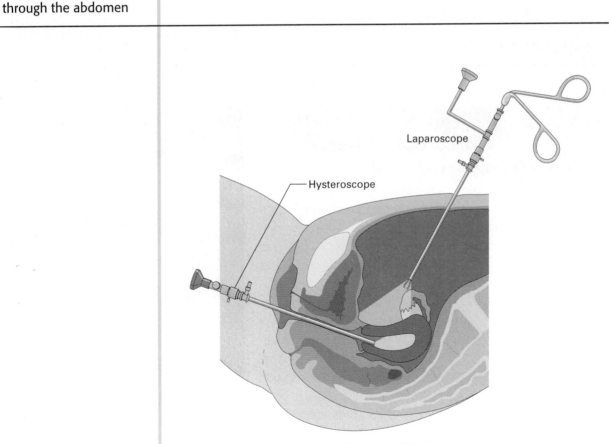

Laparoscope

Hysteroscope

Laparoscopy performed with hysteroscopy

ANSWER COLUMN

10.8

There may be longer words than this, but not many. Analyze it for fun. Think of the word parts.

Laparohysterosalpingo-oophorectomy *_____

abdomen, uterus,
  fallopian tubes,
  ovaries, excision

_____.

lap′ ə r ō **his′** ter ō sal **ping′** ō-ōō for **ek′** tō mē

10.9

pyr/o is used in words to mean heat, fever, or fire. The early Greeks and Romans burned their dead on funeral pyres. A pyr/o/maniac is one who has a madness (excessive preoccupation) for starting or seeing _____.

fires

10.10

Pyr/exia (pi **reks′** ē ə) means fever. A condition of heat (heartburn)

pyr/osis
pi **rō′** sis
hyper/pyrexia
hī′ per pī **reks′** ē ə

is _____/_____.

A condition of high fever (over 102°F) is _____/_____.

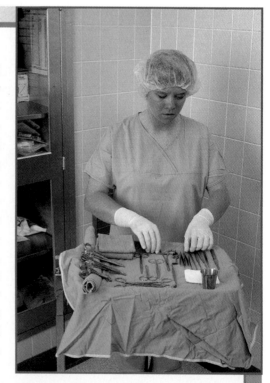

PROFESSIONAL PROFILES

Certified surgical technologists (CSTs) are an integral part of a surgical team. They prepare the operating room by selecting and opening sterile supplies; assembling, adjusting, and checking nonsterile equipment; and operating sterilizers, lights, suction machines, electrosurgical units, and diagnostic equipment. The CST most often functions as a member of the surgical team by passing instruments, sutures, and sponges during surgery, holding retractors, receiving specimens, as well as assisting other team members in gowning and gloving. They give preoperative care to surgical patients by providing physical and emotional support, checking charts, and observing vital signs. The Accreditation Review Committee on Education in Surgical Technology (ARC-ST) recommends educational standards and accredits programs. Voluntary professional certification is obtained from the Association of Surgical Technologists (AST) upon passing a CST national certification examination.

ANSWER COLUMN

10.11

Build words meaning
instrument for measuring heat (thermometer)

pyr/o/meter
pī **rô′** mə ter

_____/_____/_____;

destruction by fever

pyr/o/lysis
pī **rô′** lə sis

_____/_____/_____;

abnormal fear of fire

pyr/o/phobia
pī rō **fō′** bē ə

_____/_____/_____;

madness (obsession) for setting fires

pyr/o/mania
pī rō **mā′** nē ə

_____/_____/_____.

10.12

fever or high body
  temperature

A pyr/o/toxin is a toxin (poison) produced by

*_____.

10.13

sweat

hydro- (a combining form and prefix) means water or fluid. **hidro-** (from the Greek *hidros*) means sweat. A hidro/cyst/aden/oma is a cystic tumor of a
_____ gland.

10.14

inflammation of
  sweat glands

Hidr/aden/itis means *_____

_____.

10.15

The three words below mean sweating; define and divide them into their word parts.

hidr/osis
hī **drō′** sis
condition of sweating

hidrosis _____/_____,
*_____;

hyper/hidr/osis
hī per hī **drō** sis
  profuse sweating

hyperhidrosis _____/_____/_____,
*_____;

hidr/o/rrhea
hī drō **rē′** ə
  flow of sweat

hidrorrhea _____/_____/_____,
*_____.

10.16

absence of sweat

The word an/hidr/osis (an hī **drō′** sis) means

*_____.

ANSWER COLUMN

10.17

Both **hydro-** and **hidro-** are pronounced alike.

water or fluid

sweat

Hydro, with a *y*, means *_____.

Hidro, with an *i*, means _____.

10.18

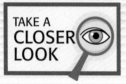

TAKE A CLOSER LOOK

glyc/o (glycos) and **gluc/o** (glucos) are different translations of Greek word parts meaning sweet or sugar. Here are some examples of sweet words:

glycogenesis/glucogenesis: formation of sugar
glycoprotein/glucoprotein: substance made of sugar and protein
glycosuria/glucosuria: (glycos/glucos) sugar in the urine
glycohemoglobin: sugar and hemoglobin

Look up terms beginning with gluco and glyco in your dictionary. They are interchangeable in some words, but notice many in which they have a unique use.

10.19

Glycogen is "animal starch" formed from simple sugars and stored as reserve fuel. The cells of the body use a simple sugar, glucose, to release energy. To use its reserve fuel supply of animal starch, the body must convert

glyc/o/gen

glī′ kō jen

_____/____/_____ to glucose.

10.20

gluc/o/gen/esis

glōō kō **jen′** ə sis

glyc/o/gen/esis

glī′ kō **jen′** ə sis

gluc/o is a combining form for glucose. The formation of glucose from glycogen stores is called _____/____/_____/_____

or

_____/____/_____/_____.

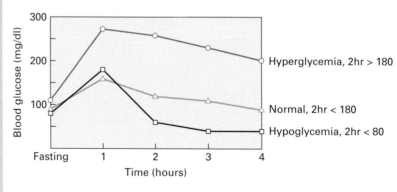

Glucose tolerance test (GTT) graph

ANSWER COLUMN

10.21

Glucose is used by the muscles to release energy. Glycogen is the reserve food supply of glucose. Glucose is the usable form of stored _____.

glycogen

10.22

Glyc/o/hem/o/globin is a combination of sugar (glucose) and hemoglobin in the blood. This substance, also called glyc/ated hem/o/globin (GHB) remains permanently in the red blood cells which live up to 90 days. If a person has experienced chronic high blood sugar levels, an increase in the level of _____/_____/_____/_____/_____ may be expected.

glyc/o/hem/o/globin
glī kō **hē**′ mə glō bin

NOTE: The hemoglobin A1c (Hb A1c or Hgb A1c) test measures the glycohemoglobin levels which indicate the average blood glucose levels during the 60 to 90 days prior to the test.

10.23

TAKE A CLOSER LOOK

Diabetes mellitus has many forms, all of which are characterized by hypoglycemia and other metabolic disturbances. Listed below are three types of diabetes mellitus and their characteristics.

Type 1 (insulin-dependent diabetes mellitus) is characterized by onset in youth, exogenous insulin dependency, tendency to ketoacidosis, viral etiology, autoimmune basis, and genetic predisposition.

Type 2 (noninsulin-dependent diabetes mellitus) is characterized by onset in adults over 40, some endogenous insulin production, obesity or normal weight, and can be treated with diet modification and oral hypoglycemic agents.

Gestational diabetes mellitus (GDM) occurs in individuals not previously diabetic who develop hyperglycemia during pregnancy. These women may progress to another diabetes mellitus or return to normal glucose levels postpartum.

10.24

Recall that **-emia** means condition in the blood. Glyc/emia means sugar in the blood. A symptom of diabetes is hyper/glyc/emia. This means
* _____
_____.

too much sugar in
the blood (high
blood sugar)

10.25

Hyper/glyc/emia means high blood sugar. The word that means low blood sugar is _____/_____/_____.

hypo/glyc/emia
hī′ pō glī **sē**′ mē ə

ANSWER COLUMN

10.26

When a person produces too much of the hormone insulin, the blood glucose
level may decrease to below normal. This is called _____.

hypoglycemia

10.27

glyc/o/gen/esis
glī′ kō **jen**′ ə sis

If glucogenesis is the formation of glucose, then the formation of glycogen from
food is _____/_____/_____/_____.

10.28

glyc/o/lysis
glī **kol**′ ə sis
glyc/o/rrhea
glī′ kō **rē**′ ə

The breakdown (destruction) of sugar is _____/_____/_____.
The discharge (flow) of sugar from the body
is _____/_____/_____.

10.29

sugar
fat

Glyc/o/lipid should make you think of two foods: _____ and _____.

10.30

immun/o/logy
im′ yoō **nol**′ ō jē

immun/o is the combining form for immune. Immun/ity is one of the body's
protections from disease. The study of the function of the immune system is
called _____/_____/_____.

10.31

immun/o/therapy
im′ yoō nō **ther**′ a pē
immun/i/zations
im′ yoō nə **zā**′ shunz

Immun/ization (vaccination) injections are given so that a person may develop
an immune response to certain diseases. The process is known as
immun/o/therapy. DPT (diphtheria, pertussis, tetanus) and IPV (inactivated
polio vaccine) are two types of _____/_____/_____
or
_____/_____/_____.

10.32

immun/o/deficiency
im′ yoō nō de **fish**′ en cē

Immun/o/logists are studying HIV (human immun/o/deficiency virus), which
causes AIDS (acquired immunodeficiency syndrome). Because it is
characterized by inability to fight off disease, AIDS is a type of
_____/_____/_____ disease.

ANSWER COLUMN

10.33

When an antigen (such as a foreign protein) invades the body, special leukocytes (lymphocytes) produce antibodies to disable the invader. This antigen-antibody reaction is called the immune response.

INFORMATION FRAME

10.34

immun/ity
im **yōo**′ ni tē

Chickenpox is caused by the virus *Varicella zoster*. When first infected, the person becomes ill. If infected again, the person will most likely not become ill due to acquired active _____/_____.

10.35

immunity

A breastfed infant receives antibodies from its mother's body through the breast milk. This type of immunity is called passive _____.

10.36

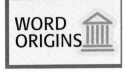

WORD ORIGINS

Vaccines are usually given by injection to stimulate the body's natural immune response. This allows us to resist an infection when exposed to that specific organism in the future. The word vaccine comes from the Latin word for cow, *vacca*. Edward Jenner first innoculated a young boy with a substance from the sore of a milkmaid infected with cowpox. At a later time, he exposed the boy to smallpox and the boy resisted the disease. This was the first vaccination (immunization).

vaccin/ation
vak sin **ā**′ shun

10.37

vaccin/e
vak **sēn**′

The inactivated polio _____ (IPV) stimulates resistance to polio.

10.38

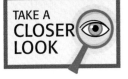

TAKE A CLOSER LOOK

Seven immunizations are typically recommended before age seven for the general population. Two others, Hepatitis A and Influenza, are recommended for selected populations. To learn about these recommendations, study the immunization schedule on page 348.

10.39

self

aut/o is a combining form that means self. You already recognize auto in such ordinary English words as aut/o/mobile (a self-propelled vehicle) and aut/o/bi/o/graphy. **aut/o** means _____.

Recommended Childhood and Adolescent Immunization Schedule
United States, 2003

- range of recommended ages
- catch-up vaccination
- preadolescent assessment

Vaccine \ Age →	Birth	1 mo	2 mos	4 mos	6 mos	12 mos	15 mos	18 mos	24 mos	4-6 yrs	11-12 yrs	13-18 yrs
Hepatitis B[1]	HepB #1	only if mother HBsAg (-)										
		HepB #2			HepB #3				HepB series			
Diphtheria, Tetanus, Pertussis[2]			DTaP	DTaP	DTaP		DTaP			DTaP	Td	
Haemophilus influenzae Type b[3]			Hib	Hib	Hib	Hib						
Inactivated Polio			IPV	IPV	IPV					IPV		
Measles, Mumps, Rubella[4]						MMR #1				MMR #2	MMR #2	
Varicella[5]						Varicella			Varicella			
Pneumococcal[6]			PCV	PCV	PCV	PCV			PCV	PPV		
Hepatitis A[7]									Hepatitis A series			
Influenza[8]					Influenza (yearly)							

Vaccines below this line are for selected populations

This schedule indicates the recommended ages for routine administration of currently licensed childhood vaccines, as of December 1, 2002, for children through age 18 years. Any dose not given at the recommended age should be given at any subsequent visit when indicated and feasible. ▭ Indicates age groups that warrant special effort to administer those vaccines not previously given. Additional vaccines may be licensed and recommended during the year. Licensed combination vaccines may be used whenever any components are not contraindicated. Providers should consult the manufacturers' package inserts for detailed recommendations.

Source: **Approved by the Advisory Committee on Immunization Practices** (www.cdc.gov/nip/acip), **the American Academy of Pediatrics** (www.aap.org), **and the American Academy of Family Physicians** (www.aafp.org).

ANSWER COLUMN

one's own skin	**10.40** Aut/o/dia/gnos/is means diagnosing one's own diseases. Aut/o/derm/ic pertains to dermat/o/plasty with *_____.
self-destruction or self-destroying aut/o/nom/ic	**10.41** Aut/o/nom/ic (aw′ tō **nom**′ ik) means self-controlling, as in the autonomic nervous system. Aut/o/lysis (aw **tol**′ ə sis) means *_____. The self-controlling part of the nervous system is the _____/_____/_____/_____ nervous system (ANS).
aut/o/immun/ity aw′ tō im yōō′ ni tē	**10.42** If one's own body produces antibodies to one's own tissues (like being allergic to oneself), _____/_____/_____/_____ has occurred. **EXAMPLE:** Rheumatoid arthritis and lupus erythematosus are often seen in the same patient and are disease conditions associated with autoimmunity.
aut/o/phobia aw tō **fō**′ bē ə aut/o/immun/ity	**10.43** Aut/o/phagia means biting one's self. A word that means abnormal fear of being alone is _____/_____/_____. _____/_____/_____/_____ is being allergic to one's own tissues.
aut/o/hem/o/therapy aw′ tō hēm′ ō **ther**′ a pē aut/o/plasty **aw**′ tō plas tē	**10.44** Build terms that mean therapy with one's own blood (transfusion) _____/_____/_____/_____/_____; surgery using grafts from one's own body _____/_____/_____.
aut/o/logous aw **tol**′ ō gus	**10.45** Aut/o/logous is an adjective meaning originating in itself or coming from one's own body. Persons anticipating surgery can have blood drawn and saved for their own use if needed. This would be an _____/_____/_____ blood transfusion.
aut/o/graft **aw**′ tō graft	**10.46** Keeping the previous frame in mind, think of what an aut/o/graft might be. A burn victim needing a skin graft may use his or her own healthy skin as an _____/_____/_____.

ANSWER COLUMN

10.47

The term aut/o/genous has a similar meaning to aut/o/logous. If a vaccine is made from a culture of a patient's own bacteria, this is called an

aut/o/gen/ous
aw **to**' jen us

_____/_____/_____/_____ vaccine.

10.48

Great! When you analyze a word, think of its meaning. If you have forgotten a part of the word, look it up. Analyze this.

aut/o/phobia
abnormal fear of one's
  self or being alone
aut/o/phagia
biting one's self

autophobia _____/_____/_____ ,

_____ ;

meaning

autophagia _____/_____/_____ ,

_____ .

meaning

Study this table. Notice the specific use of each prefix.

NUMERIC PREFIXES

Greek	Latin	Meaning	Symbol	Examples
hemi-	semi-	half	0.5 ss	hemiplegia, semiconscious
mono-	uni-	one	1.0 i	monocyte, uniparous
prot-	prim-	first		protozoan, primigravida
di(plo)-	bi-	two	2.0 ii	diplococci, bifurcation
tri-	tri-	three	3.0 iii	triglyceride, triceps
tetra-	quadr-	four	4.0 iv	tetramastia, quadriplegia
penta-	quint-	five	5.0 v	pentadactyl, quintuplets
hexa-	sex/ta-	six	6.0 vi	hexapodia, sexagenarian
hepta-	sept/a-	seven	7.0 vii	heptachromic, septuplet
octa-	oct-	eight	8.0 viii	octodont, octogenarian
enne(a)-	non(i)-	nine	9.0 ix	ennead, nonipara
deca- (10)	dec(i)- (0.1)	ten, tenth	10.0 x	decaliter, deciliter
hecto- (100)	cent(i)- (0.01)	one hundred, one hundredth		hectogram, centigram
kilo- (1,000)	mill(i)- (0.001)	one thousand, one thousandth		kilometer, millimeter

Then use this knowledge to work the rest of the frames in this unit.

ANSWER COLUMN

	10.49
one	**mono-** means one or single. You know it in the ordinary English words monorail, monopoly, and monogamy. When you see **mono-**, think of _____.
	10.50
one	A mono/graph deals with a single subject. A mono/nucle/ar cell has _____ nucleus.
	10.51
	Mono/mania is an abnormal preoccupation with one subject only. Build words meaning
mono/cyte **mon'** ō sīt	one cell _____/_____ (a type of leukocyte);
mono/oma mon **ō'** mə	one tumor _____/_____.
	10.52
	Build words that begin with **mono-**.
	paralysis of one muscle
mono/my/o/plegia mon' ō mī ō **plē'** jē ə	_____/_____/____/_____;
mono/neur/al mon ō **noor'** əl	pertaining to one nerve _____/_____/_____;
mono/cyt/osis mon' ō sī **tō'** sis	condition of increase in monocytes _____/_____/_____.
	10.53
mono/nucle/osis mon' ō noo klē **ō'** sis	Mono/nucle/osis (mono) is a condition caused by a viral infection that can damage the liver. One sign is an abnormally high monocyte count. Mono/cyt/osis may be an indication of _____/_____/_____.
	10.54
many or more than one	**multi-** means the opposite of **mono-**. **multi-** (as in multiply) means *_____.
	10.55
many	In ordinary English, you are acquainted with **multi-** in the words multiply and multitude. Something composed of multiple parts has _____ parts.

ANSWER COLUMN

	10.56
many capsules	Something that is multi/capsular has *_____.
	10.57
	Multi/glandular is an adjective meaning
many glands	*_____.
	Multi/cellular is an adjective meaning
many cells	*_____.
	Multi/nuclear is an adjective meaning
many nuclei	*_____.
	10.58
	A multi/para is a woman who has brought forth (borne) more than one child. par is one word root meaning to bear. Multi/par/ous is the adjectival form
multi/para mul **tip**′ ə rə	of _____/_____.
	10.59
	Multi/para always refers to the mother. Multi/par/ous may refer to a mother who has had many children or may mean multiple birth (twins or triplets). When desiring to indicate that a woman has borne more than one child, use the noun
multipara	_____.
	10.60
multi/para multi/par/ous mul **tip**′ ər əs	Multi/par/ous is the adjectival form of _____/_____. To indicate that twins are born, say _____/_____/_____ birth.
	10.61
multiparous multiparous	To indicate that triplets are born, say _____ birth. If ten children were born, you would still use the adjective _____.
	10.62
none	**nulli-** means *none*. To nullify something is to bring it to nothing. There are not many medical words using **nulli-**; but when you do see it, it means _____.
	10.63
a woman who has never borne a child primi/para prī **mip**′ ər ə	A nulli/para is *_____. **primi-** means first. A woman who is having her first child is a _____/_____ (noun).

ANSWER COLUMN

Identical twins

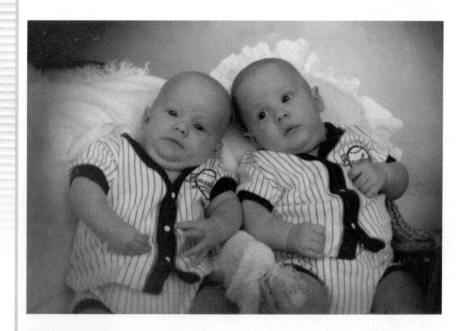

10.64

Gravida is a Latin word meaning heavy or weighted down. In medical terms it is used to mean pregnant. A woman experiencing her first pregnancy is called a

primi/gravida
prim′ i **grav**′ i da

_____/_____.

10.65

INFORMATION FRAME

Gravida refers to pregnancies, whereas para refers to live births. A woman who has been pregnant four times and had two spontaneous abortions (miscarriages) and two live births would be described on the chart as grav 4, ab 2, para 2 (G4, AB2, P2).

10.66

nulli/para
nu **lip**′ ar ə
no live births
nulli/par/ous
nu **lip**′ ar us
pertaining to no live births
primi/para
prī **mip**′ ar ə
first live birth

Analyze the following and define:
nullipara _____/_____ (noun),
*_____;

nulliparous _____/_____/_____ (adjective),
*_____;

primipara _____/_____ (noun),
*_____.

ANSWER COLUMN

10.67

Give the prefix for

nulli-

mono-

multi-

para-

primi-

none _____;

one (single) _____;

many _____;

bear _____;

first _____.

10.68

deca- and deci- both mean ten but are used differently. deca- is used in words meaning the whole number ten. deci- is used in words meaning the fraction one

ten

tenth

tenth. A decaliter (dal) is _____ liters.

A deciliter (dL) is one _____ of a liter.

10.69

kilo- and milli- both refer to thousand but are used differently. kilo- is used in words to mean one thousand. milli- is used in words to mean one thousandth.

thousand

thousandth

A kilometer (km) is one _____ meters.

A millimeter (mm) is one _____ of a meter.

10.70

Build words that mean

one thousand grams

kilo/gram

ki′ lo gram

milli/gram

mi′ li gram

kilo/meter

kil om′ ə ter

milli/meter

mil′ ə mē ter

_____/_____ (kg);

one thousandth of a gram

_____/_____ (mg);

one thousand meters

_____/_____ (km);

one thousandth of a meter

_____/_____/_____ (mm).

10.71

A volume measurement that is frequently used when giving injections is the cubic centimeter (cc). It is the amount of fluid in one centimeter cubed. If the physician writes an order to give 0.5 cc of tetanus toxoid, the medical assistant will inject

cubic centimeter

one half of a *_____.

10.72

Do the work on this frame using the table on page 350.

Build words that mean

one hundred meters

hecto/meter

hek tom′ ə ter

_____/_____ (hm);

ANSWER COLUMN

centi/meter
sen′ ti mē ter
hecto/gram
hek′ to gram
centi/gram
sen′ ti gram
milli/liter
mil′ ə lē ter

one hundredth of a meter

_____/_____ (cm);

one hundred grams

_____/_____ (hg);

one hundredth of a gram

_____/_____ (cg);

one thousandth of a liter

_____/_____;

Good work!

Prefixes representing place often cause difficulty in word building because of their similarity. Use this information carefully while working through Frames 10.73–10.104.

PREFIX	MEANING	SENSE OF MEANING
ab–	from	away from
de–	from	down from or from—resulting in less than
ex–	from	out from

10.73

from

Recall ab/duction and ad/duction. You have already learned **ab-** is the opposite of **ad-**. **ad-** means toward; **ab-** means _____.

10.74

away from

away from

Ab/duct/ion (ab **duk**′ shun) means moving away from the midline.
Ab/norm/al means going *_____ normal.
Ab/or/al means away from the mouth. Ab/errant (ab **er**′ ənt) means wandering *_____ the normal course.

10.75

ab/duct/ion
ab **duc**′ shun
ab/norm/al
ab **nor**′ m l
ab/errant
ab **air**′ ant
ab′ er ant

Swinging the arm away from the side of the body is

_____/_____/_____.

A sign or symptom that is unusual is

_____/_____/_____.

A blood vessel that is not located where it should be is an

_____/_____ vessel.

ANSWER COLUMN

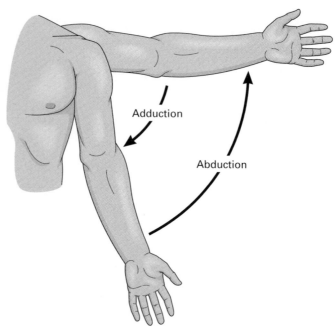

Adduction

Abduction

	10.76
away from away from	An ab/irritant is something that takes irritation *_____ the patient. Ab/lact/ation means takes the baby *_____ the breastfeeding or the cessation of milk secretion.
	10.77
ab/ort/ion a **bôr**′ shən	Ab/ort was, literally, built by joining **ab-** to a word part meaning to be born (Latin: *oriri,* to be born). A naturally occurring termination of pregnancy (miscarriage) is called a spontaneous _____/_____/_____.
	10.78
ab/ort/ed	In an induced abortion, the products of conception are taken away from the uterus or _____/_____/_____.
INFORMATION FRAME	**10.79** Three types of wounds are lacerations (cuts), contusions (bruises), and abrasions (scrapes).
	10.80
away from ab/rasion a **brā**′ shən	To ab/rade (a **brād**′) the skin is to scrape some of the skin *_____ the surface of the body. A scrape type of injury is called an _____/_____.

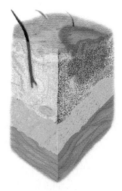

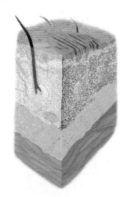

A. Bruise, also known as a contusion, results from damage to the soft tissues and blood vessels, which causes bleeding beneath the skin surface. A bruise in a light-skinned individual will change from red to purple to greenish yellow before fading. In a dark-skinned person, the bruise will first look dark red, then darker red, brown, or purple, and slowly fade.

B. Abrasion, also known as a scrape or rug burn, results when the outer layer of skin is scraped or rubbed away. Exposure of nerve endings makes this type of wound painful, and the presence of debris from the scraped surface (rug fibers, gravel, sand) makes abrasions highly susceptible to infection.

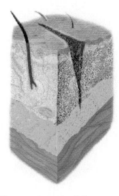

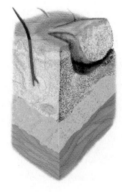

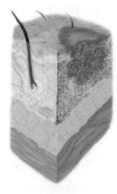

C. Laceration, cut, or incision, are caused by sharp objects such as knives or glass, or from trauma due to a strike from a blunt object that opens the skin, such as a baseball bat. If the wound is deep, the cut may bleed profusely; if nerve endings are exposed, it could also be painful.

D. Avulsion results when the skin or tissue is torn away from the body, either partially or completely. The bleeding and pain depends on the depth of tissue affected.

E. Puncture results when the skin is pierced by a sharp object such as a pencil, nail, or bullet. If a piece of the object remains in the skin, or if there is little bleeding due to the depth and location of the puncture, infection is likely.

ANSWER COLUMN

10.81

End/o/metr/ial ab/lation is a surgical procedure that destroys (takes away) the uterine lining. A special cutting instrument may be used with a hyster/o/scope to perform endometrial _____/_____.

ab/lation
ab **lā′** shun

10.82

These gynecologic procedures get pretty technical for the nonsurgeon, but remember, the part of the term ablation that means something is taken away is _____.

ab

ANSWER COLUMN

10.83

from

de- is another prefix that means _____.

10.84

down from

One who de/scends the stairs comes down from a higher level. A de/scend/ing nerve tract comes *_____ the brain.

10.85

de/cid/uous
dē **sij**′ ōō əs

De/ciduous leaves fall from a tree. "Baby teeth" that fall from a child's mouth are called _____/_____/_____ teeth.

Primary teeth (*deciduous, baby teeth*)

10.86

deciduous

There are thirty-two secondary (permanent) and twenty primary (_____) teeth.

10.87

from

When water is taken from a substance, the substance is less than it was. De/hydr/ation takes water _____ something.

ANSWER COLUMN

10.88

When water is taken from plums to make prunes, de/hydr/ation occurs. When water is taken from a cell, _____/_____/_____ also occurs.

de/hydr/ation
dē hī **drā**′ shən

10.89

When something is dehydrated, it has less water than it did before. When water is lost from the body due to excessive vomiting or diarrhea, the patient is _____/_____/_____.

de/hydr/ated
dē hī **drā**′ tid

10.90

Vomiting can cause dehydration. A high fever can also cause _____.

dehydration

10.91

When calcium is removed from the bones, there is less calcium than before. This process is called _____/_____/_____.

de/calci/fication
dē kal′ si fi **kā**′ shən

10.92

De/calci/fication can occur from many causes. When a pregnant woman does not eat enough calcium for the growing baby, her own bones will be robbed of calcium, and _____ will occur.

decalcification

10.93

Because vitamin D helps control calcium metabolism, inadequate vitamin D in the diet can account for some _____.

decalcification

10.94

Oste/o/por/osis may occur in postmenopausal women due to _____ of the bones.

decalcification

10.95

ex- also means from, but in the sense of *_____.

out from

10.96

To ex/cise is to cut _____ and remove a part. A diseased gallbladder may be _____/_____/_____.

out
ex/cis/ed
ek **sīz**′ d

ANSWER COLUMN

10.97

from

To ex/hale (ex/pire) is to breathe out waste matter _____ the body.

10.98

ex/cretion
eks **krē**′ shən

Ex/cretion is the process of ex/pelling (or getting out from the body) a substance.
Expelling urine is urinary _____/_____.

10.99

excretion
excretion

Expelling carbon dioxide is respiratory _____.
Expelling sweat is dermal _____.

10.100

excretion
excretion

Expelling menses is menstrual _____. Expelling fecal matter
is gastrointestinal (GI) _____.

10.101

SPELL
CHECK ✔

Excretions are usually waste substances. Secretions, such as hormones, are
useful substances, so do not use them as synonyms. You may think "exit—out,"
"keep the secret—in."

10.102

ex/traction
eks **trak**′ shən

An ex/traction is a procedure in which something is pulled out.
When all of a patient's teeth have to be pulled out, it is called a full-mouth
_____/_____ (FME).

10.103

ex/tends
eks **tendz**′

Recall the word flexion, meaning to bend or shorten. The opposite of flexion is
ex/tension, meaning to straighten or lengthen.
Bending flexes the arm. Straightening _____/_____ the arm.

10.104

ex/tension
eks **ten**′ shun

Contracting the biceps muscle of the upper arm causes flex/ion of the arm.
Relaxing this muscle causes _____/_____.

ANSWER COLUMN

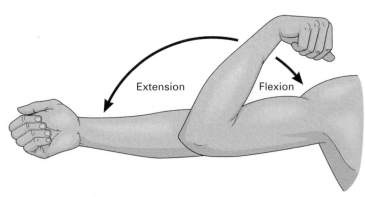

Extension   Flexion

10.105

Try to work this summary frame without referring to page 355.
Give the prefix meaning from in the following sense:

ab-   away from _____;
ex-   out from _____;
de-   down from or from, resulting in less than _____.

10.106

iso- is used in words to mean equal or the same. Something that is iso/metr/ic
equal   is of _____ dimensions.

10.107

equal   Something that is iso/cellular is composed of cells of _____ size.

10.108

An isotonic solution has the same osmotic pressure as red blood cells. Normal
iso/ton/ic   saline is an _____/_____/_____ solution.
ī sō **ton**′ ik

10.109

isotonic   Intra/ven/ous glucose is another _____ solution.

10.110

Any solution that will not destroy red blood cells because it is of equal osmotic
isotonic   pressure is an _____ solution.

10.111

higher   Hyper/tonic solutions have a _____ osmotic pressure than blood cells,
lower   hypo/tonic solutions have a _____ osmotic pressure than blood cells,
same or equal   and iso/tonic solutions have the _____ osmotic
                       pressure as blood cells.
                       Good try!

ANSWER COLUMN

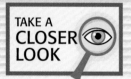

TAKE A
CLOSER
LOOK

10.112

Many physiologic processes rely on the movement of fluids and substances in and out of the cells and bloodstream. Look up diffusion, osmosis, and filtration in your dictionary or medical text and read about how each causes movement of substances. You may think it would be nice if we could learn through osmosis just by holding this book.

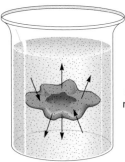
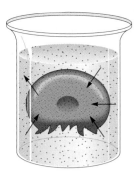
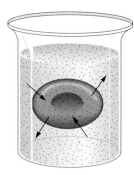

Water molecules

Hypertonic solution (sea-water) a red blood cell will shrink and wrinkle up because water molecules are moving out of the cell.

Hypotonic solution (fresh-water) a red blood cell will swell and burst because water molecules are moving into the cell.

Isotonic solution (human blood serum) a red blood cell remains unchanged, because the movement of water molecules into and out of the cell are the same.

Movement of water molecules through membranes in solutions of different osmolalities

10.113

iso/dactyl/ism
ī sō **dak′** til izm
iso/therm/al (ic)
ī sō **thûr′** məl (ik)

Build words meaning
fingers or toes of equal length
_____/_____/ism;
pertaining to equal temperature
_____/_____/_____.

10.114

an/iso
aniso

iso- is a prefix for equal. **an-** is a prefix meaning without or lack of. Something that is without equality is unequal. The combining form for unequal is _____/_____ or _____.

ANSWER COLUMN

10.115

Aniso/mastia means that a woman's breasts are of _____ size.

unequal

10.116

Mastos (or *mazos*) is the Greek word for breast. Inflammation of the breast is mast/itis. Surgical excision of part or all of the breast is

a _____/_____.

mast/ectomy
mast **ek**′ tōm ē

10.117

Radical and simple are the two main types of surgery for excising diseased breast tissue or _____.

mastectomy

10.118

Build a term that means a cancerous tumor of the breast
_____/_____/_____/_____. See the case study on
mastectomy at the end of this unit.

mast/o/carcin/oma
mast′ ō kär sin **ō**′ mə

10.119

WORD
ORIGINS

A legendary tribe of female warriors in Asia Minor were known to have removed one breast so that they could more powerfully draw their bows. They were named the Amazons, meaning without a breast (a, *without;* mazos, *breast*). In the 1500s, a Spanish explorer named a river the Amazon after doing battle with a South American tribe that included its women in the fight.

10.120

Aniso/cyt/osis means that cells are of unequal sizes. This word is commonly limited to red blood cells in medical usage. A word indicating a condition of inequality in cell size is _____/_____/_____.

aniso/cyt/osis
an ī′ sō sī **tō**′ sis

10.121

Normal red blood cells are the same size (7.2 μm). An abnormal condition resulting in unequal size of red blood cells is _____.

anisocytosis

10.122

Red blood cells are formed in the bone marrow. An unhealthy bone marrow can result in unequal red blood cells, or _____.

anisocytosis

ANSWER COLUMN

Use the following information to work Frames 10.123–10.146. This is another group of prefixes of place.

PREFIX	MEANING	DIFFERENTIATION
dia-	through, complete	used with the combining forms for medical terminology
per-	through	prefix from Latin used more often in ordinary English
peri-	around	prefix from Greek used with the combining forms for medical terminology
circum-	around	Latin prefix used more often in ordinary English

10.123

Peri/articular means around articulations or joints. Peri/tonsill/ar means

around the tonsil

*_____.

10.124

around the colon or
pertaining to around the
colon

Peri/col/ic means *_____
_____.

10.125

Peri/odont/al means pertaining to diseases of the support structures around
(**peri-**) the teeth (**odont/o**). A word that means around a cartilage is

peri/chondr/al
per i **kon**′ drəl
peri/odont/al
per i ō **don**′ təl

_____/_____/_____. Gum disease may require

_____/_____/_____ surgery.

10.126

Build words meaning
inflammation around a gland

peri/aden/itis
per′ i ad en **ī**′ tis
peri/colp/itis
per′ i kol **pī**′ tis
peri/hepat/itis
per′ i hep ə **tī**′ tis
peri/cardi/ectomy
per′ i kär′ dē **ek**′ tō mē

_____/_____/_____;
inflammation around the vagina
_____/_____/_____;
inflammation around the liver
_____/_____/_____;
excision of tissue (pericardium) around the heart
_____/_____/_____.

ANSWER COLUMN

SPELL
CHECK ✓

10.127

para- and peri- are similar prefixes. They are often confused as homonyms (sound alike) and as synonyms (mean the same). They are seldom interchangeable and you should look up terms that begin with **para-** and **peri-** in your medical dictionary before you use them, just to make sure. Here are some patterns that may help.

para- is used more often for conditions with **-ia**, **-osis**, **-itis**, and **-oma** suffixes, as in paranoia and para-appendicitis.

para- is also used as a chemical name prefix in para-aminobenzoic acid.

peri- is a common anatomic term prefix as in peri/cardium, peri/toneum, and peri/osteum.

10.128

circum-

Another prefix that means around is _____.

10.129

around

Circum/ocular means _____ the eyes.

10.130

around

Circum/or/al means _____ the mouth.

10.131

circum/scribed
sûr′ kəm skrīb′d

Circumscribed means limited in space (as though a line were drawn around it). A hive is limited in space—does not spread. A hive may be called a _____/_____ wheal.

10.132

circumscribed

A boil is also limited in the space it covers. A boil is a _____ lesion.

10.133

circumscribed

Pimples and pustules are also _____ lesions.

10.134

circum/duction
sûr kəm **duk′** shən

Moving toward is ad/duction. Moving away is ab/duction.
Moving around (circular motion) is _____/_____.

SURFACE LESIONS

A.

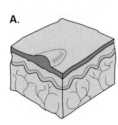

Papule
  Solid, elevated lesion less than 0.5 cm in diameter
Example
  Warts, elevated nevi

B.

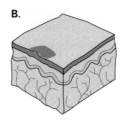

Macule
  Localized changes in skin color of less than 1 cm in diameter
Example
  Freckle

C.

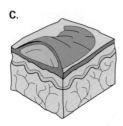

Wheal
  Localized edema in the epidermis causing irregular elevation that may be red or pale
Example
  Insect bite or a hive

D.

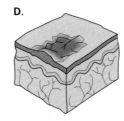

Crust
  Dried serum, blood, or pus on the surface of the skin
Example
  Impetigo

FLUID FILLED

E.

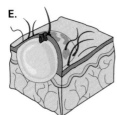

Boil (Furuncle)
  Skin infection originating in gland or hair follicle
Example
  Furunculosis

F.

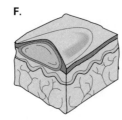

Bullae
  Same as a vesicle only greater than 0.5 cm
Example
  Contact dermatitis, large second-degree burns, bulbous impetigo, pemphigus

G.

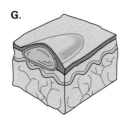

Pustule
  Vesicles or bullae that become filled with pus, usually described as less than 0.5 cm in diameter
Example
  Acne, impetigo, furuncles, carbuncles, folliculitis

H.

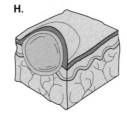

Cyst
  Encapsulated fluid-filled or a semi-solid mass in the subcutaneous tissue or dermis
Example
  Sebaceous cyst, epidermoid cyst

Lesions

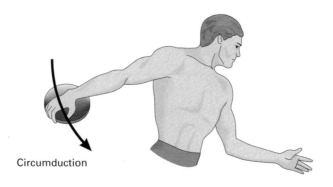

Circumduction

ANSWER COLUMN

10.135

From the word parts you have already learned, think of the meaning for the following term and write it below.

to cut around (actually a surgical procedure for removing the foreskin of the penis)

circum/cision *_____

_____

_____

10.136

circum/cision
sûr′ kum si shun

The pediatrician performed a _____/_____ on the new baby boy soon after birth.

10.137

dia

There are two prefixes that mean through. The one that you would expect to use more often in medical terminology is _____.

10.138

through
through

dia/rrhea
dia/thermy
dī′ ə thûr mē

You have already learned dia/gnosis, which means knowing _____, and dia/thermy, which means heating

_____.
Build a term that means
flow through _____/_____;
heat through _____/_____.

10.139

dia/phor/esis
dī ə fôr ē′ sis

-**esis** is a suffix meaning action or process. Dia/phor/esis is an action of profuse sweating. Diaphoretic is the adjectival form. Can you think of the reason for using **dia-** as the prefix in these terms?

10.140

di/ur/esis
dī yōōr ē′ sis

Arthr/o/desis is the action of immobilizing (binding) a joint.
Hemat/o/poi/esis is the process of forming blood. The process of causing urine to flow through more rapidly is _____/_____/_____.

NOTE: In the term diuretic the **dia-** is shortened to **di-** and still means through.

ANSWER COLUMN

10.141

A substance that causes increase in urine output (water excretion) is called

di/ur/etic
di yōōr ē′ tik

a _____/_____/_____.

10.142

From what you have just learned in the past few frames, decipher and recall the meaning of this condition.

noct/urnal en/ur/esis

nighttime bedwetting

*_____

10.143

Per/for/ation (noun) means puncture or hole.

through

Per/for/ate (verb) means the act of puncturing _____ something.

10.144

The past tense verb of per/for/ate is per/for/ated.
An ulcer that has eaten a hole through the stomach wall is

per/for/ated
per′ fôr ā t′d
per/for/ate
per′ fôr āt

a _____/_____/_____ ulcer.

An ulcer may also _____/_____/_____ (present tense verb) the stomach wall.

10.145

per/for/ation
per fôr ā′ shən

When ulcers perforate an organ, a _____/_____/_____ (noun) is formed.

10.146

Percussion (noun) means a striking through. Read the section on percussion in a dictionary. Analyze the word here.

per/cussion
per **kush**′ ən

_____/_____

NOTE: A drum is a percussion instrument.

10.147

Supplying tissues with oxygen and nutrients through the blood supply or other tissue fluids is called perfusion. The passage of blood through the arteries of the heart is called coronary _____/_____.

per/fusion
per **fyōō**′ shun

10.148

per/fuse
per **fyōōz**′

A perfusate is a fluid used to _____/_____ (verb form) tissues.

ANSWER COLUMN

1. stethoscope
2. penlight
3. guaiac/occult blood test developer
4. guaiac/occult blood test
5. flexible tape mearuse
6. urine specimen container
7. metal nasal speculum
8. tuning fork
9. percussion hammer
10. tongue depressor
11. ophthalmoscope head
12. okastic ear/nose speculum
13. otoscope head attached to base handle
14. sphygmomanometer
15. latex gloves

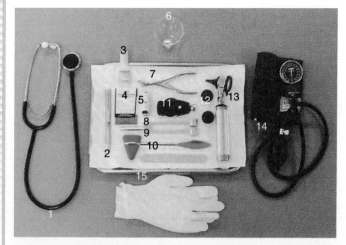

Instruments and supplies used in the physical examination for auscultation, percussion, inspection, and palpation

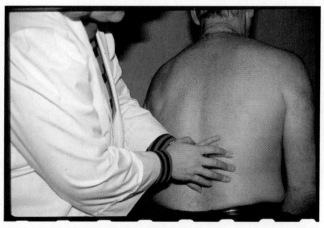

The examiner uses blunt percussion to examine the kidney

---

per, dia circum, peri	**10.149** Summarize. Two prefixes meaning through are _____ and _____. Two prefixes meaning around are _____ and _____.

	10.150 Look up the following terms in your dictionary. Notice that medical specialists use the word-building system to name new procedures. Write the meaning of each term.
through the skin across the lumen heart vessel repair	per/cutaneous *_____; trans/luminal *_____; coronary *_____; angi/o/plasty *_____; (abbreviation: PTCA).

10.151

Necros is a Greek word meaning corpse. **necr/o** is used in words pertaining to death. Necr/o/cyt/osis is cellular _____.
A necr/o/parasite is one that lives on _____ organic matter.

death
dead

10.152

Necr/osis refers to a condition in which dead tissue is surrounded with healthy tissue. Certain diseases can cause _____/_____ of the bones.
When blood supply is cut off from an arm, gangrene sets in. This results in _____ (death) of the arm tissue.

necr/osis
ne **krō**′ sis
necrosis

10.153

Build words meaning
excision of dead tissue
_____/_____;
incision into (dissection of) a dead body
_____/_____/_____;
abnormal fear of death
_____/_____/_____.

necr/ectomy
ne **krek**′ tō mē
necr/o/tomy
ne **krot**′ ō mē
necr/o/phobia
ne krō **fōb**′ ē ə

10.154

There are three ways of saying postmortem (after death) examination. One is aut/o/psy. Another is _____/_____/psy and the third is necr/o/scopy.

necr/o
nek′ rop sē

10.155

If the cause of death is unknown, an _____/_____/_____ may be required to examine the body.

aut/o/psy
aw′ top sē   or
necropsy   or
postmortem exam   or
necr/o/scopy
ne **kros**′ kō pē

10.156

Cyan/o/tic is the adjectival form of cyanosis. Build the adjectival form of necrosis:
_____/_____/_____.

necr/o/tic
ne **kro**′ tik

10.157

De/bride/ment (dā brēd **mən**′) of dead tissue is often done for patients with severe burns. The _____/_____/_____ (dead) tissue is removed.

necr/o/tic
ne **kro**′ tik

ANSWER COLUMN

INFORMATION
FRAME

10.158

-philia is the opposite of **-phobia**. **-phobia** is abnormal fear of; **-philia** is abnormal or unusual attraction to.

10.159

Words that can end in **-phobia**, can also end in **-philia**.
Necr/o/phobia is an abnormal fear of dead bodies. Necr/o/philia is

abnormal attraction to
  dead bodies

* _____.

Morbid fear of water is

hydro/phobia

_____/_____.

(You pronounce)

Strong attraction to water is

hydro/philia

_____/_____.

hī drō **fil′** ē ə

10.160

Think of the meaning while building words opposite of

hemat/o/philia   hemat/o/phobia _____/_____/_____;

pyr/o/philia   pyr/o/phobia _____/_____/_____;

aer/o/philia   aer/o/phobia _____/_____/_____;

aut/o/philia   aut/o/phobia _____/_____/_____.

(You pronounce)

10.161

phil/o is the combining form that means

attraction to, liking, loving

* _____.

10.162

Can you think of a nonmedical word that involves **phil/o**? If so, write it here:

philosopher, philosophy,

_____.

  Philadelphia, etc.

Abbreviation	Meaning
+	death
μm	micrometer
2 h pc, 2 hr pc, 2° pc	two hours postcibum (after meal)
2 h pg, 2 hr pg, 2° pg	two hours postglucose (after drinking glucose)
2 h pp, 2 hr pp, 2° pp	two hours postprandial (after meal)
Ab 1,2,3, AB	abortion (number of)

(continues)

Abbreviation	Meaning
AIDS	acquired immunodeficiency syndrome
bid	*bis in die*, twice a day
Ca	calcium
cc	cubic centimeter(s)
cm	centimeter
CST	certified surgical technologist
D/W	dextrose in water
DPT, DTP, DTaP	diphtheria, pertussis, tetanus (vaccine)
exc	excision
FBS	fasting blood sugar
FME	full mouth extraction
grav 1,2,3	pregnancy (number of)
GHB	glycated hemoglobin
GTT	glucose tolerance test (3 hr–5hr)
Hb A1c, Hgb A1c	Hemoglobin A1c (test)
HepB, hBv	hepatitis B vaccine
Hib	*Haemophilus influenzae* vaccine
HIV	human immunodeficiency virus
hs	hour of sleep, bed time
IPV	inactivated poliovirus vaccine (injectable)
kg	kilogram
LAVH	laparoscopically assisted vaginal hysterectomy
mcg, μg	microgram
mg	milligram
mg/dl	milligram/deciliter(s)
ml	milliliter
mm	millimeter
MMR	measles, mumps, rubella (vaccine)
mono	mononucleosis
NS	normal saline (isotonic saline)
para 1,2,3	live births past 20 months' gestation (numbers of)
PCV	pneumococcal vaccine
PTCA	percutaneous transluminal coronary angioplasty
q 2 h, q 2 hr, q 2°	*quaque 2 hora*, every 2 hours
qid	*quarter in die*, four times a day
S/A, S&A	sugar and acetone
Td	Tetanus toxoid (vaccine)
tid	*ter in die*, three times a day
Var	chickenpox vaccine (*Varicella zoster*)

Also, study the weights and measures abbreviations in Appendix B.

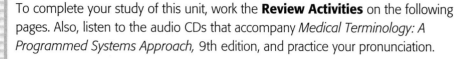

ANSWER COLUMN

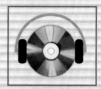

To complete your study of this unit, work the **Review Activities** on the following pages. Also, listen to the audio CDs that accompany *Medical Terminology: A Programmed Systems Approach,* 9th edition, and practice your pronunciation.

Additional practice exercises for this unit are available on the Learner Practice CD-ROM found in the back of the textbook.

REVIEW ACTIVITIES

PREFIX AND WORD

Write the prefix that represents the direction, then build a word using that prefix.

Prefix			Word
_____	1.	away from	move away from the body
_____	2.	down from	part of the aorta that moves down from the heart
_____	3.	out of	to cut out
_____	4.	equal/same	equal osmotic pressure (solution)
_____	5.	unequal	condition of unequal sized cells
_____	6.	through	treatment by heating through tissues
_____	7.	through	to strike through (part of physical examination)
_____	8.	around	membrane around the heart
_____	9.	around	circular motion
_____	10.	under	below the tongue

REVIEW ACTIVITIES

CIRCLE AND CORRECT

Circle the correct answer for each question. Then, check your answers in Appendix A.

1. Word root for abdominal wall
   a. abdomeno   b. lapar
   c. hepar   d. hyster

2. Suffix for destruction
   a. -tripsy   b. -stasis
   c. -pexy   d. -lysis

3. Combining form for sweat
   a. hidro   b. hydro
   c. sudoriferous d. hyper

4. Suffix meaning in the urine
   a. -urea   b. -uria
   c. -uric   d. -uro

5. Term indicating high blood sugar
   a. glycogen   b. hypoglycemia
   c. hypertension d. hyperglycemia

6. Suffix meaning producing or generating
   a. -lysis   b. -trophy
   c. -genesis   d. -stasis

7. Physician specialist in immunity
   a. immunology b. immunologist
   c. immunization d. immunotherapist

8. An autologous donor gives blood
   a. to a family member b. to self
   c. to a friend d. frequently

9. The opposite of -philia
   a. hemato   b. genesis
   c. phobia   d. phagia

10. Word part indicating pregnancy
   a. para   b. genesis
   c. partum   d. gravida

COUNT WITH PREFIXES

Count and write the prefix. Then build a word using that prefix.

Prefix			Word
_____	1.	none	no pregnancies	_____
_____	2.	first	first live birth	_____
_____	3.	one	one cell	_____
_____	4.	two	two branches (use your dictionary)	_____
_____	5.	three	three sided	_____
_____	6.	four	paralysis, four limbs	_____
_____	7.	five	five infants born at the same time (use your dictionary)	_____
_____	8.	six	sixth pregnancy	_____

REVIEW ACTIVITIES

Prefix			Word
_____ 9.	seven	seventh live birth	_____
_____ 10.	eight	person 80 years old (use your dictionary)	_____
_____ 11.	nine	ninth pregnancy	_____
_____ 12.	ten	ten liters	_____
_____ 13.	one hundred(th)	1/100th of a meter	_____
_____ 14.	one thousand(th)	1,000 calories	_____
_____ 15.	many	many glands	_____

SELECT AND CONSTRUCT PART I

Select the correct word parts from the following list and construct medical terms that represent the given meaning.

cyst/o/ic	deca	deci	emia	enter(o)(y)	gluco
glyco	gram	hecto	hidro	hyper	hypo
itis	kilo	laparo	lipid	lysis	mammary
meter	milli	(o)sis	ous	para	plasm
pyro	retro	rrhea	scope (ic)		

1. instrument for looking into the abdomen _____
2. condition of heat (fever) _____
3. excessive sweating _____
4. breakdown of sugar _____
5. inflammation around the bladder _____
6. low blood sugar _____
7. containing sugar and fat _____
8. ten grams _____
9. one thousandth of a meter _____
10. behind the breast _____

REVIEW ACTIVITIES

SELECT AND CONSTRUCT PART II

Select the correct word parts from the following list and construct medical terms that represent the given meaning.

a(b)	aden	a(n)	aniso	a/t/ion	blat	bort
brade	bras	calcific	carcin	cardium	circum	cision
coction	cre(t)	cussion	cyt	de	dia	duct
ecto	ex	fusion	hale	hepat	hydr	irritant
iso	itis	lact/ation	lation	lepsy	mast/o	narco
oma	osis	per	peri	rade	tic	tion
tonic						

1. removal of waste from the body _____

2. to take away the products of conception _____

3. sleep attacks (seizures) _____

4. cancer of the breast _____

5. take away skin by scraping (verb) _____

6. inflammation around the liver _____

7. drug that produces sleep _____

8. process of taking calcium from bone _____

9. IV solutions are _____
   compared to blood cells _____

10. process of cutting around (usually the foreskin for removal) _____

11. take away tissue (i.e., endometrial
    _____) _____

12. striking through (i.e., hammer) _____

13. condition of cells of unequal size _____

14. taking the baby away from the breast (weaning) _____

15. condition of water taken away from the body _____

16. process of supplying blood through tissue _____

17. circular motion _____

18. breathe out _____

19. destroying and scraping away _____

20. membrane around the heart _____

REVIEW ACTIVITIES

DEFINE AND DISSECT

Give a brief definition, and dissect each term listed into its word parts in the space provided. Check your answers by referring to the frame listed in parentheses and your medical dictionary. Then listen to the CDs to practice pronunciation.

1. laparotomy (10.6)

_____/_____/_____
rt   v   suffix

_____
definition

2. laparohepatotomy (10.7)

_____/_____/_____/_____/_____
rt   v   rt   v   suffix

_____

3. pyrolysis (10.11)

_____/_____/_____
rt   v   suffix

_____

4. pyrexia (10.10)

_____/_____
rt   suffix

_____

5. glucogenesis (10.20)

_____/_____/_____/_____
rt   v   rt   suffix

_____

6. glycogenesis (10.20)

_____/_____/_____/_____
rt   v   rt   suffix

_____

7. hypoglycemia (10.25)

_____/_____/_____
pre   rt   suffix

_____

8. glucosuria (10.18)

_____/_____/_____
rt   v   rt/suffix

_____

9. laparoscopic (10.5)

_____/_____/_____/_____
rt   v   rt   suffix

_____

10. glycoprotein (10.18)

_____/_____/_____
rt   v   rt

_____

11. glycolipid (10.29)

_____/_____/_____
rt   v   rt

_____

REVIEW ACTIVITIES

12. immunology (10.30)

_____ / _____ / _____
rt   v   suffix

13. immunodeficiency (10.32)

_____ / _____ / _____
rt   v   rt/suffix

14. autoimmunity (10.42)

_____ / _____ / _____ / _____
pre   v   rt   suffix

15. autophagia (10.43)

_____ / _____ / _____
pre   v   rt/suffix

16. mononucleosis (10.53)

_____ / _____ / _____
pre   rt   suffix

17. multiparous (10.60)

_____ / _____ / _____
pre   rt   suffix

18. primigravida (10.64)

_____ / _____
pre   rt/suffix

19. kilometer (10.69)

_____ / _____
pre   suffix

20. centigram (10.72)

_____ / _____
pre   rt

21. quadriplegia (table)

_____ / _____
pre   rt/suffix

22. sexagenarian (table)

_____ / _____
pre   rt/suffix

23. septuplets (table)

_____ / _____
pre   rt/suffix

24. immunization (10.31)

_____ / _____ / _____
rt   v   suffix

25. autohemotherapy (10.44)

_____ / _____ / _____ / _____ / _____
pre   v   rt   v   suffix

REVIEW ACTIVITIES

26. monocytosis (10.52)

_____/_____/_____
pre   rt   suffix

_____

27. hemiplegia (table)

_____/_____
pre   suffix

_____

28. deciliter (table)

_____/_____
pre   rt

_____

29. nullipara (10.66)

_____/_____
pre   rt/suffix

_____

30. bifurcation (table)

_____/_____/_____
pre   rt   suffix

_____

31. aberrant (10.75)

_____/_____
pre   rt/suffix

_____

32. abrasion (10.80)

_____/_____
pre   rt/suffix

_____

33. deciduous (10.85)

_____/_____
pre   rt/suffix

_____

34. dehydrated (10.89)

_____/_____/_____
pre   rt   suffix

_____

35. decalcification (10.91)

_____/_____/_____
pre   rt   suffix

_____

36. excised (10.96)

_____/_____/_____
pre   rt   suffix

_____

37. isotonic (10.108)

_____/_____/_____
pre   rt   suffix

_____

38. anisocytosis (10.120)

_____/_____/_____
pre   rt   suffix

_____

REVIEW ACTIVITIES

39. mastectomy (10.116)

_____/_____
rt   suffix

40. circumscribed (10.131)

_____/_____
pre   rt/suffix

41. perforated (10.144)

____/_____/_____
pre   rt   suffix

42. diaphoresis (10.139)

_____/_____/_____
pre   rt   suffix

43. percutaneous (10.150)

_____/_____/_____
pre   rt   suffix

44. necrotic (10.156)

_____/___/_____
rt   v   suffix

45. necrophobia (10.153)

_____/___/_____
rt   v   suffix

46. circumcision (10.136)

_____/_____
pre   rt/suffix

47. extension (10.104)

___/_____
pre   rt/suffix

48. flexion (10.104)

_____/_____
rt   suffix

49. diuresis (10.140)

___/___/_____
pre rt suffix

50. percussion (10.146)

_____/_____
pre   rt/suffix

51. pericardiectomy (10.126)

_____/_____/_____
pre rt suffix

REVIEW ACTIVITIES

52. ablation (10.81)

_____/_____
 pre   rt/suffix

_____

53. perfusion (10.147)

_____/_____
 pre   rt/suffix

_____

ABBREVIATION MATCHING

Match the following abbreviations with their definition.

_____ 1. 2 h pc
_____ 2. GTT
_____ 3. FBS
_____ 4. Type II diabetes
_____ 5. S&A
_____ 6. IDDM
_____ 7. ab 2
_____ 8. IPV
_____ 9. mono
_____ 10. HepB
_____ 11. AIDS
_____ 12. para 2
_____ 13. DPT

a. sugar and acetone
b. NIDDM
c. IDDM
d. two hours after meal
e. acid-fast bacillus
f. fasting blood sugar
g. glucose tolerance test
h. type 1 diabetes mellitus
i. human immunodeficiency virus
j. diphtheria, pertussis, tetanus
k. one
l. oral poliovirus vaccine
m. acute autoimmune disease
n. herpes influenza virus
o. two abortions
p. acquired immunodeficiency syndrome
q. mononucleosis
r. hepatitis B vaccine
s. two live births (viable)
t. inactivated poliovirus vaccine

ABBREVIATIONS—WEIGHTS AND MEASURES

State the correct abbreviation for the following weights and measures.

_____ 1. kilogram
_____ 2. milligram
_____ 3. cubic centimeter
_____ 4. deciliter
_____ 5. millimeter
_____ 6. microgram

REVIEW ACTIVITIES

ABBREVIATION MATCHING

Match the following abbreviations with their definition.

_____ 1. bid   a. every night

_____ 2. q2h   b. micrometer

_____ 3. PTCA   c. three times a day

_____ 4. exc   d. normal saline

_____ 5. hs   e. parent-teacher agency

_____ 6. Ca   f. at bedtime

_____ 7. tid   g. twice a day

_____ 8. μm   h. every two hours

i. excision

j. calcium

k. full-mouth extraction

l. dextrose in water

m. percutaneous transluminal coronary angioplasty

n. millimeter(s)

ABBREVIATION FILL-INS

Fill in the blank with the correct abbreviation.

9. every four hours   _____

10. dextrose in water   _____

11. normal saline   _____

12. four times a day   _____

13. death (symbol)   _____

CASE STUDIES

Write the term next to its meaning given below. Then draw slashes to analyze the word parts. Note the use of medical abbreviations. Look these up in your dictionary or find them in Appendix B. If you have any questions about the answers, refer to your medical dictionary or check with your instructor for the answers in Appendix A.

CASE STUDY 10-1

Mastectomy

Pt: 50-year-old female

Surgeon: Sharon Rooney-Gandy, D.O.

Preoperative Dx: **Multifocal** ductal **carcinoma in situ**, left breast

Postoperative Dx: Multifocal ductal carcinoma in situ, left breast, pathology pending

REVIEW ACTIVITIES

Operation performed: Left simple **mastectomy**

Preop History: The patient was noted to have calcifications on routine **mammogram**. She does not practice breast self-exam and felt no lumps herself. Upon needle localization left breast **biopsy**, she was found to have multifocal ductal carcinoma in situ, noncomedo type with tumor extending to margin of excision and **microcalcifications**. *Hx:* Grav 0, Para, AB 0, and is in **menopause** with history of ependymoma and radiation of her spine, paternal grandmother with **bilateral** breast cancer, paternal aunt with bilateral breast cancer. Physical examination of the right breast was essentially unremarkable. The left breast revealed a well-healed upper medial quadrant curvilinear **incision** from previous biopsy. There was no **retraction**, discharge, masses, or **axillary** nodes. After biopsy she was evaluated by an oncologist for treatment of carcinoma in situ. Dr. Peter, radiation oncologist, evaluated her for radiation therapy. It was felt best that the patient undergo simple mastectomy, not so much because of previous radiation therapy, but because of the residual multicalcifications remaining in her left breast. The patient did understand this. Because of her small breasts, we thought she would be best treated cosmetically with a left simple mastectomy. The patient tolerated the procedure well and was taken to the recovery room in satisfactory condition.

Procedure: The patient was taken to the operating room, given general **anesthesia**, prepped and draped in a **sterile** manner. Elliptical incisions were made in a horizontal fashion incorporating the previous biopsy site. The skin was incised with minor bleeding controlled using Bovie cautery. The breast tissue was **dissected** down to the pectoral fascia and up to the clavicle, elevating the **superior** skin flap. The lower skin flap was developed using Bovie cautery down to the pectoral fascia. The breast was excised using Bovie cautery, **hemostasis** secured with Bovie cautery. The incision was irrigated with saline. No other masses or **axillary** nodes could be palpated. The skin was closed with interrupted 4-0 Vicryl followed by a continuous **subcuticular** 4-0 Prolene. Prior to closing the skin a JP drain was placed through a separate stab incision. Steri-strips were applied and the drain was sutured in place. A sterile pressure dressing was applied. **Postoperative** condition was stable. The case was clean and elective.

1. pertaining to below the epidermis _____
2. condition creating no sensation _____
3. having more than one focus (location) _____
4. type of cancer in one location _____
5. was cut apart _____
6. area under the arm _____
7. control of blood flow _____
8. excision of the breast _____
9. breast x-ray _____
10. absence of organisms _____
11. pulling and holding back _____
12. small calcium deposits _____
13. examination of living tissue _____

REVIEW ACTIVITIES

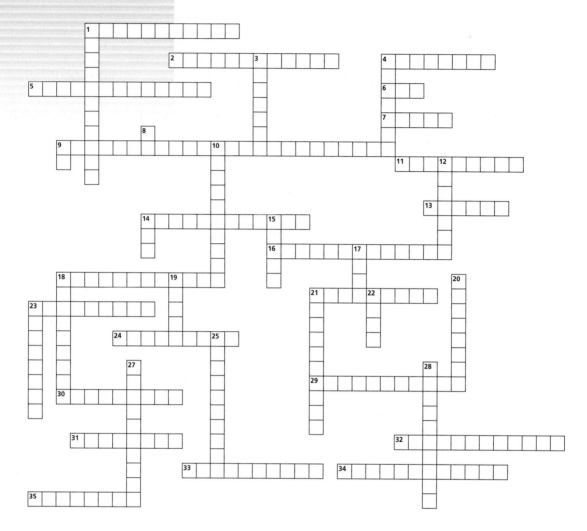

Across

1. condition of increase in monocyes
2. fear of water (rabies)
4. surgical destruction by scraping layers of tissue
5. pertaining to many capsules
6. three time a day
7. prefix for first
9. x-ray process, biliary and pancreatic vessels
11. make a hole (verb)
13. breathe out
14. across the lumen (blood vessel)
16. movement in a circle
18. immune response to one's self
21. teeth that fall out (primary)
23. movement toward the midline
24. 0.01 gram
29. loss of water
30. night (adjective)
31. removal
32. attraction to blood
33. excision of a breast
34. same length fingers or toes
35. scraping wound

Down

1. pertaining to many live births
3. fever
4. exam of a dead body
8. kilogram
9. symbol for calcium
10. seizures of sleep
12. bending
14. prefix for three
15. combining form for dead
17. prefix for one tenth
18. movement away from the body
19. prefix for none
20. termination of pregnancy
21. The _____ colon moves down.
22. prefix for ten
23. wandering from the norm
25. pertaining to self generating
27. striking or tapping
28. 0.001 meter

REVIEW ACTIVITIES

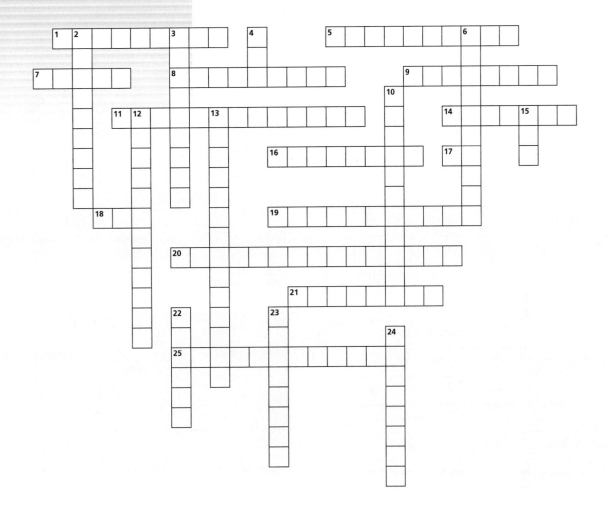

Across

1. make a hole in (verb)
5. seizures of sleep
7. combining form for dead
8. teeth that fall out (primary)
9. agent that causes diuresis
11. encircled
14. synonym for necropsy
16. seizure disorder
17. hour of sleep, at bedtime (abbreviation)
18. excision (abbreviation)
19. water loss (noun)
20. excision of the pericardium
21. wandering from the norm
25. loves blood

Down

2. waste removal
3. movement away from the midline
4. twice a day (abbreviation)
6. striking to examine
10. different size breasts
12. same size digits
13. breast cancer
15. percutaneous transluminal coronary angioplasty (abbreviation)
22. breathe out
23. termination of pregnancy
24. sleeping drug

REVIEW ACTIVITIES

GLOSSARY

abduction	movement away from the midline	autophobia	abnormal fear of one's self, being alone
aberrant	wandering away from the norm	autopsy	necropsy, postmortem examination
ablactation	weaning a baby from the breast	centigram	one hundredth of a gram (0.01 g)
ablation	takes away a layer or destroys a tissue layer	centimeter	one hundredth of a meter (0.01 g)
abnormal	unusual (not normal)	cholangio-pancreatography	X-ray of bile ducts and pancreatic ducts using contrast medium
aboral	away from the mouth		
abortion	termination of pregnancy	circumduction	moving as to describe a circle with a body part
abrasion	scraping		
adduction	movement toward the midline	circumocular	encircling the eye
aerophilia	attraction to air	circumscribed	encircling or in the shape of a circle
anhidrosis	absence of sweating		
anisocytosis	cells of unequal sizes	cytoplasm	substance within the cell (endoplasm)
anisomastia	breasts of unequal size	decagram	ten grams
autodermic	plastic surgery and grafting using one's own skin (dermatoplasty)	decalcification	calcium loss (from bone)
		decaliter	ten liters
autodiagnosis	diagnosing one's self	deciduous	falls down (primary teeth that come out)
autogenous	made by or from one's own tissues (adjective)	decigram	one tenth of a gram (0.1 g)
autograft	graft of tissue from one's own body	deciliter	one tenth of a liter (0.1 L)
		dehydration	water loss
autohemotherapy	transfusion with one's own blood (autologous donor)	descending	moving downward
autoimmunity	reaction of immune response to one's own tissues	diaphoresis	profuse sweating
		diuresis	increase in urine output
autonomic	self-controlling part of the nervous system (adjective)	diuretic	agent that causes diuresis
		epilepsy	disorder characterized by seizures
autophagia	biting one's self		
autophilia	attraction to one's self	excision	removing a body part

REVIEW ACTIVITIES

excretion	removal of waste (urination, defecation)	multicellular	having or involving many cells (adjective)
exhale	breathe out (expire)	multiglandular	having or involving many glands (adjective)
extension	to straighten or lengthen a body part	multinuclear	a cell having more than one nucleus (adjective)
extraction	removal or pulling out of a body part	multipara	having many live births (born in third trimester)
flexion	to shorten or bend a body part	necrectomy	excision of dead tissue
hematophilia	attraction to blood	necrocytosis	condition of cell death or decomposition
hydrophilia	attraction to water		
hydrophobia	fear of water (symptom of rabies)	necroparasite	organism that lives off dead tissue
isocellular	equal size cells	necrophobia	abnormal fear of dead bodies
isodactylism	digits the same length	necrotic	pertaining to necrosis (condition of dead tissue)
isometric	measures the same on all sides	necrotomy	incision into dead tissue
isotonic	osmotic pressure equal to the inside of a cell	nocturnal enuresis	bedwetting
		nullipara	having no pregnancies carried to the third trimester
mastectomy	excision of breast tissue		
mastocarcinoma	breast cancer	percussion	striking or tapping
millimeter	one thousandth of a meter (0.001 m)	percutaneous	through the skin
monocyte	one cell (type of leukocyte)	perforation	puncturing
monocytosis	increase in the number of monocytes	periarticular	area surrounding a joint
		pericardiectomy	excision of the membrane around the heart
monoma	a single tumor	pericolic	area surrounding the colon
monomyoplegia	paralysis of one muscle	perihepatitis	inflammation around the liver
mononeural	involving one nerve	peritonsillar	area surrounding the tonsils
mononuclear	having one nucleus	primigravida	first pregnancy
mononucleosis	viral infection causing monocytosis	primipara	first live birth
multicapsular	having more than one capsule (adjective)	pyrexia	fever (hyperthermia)

REVIEW ACTIVITIES

pyrolysis	destruction of tissue caused by fever
pyromania	compulsion (madness) for setting fires
pyrometer	thermometer
pyrophilia	attraction to fire

pyrophobia	abnormal fear of fire
pyrosis	heartburn
pyrotoxin	poisonous by-product of metabolism created during fever
transluminal	across the lumen

UNIT 11

Descriptive Prefixes, Asepsis, and Pharmacology

ANSWER COLUMN	
	11.1
	homo- means same. Homo/genized milk has the same amount of cream throughout. Homo/gland/ular means pertaining to the
same gland	*_____.
	11.2
same	Homo/therm/al means having the _____ body temperature all the time (i.e., 98.6°F).
	11.3
same	Homo/later/al means pertaining to the _____ side.
	11.4
	Homo/sex/ual means being attracted to the same sex. When men are sexually attracted to men, they are said to be _____/_____/_____.
homo/sex/ual hō′ mō **sek**′ shōō əl	
	11.5
	When women are attracted to women rather than to men, they too are called
homosexual	_____.
	11.6
	hetero- is the opposite of **homo-**. **hetero-** means
different	_____.
	Heter/opsia (het ûr **ō**′ pē ə) means
different	_____ vision in each eye.

389

ANSWER COLUMN

different

11.7

Hetero/sex/ual means being attracted to a _____ sex.

INFORMATION TABLE SEXUALITY TERMS

Sexual Orientation	Sexual Preference
Heterosexual:	Person whose predominant physical or sexual attraction is to the opposite sex; also known as "straight"
Homosexual:	Person whose predominant physical or sexual attraction is to the same sex; also known as gay (homosexual men or women, mostly men) or lesbian (homosexual women)
Bisexual:	Someone who has a physical or sexual attraction to both sexes
Transgender	**Umbrella Term for all Gender Variant People**
Cross-Dresser:	Person who wears clothing typically worn by the opposite sex; also known as "transvestite"
Transsexual:	Person in the process of physically altering his or her sex to be more like the opposite sex; may be by use of hormones, implants, or surgery. (male-to-female = mtf) (female-to-male = ftm).
Intersex:	Person born with a body not clearly male or female; may be caused by any of several medical conditions including genetic or chromosomal anomalies which interfere with sexual differentiation during gestation. Intersex is the preferred term over "Hermaphrodite"

11.8

Look up the meanings of homogeneous and heterogeneous. Draw the slashes and write the definitions below

homo/gen/eous
hō′ mō **jē**′ nē us
pertaining to the same
  throughout
hetero/gen/eous
het′ ûr ō **jē**′ nē us
pertaining to different
  throughout

* _____ ,
   _____ .

* _____ ,
   _____ .

ANSWER COLUMN

11.9

Open your dictionary and look up these terms. While you think of their meanings, form *opposites* of the following.

homo/gen/esis

hetero/gen/esis
het′ ûr ō **jen**′ ə sis

_____/_____/_____

hetero/sex/ual
het′ ûr ō **seks**′ ū əl

homo/sex/ual

_____/_____/_____

11.10

Think of their meanings while you recall these or other opposites

anterior

posterior _____;

iso

aniso- (prefix) _____;

hyper

hypo- (prefix) _____;

adduction

abduction _____.

11.11

Good. Now you'll study **syn-** and **sym-**. They are different forms of the same prefix. **syn-** and **sym-** mean

together or joined

*_____.

11.12

Review: You have already learned **syn-** in the words syndactylism, synergetic, synarthrosis, and syndrome.

11.13

sym-

syn- is the form of the prefix that is used to mean fixed or joined, except when it is followed by the sound of "b," "m," "f," "ph," or "p." Then, _____ is used.
EXAMPLE: symbol, symphony, sympathy

11.14

suffering (medical) or
feeling (standard)

Sym/pathy is an ordinary word that has a special medical meaning. From either a medical or regular English dictionary, find what it takes to fill this blank:
sym- + path/os, the Greek word for _____.

11.15

eyelids have grown
together, or adhesions
of the eyelids

blephar/o means eyelid. A sym/physis is a growing together of parts.
Sym/blepharon means *_____
_____.

ANSWER COLUMN

11.16

pod/o is one combining form for foot. Build words meaning lower extremities are grown together (united)

_____/_____;

sym/podia
sim **pō**′ dē ə

excision of a sympathetic nerve

_____/_____;

sym/path/ectomy
sim pa **thek**′ tō mē

tumor of a sympathetic nerve

_____/_____/_____.

sym/path/oma
sim path **ō**′ mə

11.17

Find a fairly common word in your medical dictionary in which **sym-** is followed by *m*. (There are only two or three choices.)

symmetry, symmetric,
  or symmetrical

One is _____.

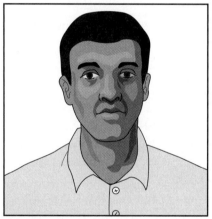

Symmetry

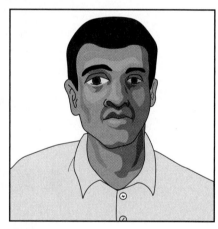

Asymmetry

11.18

Find a common word in your medical dictionary that is used in ordinary English in which **sym-** is followed by "b"

symbol or symbolism

*_____.

11.19

syn- and **sym-** both mean together. **sym-** is used when followed by the sound of the letters _____, _____, _____, _____, and _____. **syn-** is used in other medical words.

b
m
p
f
ph

ANSWER COLUMN

TAKE A
CLOSER
LOOK

11.20

super- and **supra-** are both prefixes that mean above or beyond. Analyze the following words in which **super-** and **supra-** are used. Write the meaning of the word as you analyze it. If necessary, consult a dictionary.

11.21

super/fici/al
super/cili/ary
super/infect/ion
super/ior/ity
super/leth/al
super/numer/ary

Draw the slashes as you write the following
superficial _____;
superciliary _____;
superinfection _____;
superiority _____;
superlethal _____;
supernumerary _____.
Look up their meanings in your dictionary.

11.22

supra/lumb/ar
supra/pub/ic
supra/mammary
supra/ren/al
supra/inguin/al
supra/ren/o/pathy

Draw the slashes as you write the following
supralumbar _____;
suprapubic _____;
supramammary _____;
suprarenal _____;
suprainguinal _____;
suprarenopathy _____.
Look up their meanings.

11.23

used more frequently in
  modern English
used more frequently in
  medical words

Draw a conclusion about **super-** and **supra-** from your answers in the last two frames
super- is *_____
_____.
supra- is *_____
_____.

a- and **an-** are prefixes that mean without or lack of. Examine the following list of words.

an/algesia	an/esthesia	an/onychia	a/biotic	a/febrile	a/phasia
ana/phylaxis	an/isocytosis	an/orexia	a/blastemic	a/galactia	a/pnea
an/emia	an/hidrosis	an/uria	a/cholia	a/kinesia	a/sepsis
an/encephalus	an/iridia	an/uresis	a/dermia	a/menorrhea	a/symmetry

ANSWER COLUMN

11.24

consonant

Draw a conclusion.
Use **a-** if it is followed by a (choose one) _____ (vowel/consonant).

vowel

Use **an-** if it is followed by a (choose one) _____ (vowel/consonant).

More prefixes! Use this table to work Frames 11.25–11.62.

Prefix	Meaning	Special Comment
epi-	over, upon	epicenter of an earthquake
extra-	outside of, beyond, in addition to	extracurricular activities
infra-	below, under	almost always below a part of the body; almost always adjectival in form; there are fewer words beginning with **infra-** than with **sub-**
sub-	under, below	many words of all kinds begin with **sub-**
meta-	beyond, after, occurring later in a series	also used with chemical names

Directional prefixes

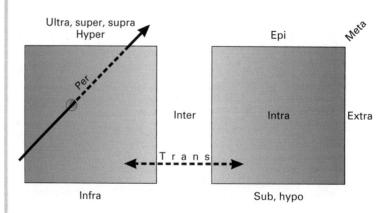

11.25

over the stomach

epi- means upon or over. The epi/gastr/ic region is the region
* _____ .

ANSWER COLUMN

11.26

Epi/splen/itis means inflammation of the tissue

over the spleen

*_____.

11.27

Build words meaning
inflammation of the area over the bladder

epi/cyst/itis
ep' i sis **tī**' tis

_____/_____/_____;

epi/nephr/itis
ep' i nef **rī**' tis

inflammation (of the tissue) upon the kidney

_____/_____/_____.

11.28

Build words meaning
excision of the tissue upon the kidney

epi/nephr/ectomy
ep' i nef **rek**' tə mē
epi/gastr/o/rrhaphy
ep' i gas **trôr**' ə fē

_____/_____/_____;

suture of the region over the stomach

_____/_____/____/_____.

11.29

Build words meaning pertaining to (the tissue) upon the skin (outermost layer)

epi/derm/al

_____/_____/_____;

(the tissue) covering the cranium

epi/crani/al

_____/_____/_____;

the area above the stern/um

epi/stern/al

_____/_____/_____;

the tissues upon the heart

epi/card/ium
(You pronounce)

_____/_____/_____.

11.30

INFORMATION
FRAME

Didymos is another Greek word for testis. The epi/didymis is a small oblong body resting upon the testicle, containing convoluted tubules. The epididymis is involved in sperm production and transportation.

11.31

Build words that mean
inflammation of the epididymis

epi/didym/itis
ep' i did i **mī**' tis
epi/didym/ectomy
ep' i did i **mek**' tōm ē

_____/_____/_____;

excision of the epididymis

_____/_____/_____.

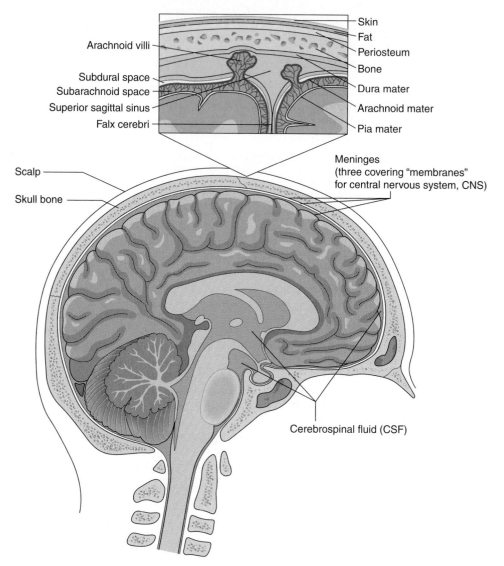

Arachnoid villi
Subdural space
Subarachnoid space
Superior sagittal sinus
Falx cerebri

Skin
Fat
Periosteum
Bone
Dura mater
Arachnoid mater
Pia mater

Meninges
(three covering "membranes"
for central nervous system, CNS)

Scalp
Skull bone

Cerebrospinal fluid (CSF)

The meninges

ANSWER COLUMN	
	11.32
upon	Recall your previous study of the meninges, the membranes that surround the brain and spinal cord. The dura (dur) mater is a layer of the meninges. The epi/dur/al layer is located _____ the dura.
	11.33
epi/dur/al ep′ i **dur**′ əl	Anesthetic can be administered in the layer or space upon the dura. This is _____/_____/_____ anesthesia.

11.34

Using dur/al build words meaning
below the dura mater

sub/dur/al
sub **dur**′ əl
epi/dur/al
ep′ i **dur**′ əl

_____/_____/_____;

upon the dura mater

_____/_____/_____.

11.35

SPELL CHECK ✓

derm/al and dur/al look and sound similar but have completely different meanings. The derm/is is the middle layer of the skin, and the **dura mater** is the outer layer of the meninges. Look up the following terms in your dictionary, and be watchful of their use and spelling.

epi/derm/al _____

epi/dur/al _____

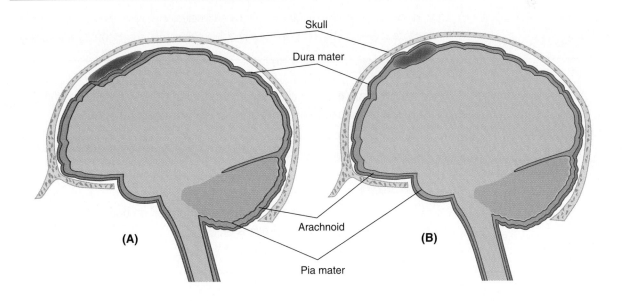

Cranial hematomas: (A) epidural, (B) subdural

11.36

outside of or beyond

extra- means outside or beyond. Think of extraterrestrial. Extra/nuclear (eks tra **noo**′ klē är) means *_____ the nucleus of a cell.

11.37

outside of or beyond

Extra/uterine is an adjective meaning *_____ the uterus.

ANSWER COLUMN

11.38

Build words meaning outside of the joint

extra-/articul/ar
eks′ trə är **tik**′ yə lər

_____/_____/_____;

urinary bladder

extra/cyst/ic
eks′ trə **sis**′ tik

_____/_____/_____;

dura mater (meninges)

extra/dur/al
eks′ trə **dōor**′ əl

_____/_____/_____;

genitals

extra/genit/al
eks′ trə **jen**′ i təl

_____/_____/_____;

liver

extra/hepat/ic
eks′ trə hep **at**′ ik

_____/_____/_____;

cerebrum

extra/cerebr/al
eks′ trə ser ē′ brəl

_____/_____/_____.

11.39

adjectives

Look at the words in the last frame. Draw a conclusion. **extra-** is used as a prefix in words that are usually (choose one) _____ (nouns/adjectives).

11.40

mamm/o/graphy
mam **og**′ raf ē

Recall that **mamm/o** is one combining form for breast. An x-ray picture of the breast is a mammogram. The process of taking this x-ray is called
_____/_____/_____.

11.41

both sides
both breasts

bi- means both or two. When a procedure is performed on both sides, it is said to be bilateral. A bilateral hernia repair is on *_____.
A bilateral mammogram is a radiograph of *_____.

11.42

bi/later/al
bī **lat**′ er əl

In humans, because most body parts are in pairs, the opposite of unilateral is
_____/_____/_____.

11.43

below or under

infra- means below or under. Infra/mammary means
*_____ the mammary gland.

11.44

below or under

Infra/patell/ar means *_____ the patella (kneecap).

During a mammography, the breast is gently flattened and then radiographed

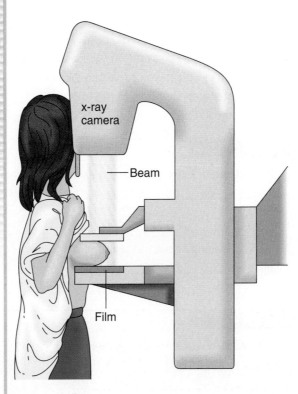

x-ray camera

Beam

Film

11.45

sub

Below the tongue is _____/lingual.

11.46

under or below
under

sub- is a prefix that means *_____.
A sub/dural hematoma is a mass of clotted blood _____ the dura mater.

11.47

under
below
below

Sub/abdominal means _____ the abdomen. aur from the Latin word *auris* is one word root for ear. Sub/aur/al means _____ the ear. Sub/cutaneous (subcu, subq, s.c) means _____ the skin.

11.48

Build words that mean below or under the dura mater

sub/dur/al

_____/_____/_____;

ear

sub/aur/al

_____/_____/_____;

skin

sub/cutan/eous

_____/_____/_____.

ANSWER COLUMN

11.49

The prefixes **infra-** and **sub-** are sometimes confusing in word building. For that reason, you will build words that can take either prefix. When you see **sub-** or **infra-**, you will think of _____ or _____.

under
below

11.50

Using **stern/o**, build two words meaning below the sternum

_____/_____/_____

and

_____/_____/_____.

A word meaning above the sternum is

supra/_____/_____.

infra/stern/al
in' fra stûr' nəl
sub/stern/al
sub' stûr' nəl
supra/stern/al
sōō' pra stûr' nəl

11.51

Using **cost/o**, build two words meaning under the ribs

_____/_____/_____;

_____/_____/_____.

A word meaning above the ribs is _____/_____/_____.

The _____/_____/_____ muscles are between the ribs.

infra/cost/al
sub/cost/al
supra/cost/al
inter/cost/al
(You pronounce)

11.52

Using **pub/o**, build two words meaning under the pubis:

_____/_____/_____ and

_____/_____/_____.

A word meaning above the pubis is _____/_____/_____.

infra/pub/ic
sub/pub/ic
supra/pub/ic
(You pronounce)

11.53

INFORMATION FRAME

meta- is a prefix used in many ways. Look at the table on page 394 to discover its meanings.

11.54

Analyze the term metaphysics. It is the study of things

*_____.

beyond the physical
  or of the spirit

Bones of the wrist and hand

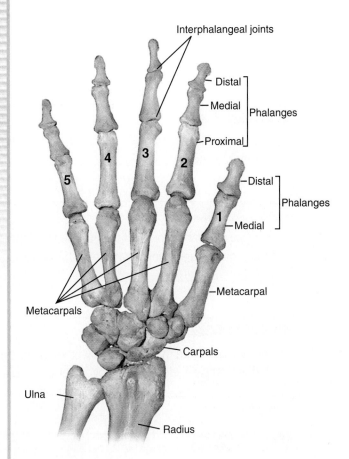

Interphalangeal joints

Distal ⎤
Medial ⎬ Phalanges
Proximal ⎦

Distal ⎤
⎬ Phalanges
Medial ⎦

Metacarpal

Metacarpals

Carpals

Ulna

Radius

11.55

The bones of the hand that are beyond the carpals (wrist) are the

meta/carpals
me′ tə **kar**′ palz

_____/_____.

11.56

The bones of the foot that are beyond the tarsals (ankle) are the

meta/tarsals
me′ tə **tar**′ salz

_____/_____.

11.57

A meta/stasis occurs when a disease spreads beyond its point of origin. A
meta/static (adjective) tumor is a secondary growth from a malignant tumor. This
secondary growth is a _____/_____ (singular noun).
The plural form of this word is
_____/_____.

meta/stasis
me **tas**′ tə sis
meta/stases
me **tas**′ tə sēs

ANSWER COLUMN

11.58

metastasis

The area of the origin of cancer or the first discovered site in a patient is said to be the primary site. If a secondary site is found, it is a _____.

11.59

ultra/violet
ul′ tra **vī** ō let

ultra- is a prefix meaning beyond or in excess. Light waves that are beyond the violet frequency are _____/_____ (UV).

11.60

ultra/son/o/graphy
ul′ tra son **og**′ raf ē

Sound waves that are beyond the audible frequency are ultra/son/ic. The process of making an image using ultrasound (US) is called
_____/_____/____/_____ or sonography.

11.61

ultrasonography
ultrasonography

Ultra/sound may be used for therapy or for diagnostic testing. To detect gallstones in a diseased gallbladder, the sonographer uses diagnostic
_____. To treat a patient with kidney stones, the sonographer uses therapeutic _____.

11.62

Do it

You have now learned many prefixes of location. Review them by making a list with their meaning plus anything special about them.

11.63

a/seps/is
ə **sep**′ sis, ā **sep**′ sis

Recall that path/o/genic refers to disease production. Sepsis is a noun meaning a poisoned state or infection caused by absorption of pathogenic bacteria and their products into the bloodstream. A noun meaning a state without (or lack of) sepsis
____/_____.

11.64

a/sept/ic
ə **sep**′ tik, ā **sep**′ tik

Sept/ic is the adjectival form of sepsis. The adjectival form for the word meaning free from infection is ____/_____/_____.

11.65

infection with pus in
  the bloodstream

Sept/i/cemia is an infection (poisoned state) in the bloodstream. Septic/o/py/emia means *_____

_____.

Note: sept/i, sept/o, and septic/o are combining forms for infection.

PROFESSIONAL PROFILES

Registered diagnostic medical sonographers (RDMSs) are highly skilled allied health professionals who use ultrasound (high-frequency sound) to create images of organs and tissues that are displayed on a computerized monitor in real time and on still films (sonograms). Knowledge of sectional anatomy, pathology, computer technology, and medical ethics is essential. The American Registry of Diagnostic Medical Sonographers (ARDMS) determines educational requirements and criteria for registration of diagnostic medical sonographers.

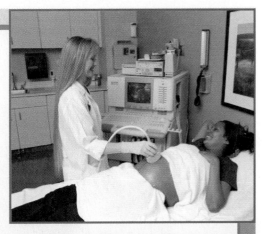

Sonographer performing fetal ultrasound

ANSWER COLUMN

Fetal ultrasound (Prepared by Lynne Schreiber, MA, RDMS, RT[R])

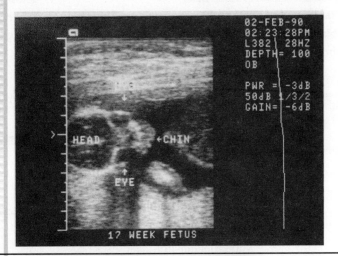

Urinary catheterization requires strict asepsis

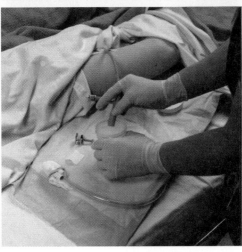

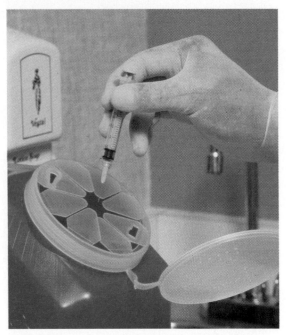

Proper disposal of contaminated needles and syringes (sharps) into biohazard containers prevents accidental exposure to potentially infectious body fluids

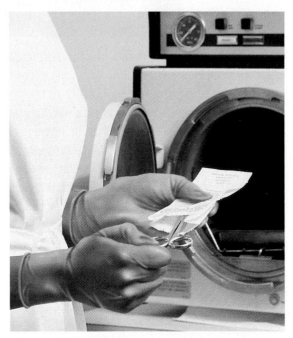

This medical assistant places an instrument into an envelope package for sterilization using an autoclave

ANSWER COLUMN	
	11.66
sept/o (used most often) or seps/o	Study the last two frames. A combining form for infection is _____/_____.
	11.67
	Review the material from Frames 11.63–11.66. Give words that mean
seps/is	noun for infection _____/_____;
sept/ic	adjective for infected _____/_____;
a/seps/is	noun for state free from infection ____/_____/_____;
ā **sep**′ sis	adjective for free from infection ____/_____/_____.
a/sept/ic	
ā **sep**′ tik	
	11.68
	anti- is a prefix meaning against. An anti/pyretic is an agent that
against	works _____ a fever. An anti/toxin is an agent that
against	works _____ a toxin. A pyr/o/toxin

toxin

is a _____ produced by fever (heat).

NOTE: A toxin is a poisonous substance produced by an organism.

The following table lists categories of drugs that work against something.

Drug Category	Works Against
ant/acid	acid
anti/anemic	anemia
anti/arrhythmic	irregular heartbeats
anti/arthritic	arthritis
anti/biotic	bacteria
anti/cholinergic	parasympathetic impulses
anti/coagulant	clotting
anti/convulsant	seizures
anti/depressant	depression
anti/diarrheal	diarrhea
anti/emetic	vomiting
anti/fungal	fungi
anti/histamine	histamine (allergic reactions)
anti/hypertensive	high blood pressure
anti-/inflammatory	inflammation
anti/manic	manic-depression
anti/narcotic	narcotics
anti/neoplastic, anti/tumor	tumors
anti/pruritic	dry skin (itching)
anti/psychotic	psychosis
anti/pyretic	fever
anti/spasmodic	muscle spasms
anti/toxin	poisons (toxins)
anti/tussive	coughs

11.69

against

An anti/narcotic is an agent that works _____ narcotics.

11.70

against

An anti/biotic is an agent that works _____ living bacterial infections.

11.71

Erythromycin is prescribed to fight bacteria and is one type of

anti/biotic
an′ ti bī **ot**′ ik

_____/_____.

Culture and Sensitivity (C&S)
Antibiotic susceptibility test plate

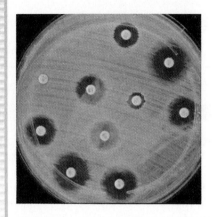

Confused about agents that fight pathogenic organisms? Study the following table.

AGENTS THAT FIGHT PATHOGENIC ORGANISMS

Antiseptics are agents that prevent sepsis by inhibiting growth of causative organisms. They may be inorganic, such as mercury and iodine preparations, or organic, such as carbolic acid (phenol) and alcohol.

Antibiotics are mostly prescription drugs that inhibit growth or destroy microorganisms, especially bacteria. Antibiotics can be used topically or taken internally for a systemic effect. Examples: penicillin, Keflex, erythromycin. Antibiotics can be bacteriocidal (kill bacteria) or bacteriostatic (inhibit growth, keep the numbers down).

Disinfectants are chemical or physical agents that prevent infection by killing microorganisms. They are used to clean equipment or surfaces rather than in or upon the body (i.e., Virex, bleach).

Sterilization is a process that kills organisms of all sorts. An autoclave uses pressure and steam and is the most effective form of sterilization. Chemical sterilization using disinfectants such as bleach kills most organisms but not the ones that form spores.

11.72

Now, build words describing the agents that work against
rheumatic disease

anti/rheumatic
an' ti rōō **ma**' tik

_____/_____ ;

spastic muscle

anti/spasmodic
an' ti spaz **mod**' ik

_____/_____ ;

toxins

anti/toxin
an' ti **toks**' in

_____/_____ .

ANSWER COLUMN

11.73

Build adjectives describing the agents that work against
convulsive states

anti/convulsive
an′ ti kon **vul**′ siv

_____/_____;

arthritic diseases

anti/arthritic
an′ ti ar **thri**′ tik

_____/_____;

toxic states

anti/toxic
an′ ti **toks**′ ik

_____/_____;

sepsis

anti/septic
an′ ti **sep**′ tik

_____/_____.

11.74

contra- is a prefix that means against. **contra-** is usually used with modern
English words. To contra/dict someone is to speak _____ what the
person is saying.

against

11.75

Contra/ry things are _____ each other. A contra/ry person is one who
is _____ your wishes.

against
against

11.76

Analyze these three words
contraindication

contra/indication
kon′ tra in di **kā**′ shun

_____/_____;

contraceptive

contra/ceptive
kon′ tra **sep**′ tiv

_____/_____;

contralateral

contra/later/al
kon′ tra **lat**′ ur əl

_____/_____/_____.

11.77

Using the words in Frame 11.76, fill the following blanks with a word whose literal
meaning is

contraindication
contraceptive
contralateral

against indication _____;
against conception _____;
opposite (against) side _____.

11.78

Using the noun contra/indication, build other parts of the same word

contra/indicate
contra/indicated
(You pronounce)

_____/_____ (present tense verb);
_____/_____ (past tense verb).

ANSWER COLUMN

11.79

Before beginning a drug therapy of any kind on a patient who is pregnant, a physician will consult a drug reference guide to see if the medication is safe to use during pregnancy. If it is not, the guide will say the medication is contra/indicated during pregnancy. Narcotic medications are not advisable during pregnancy; therefore, they are _____/_____.

contra/indicated
kon′ tra **in**′ di kā ted

Study the following list of drug categories that do not begin with **anti-**. Can you analyze their meaning from word parts you have already learned? If not, look them up in your dictionary for more information.

Drug	Action
bronch/o/dilat/or	dilates or enlarges bronchi
de/congest/ant	reduces respiratory congestion
di/ur/etic	increases urine flow
ex/pector/ant	assists in removing respiratory secretions
hem/o/stat/ic	controls bleeding
hormon/es	endocrine secretions that affect control mechanisms
hypn/o/tic	sleep agent, produces state of hypnosis
hypo/glyc/em/ic	agent that lowers blood sugar (glucose)
lax/a/tive	loosens or liquifies stool for relief of constipation
muscle re/lax/ant	relieves tension in skeletal muscle
sed/a/tive	calms nervous excitement
tran/quiliz/er	lowers anxiety and mental tension
vas/o/dilat/or	dilates blood vessels
vas/o/press/or	constricts blood vessels, increases blood pressure

11.80

across or over

trans- is a Latin prefix meaning across or over. To trans/port a cargo is to carry it
* _____ the ocean or land.

11.81

across or over

Trans/position means literally position * _____.

11.82

trans/position
trans′ pə **zish**′ ən

When an organ is placed across to the other side of the body from where it is normally found (e.g., liver on the left side), _____/_____ occurs.

ANSWER COLUMN

11.83

Cardi/ac transposition means that the heart is on the right side of the body. If the stomach is on the right side of the body, the condition is gastr/ic

transposition

_____.

11.84

When a trans/fusion is given, blood is passed

across or over

*_____ from one person to another.

11.85

Recall that the procedure performed across the lumen of an artery of the heart

trans-

is percutaneous _____/luminal angioplasty (PTA).

Transurethral resection of the prostate (TURP)

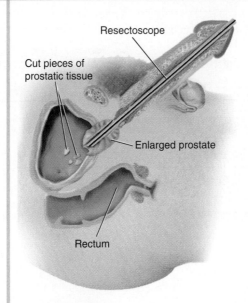

Resectoscope

Cut pieces of
prostatic tissue

Enlarged prostate

Rectum

11.86

Analyze the following by drawing the slashes and writing the meaning

trans/sex/ual

transsexual _____, _____
meaning

trans/illumin/ation

transillumination _____, _____
meaning

trans/vagin/al

transvaginal _____, _____
meaning

trans/thorac/ic

transthoracic _____, _____
meaning

trans/urethr/al

transurethral _____, _____
meaning

trans/fusion

transfusion _____, _____
meaning

(You pronounce)

ANSWER COLUMN

11.87

| INFORMATION FRAME | A catheter (**kath'** e ter) is a flexible tube. When a sterile urine specimen is needed, the urologist may introduce a catheter through the urethra into the bladder to obtain the specimen. |

11.88

| INFORMATION FRAME | A procedure for enlarging heart vessels is called trans/catheter therapy or angioplasty. It is possible to introduce an intravascular occlusion balloon "through" a catheter. Look up these terms in your dictionary and note the use of the prefix **trans-**. |

11.89

Inserting a catheter for urine collection is called

catheterization

_____/_____.

11.90

Cardiac catheterization allows the physician to view the inside of the vessels

heart

of the _____.

Abbreviation	Meaning
A, B, O, AB	blood types
AAMA	American Association of Medical Assistants
ARDMS	American Registry of Diagnostic Medical Sonographers
c̄	with
cath	catheter
cm	centimeter
CMA	certified medical assistant
C&S	culture and sensitivity (antibiotic)
ftm	female to male
inf	infusion
met., metas./mets.	metastasis/metastases
mtf	male to female
RDMS	registered diagnostic medical sonographer
s̄	without
subcu, subq, sc	subcutaneously
trans	transverse
TURP	transurethral resection of the prostate
US	ultrasound
UV	ultraviolet
XM	cross match (as in blood type and cross match)

ANSWER COLUMN

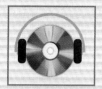

To complete your study of this unit, work the **Review Activities** on the following pages. Also listen to the audio CDs that accompany *Medical Terminology: A Programmed Systems Approach,* 9th edition, and practice your pronunciation.

Additional practice exercises for this unit are available on the Learner Practice CD-ROM found in the back of the textbook.

REVIEW ACTIVITIES

CIRCLE AND CORRECT

Circle the correct answer for each question. Then check your answers in Appendix A.

1. Heteropia indicates _____ visual acuity in each eye.
   a. the same   b. blurred
   c. different   d. changed

2. If a substance is blended or the same throughout, it is _____
   a. homozygous   b. hypertrophic
   c. isocellular   d. homogenous

3. If the next letter is b, m, f, or ph, use _____ as the prefix for joined.
   a. sym-   b. syn-
   c. iso-   d. inter-

4. In anatomic terms indicating a location above, use _____ as a prefix.
   a. hydro-   b. antero-
   c. superio-   d. supra-

5. The fluid outside of the cell is _____ cellular fluid.
   a. extra-   b. intra-
   c. sub-   d. exo-

6. If the next letter is a vowel, use _____ as the prefix meaning not or lack of
   a. a   b. an
   c. either a or an

7. Epicystitis is inflammation _____ the urinary bladder.
   a. in   b. outside of
   c. upon   d. under

8. Which of the following is spelled correctly?
   a. extra-articular   b. extra-genital
   c. extra-cerebral   d. extra-hepatic

9. Which of the following refers to a layer of the meninges?
   a. dermal   b. pneumonic
   c. myelo   d. dural

10. If a procedure is performed on both sides it is
   a. diplocellular   b. bilateral
   c. laterodiploid   d. bifurcated

REVIEW ACTIVITIES

SELECT AND CONSTRUCT

Select the correct word parts from the following list and construct medical terms that represent the given meaning.

a(an)	algesia	aniso	anti	bi
ceptive	contra	cyst/o(ic)	cyt(o)(ic)	derm/o(al)
didym/o(is)	dur/a(al)	ectomy	epi	extra
gastr/o	graph/o(y)(er)	hetero	homo	infra
iso	itis	later/o(al)	lumb/ar	mamm/o
meta	oma	osis	otic	path(o)(y)
pod/o(ia)	ren/o(al)	rrhaphy	sept/o(ic)	sex(ual)
son/o	stasis	stern/o(al)	sub	sym
syn	tox/o(in)(ic)	tri	ultra	

1. agent that works against infection   _____
2. agent that works against fertilization of an ovum   _____
3. attracted to the same sex   _____
4. cells of different sizes   _____
5. feet joined (grown) together   _____
6. below the sternum   _____
7. breast x-ray procedure   _____
8. one who uses reflected sound to make images   _____
9. upon the dura mater   _____
10. outside of the urinary bladder   _____
11. three sides   _____
12. disease that goes beyond its original growth   _____

PREFIX AND WORD

Write the prefix that represents the direction. Then build a word using that prefix.

Prefix   Word

_____ 1. same   attracted to the same sex   _____

_____ 2. different   made of different
                                substances   _____

_____ 3. join   feet grown together
                                (followed by b, m,
                                f, ph, p)   _____

REVIEW ACTIVITIES

_____ 4. above   above the surface   _____

_____ 5. above   above the kidneys   _____

_____ 6. without   absence of menstruation   _____

_____ 7. without   without feeling or sensation _____

_____ 8. upon/over   upon the stomach (adjective) _____

_____ 9. outside of   outside of the cell (adjective) _____

_____10. below/under below the sternum (adjective) _____

_____11. beyond   bones beyond the carpals _____

_____12. beyond   beyond audible sound waves _____

_____13. both   including both sides (adjective) _____

_____14. against   against arthritis (adjective) _____

_____15. against   against indications(not indicated) _____

_____16. across   across the urethra (adjective) _____

DEFINE AND DISSECT

Give a brief definition and dissect each term listed into its word parts in the space provided. Check your answers by referring to the frame listed in parentheses and your medical dictionary. Then listen to the CDs to practice pronunciation.

1. homolateral (11.3)   _____/_____/_____
                                              pre   rt   suffix

_____
                              definition

2. heterosexual (11.9)   _____/_____/_____
                                              pre   rt   suffix

_____

3. sympathectomy (11.16)   _____/_____/_____
                                            pre   rt   suffix

_____

4. symmetrical (11.17)   _____/_____/_____
                                              pre   rt   suffix

_____

5. superinfection (11.21)   _____/_____/_____
                                              pre   rt   suffix

_____

REVIEW ACTIVITIES

6. suprarenopathy (11.22)

_____/_____/_____/_____
pre   rt   v   suffix

7. analgesia (table)

_____/_____
pre   rt/suffix

8. asepsis (11.63)

_____/_____
pre   rt/suffix

9. episplenitis (11.26)

_____/_____/_____
pre   rt   suffix

10. extra-articular (11.38)

_____/_____/_____
pre   rt   suffix

11. extracerebral (11.38)

_____/_____/_____
pre   rt   suffix

12. inframammary (11.43)

_____/_____
pre   rt/suffix

13. mammography (11.40)

_____/_____/_____
rt   v   suffix

14. metastasis (11.57)

_____/_____
pre   rt/suffix

15. ultrasonography (11.60)

_____/_____/_____/_____
pre   rt   v   suffix

REVIEW ACTIVITIES

16. anti-inflammatory (table)

_____/_____/_____/_____

      pre   pre   rt   suffix

17. contraceptive (11.76)

_____/_____

       pre   rt/suffix

18. transcatheter (11.88)

_____/_____

       pre   rt/suffix

19. homogeneous (11.8)

_____/_____/_____

      pre   rt   suffix

20. antiseptic (11.73)

_____/_____/_____

      pre   rt   suffix

21. antibiotic (11.71)

_____/_____/_____

       pre   rt   suffix

22. bacteriostatic (table)

_____/_____/_____/_____

        rt   v   rt   suffix

23. epididymitis (11.31)

_____/_____/_____

      pre   rt   suffix

24. epidural (11.33)

_____/_____/_____

      pre   rt   suffix

25. contraindication (11.76)

_____/_____/_____

      pre   rt   suffix

REVIEW ACTIVITIES

ABBREVIATION MATCHING

Match the following abbreviations with their definition.

_____ 1. c̄
_____ 2. trans
_____ 3. C&S
_____ 4. CMA
_____ 5. UV
_____ 6. mets.
_____ 7. RDMS
_____ 8. A, B, O, AB

a. ultraviolet
b. transurethral
c. blood group types
d. catheter
e. fractured metatarsals
f. transverse
g. with
h. certified medical assistant
i. culture and sensitivity
j. metastases
k. registered dietitian
l. registered diagnostic medical sonographer
m. without
n. infrared
o. certified physicians' assistant

ABBREVIATION FILL-INS

Fill in the blank with the correct abbreviation.

9. American Association of Medical Assistants _____

10. without _____

11. infusion _____

12. crossmatch _____

13. subcutaneously _____

14. female to male _____

15. transurethral resection
    of the prostate _____

REVIEW ACTIVITIES

CASE STUDIES

Write the term next to its meaning given below. Then draw slashes to analyze the word parts. Note the use of medical abbreviations. Look these up in your dictionary or find them in Appendix B. If you have any questions about the answers, refer to your medical dictionary or check with your instructor for the answers in Appendix A.

CASE STUDY 11-1

NEUROLOGY OPERATIVE REPORT

Pt: Male, age 46

Preoperative diagnosis: Left **hemiparesis** with right **subdural** hygroma Postoperative

Dx: Left hemparesis with right subdural hygroma

Procedure: Bur hole with evacuation of subdural fluid

Anesthesia: 1% Xylocaine with standby **anesthesiologist**

Having shaved his head and properly positioned him, the patient was turned slightly to the left. IV Valium was given by the anesthetist who was monitoring his vital signs, including oxygenation.

The right temporoparietal region was prepared and draped in the usual fashion. Xylocaine 1% was administered locally and thereafter a scalp **incision** was carried out, which was deepened down through the **subcutaneous** tissue. The galea was incised. **Hemostasis** was achieved. The muscle fascia and muscle fibers were incised; thereafter, the wound was retracted, and the **pericranium** was thus opened and incised. Using McKenzie's **perforator**, a bur hole was made, which was widened and thereafter the **dura mater** was thus exposed. **Cauterization** was carried out. Bone wax was applied to the scalp margin, and thereafter a cruciate incision was carried out. Clean fluid with pressure was obtained, however, there was no evidence of any blood. The fluid was allowed to seep out, was suctioned out, and a small amount of dura was removed, using Kerrison rongeur. I felt no drain would be necessary in the absence of blood. The wound was closed in layers, closing the temporalis muscle fascia, the galea and skin. Steri-strips were applied and the patient was **transferred** to his room in stable condition.

1. below the dura mater _____
2. physician specializing in painless surgery _____
3. making a cut into (noun) _____
4. controlling blood flow _____
5. below the skin _____
6. membrane surrounding the skull _____
7. pulled back _____
8. instrument used to make a hole _____
9. outermost layer of the meninges _____
10. placed in another location _____
11. half (partially) paralyzed _____
12. pertaining to the temporal and parietal region _____

REVIEW ACTIVITIES

CROSSWORD PUZZLE

Check your answers by going back through the frames or checking the solutions in Appendix C.

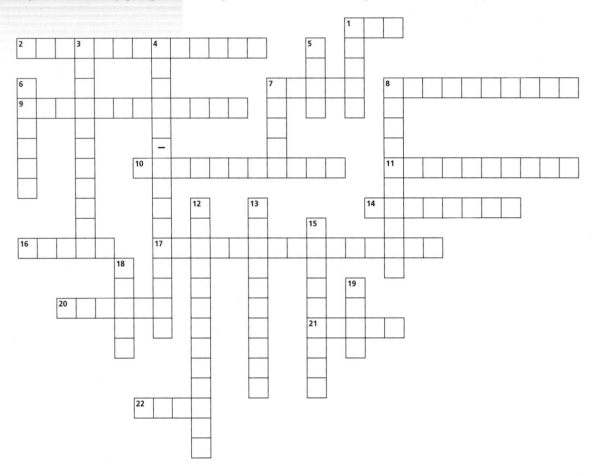

Across

1. synonym for syn-
2. prevents pregnancy
7. prefix meaning between
8. toxins in the blood from infection
9. inflammation upon the kidney
10. x-ray of the breast (process)
11. agent that fights bacteria
14. below the dura mater
16. prefix meaning across
17. used to obtain a sterile urine specimen
20. prefix meaning against
21. prefix meaning outside
22. prefix meaning same

Down

1. prefix meaning above
3. Donors give blood for _____.
4. outside of a joint
5. prefix meaning against
6. prefix meaning different
7. prefix meaning within
8. above the pubic bone
12. made of different substances or tissues
13. cleans the skin before surgery
15. both sides
18. prefix meaning beyond
19. prefix meaning beyond

REVIEW ACTIVITIES

GLOSSARY

antiarthritic	agent that works against arthritis	epigastric	upon the stomach
antibiotic	agent that works against organisms, especially bacteria	epigastrorrhaphy	suturing of tissue in the region upon the stomach
anticonvulsant	agent that prevents seizures	epinephrectomy	excision of tissue upon the kidney
antinarcotic	agent that works against the effects of narcotics	epinephritis	inflammation upon the kidney
antipyretic	agent that works against fever	episplenitis	inflammation upon the spleen
antirheumatic	agent that works against rheumatic disease	extra-articular	outside of a joint (adjective)
antiseptic	agent that protects against infection (external cleaner)	extracerebral	outside of the cerebrum (adjective)
antispasmodic	agent that prevents muscle spasms	extracystic	outside of the bladder (adjective)
antitoxin	agent that works to destroy toxins	extradural	outside of the dura mater (adjective)
asepsis	without poisons or infection	extragenital	outside of the genital area (adjective)
bilateral	including both sides (adjective)	extranuclear	outside of the nucleus (adjective)
catheterization	using a tube (catheter) inserted into the bladder or vessels to obtain specimens, to look, or to keep the vessel open	heterogeneous	different throughout (adjective)
		heteropsia	different vision in each eye
		heterosexual	attracted to the opposite sex (adjective)
contraceptive	agent that prevents conception	homogeneous	the same throughout (adjective)
contraindicated	not recommended under these circumstances	homoglandular	same gland (adjective)
contravolitional	against one's will	homosexual	attracted to the same sex (adjective)
disinfectants	chemical or physical agents that kill organisms; not used on the human body	infracostal	below the ribs (adjective)
		inframammary	below the breast (adjective)
epicystitis	inflammation upon the urinary bladder	infrapatellar	below the patella (adjective)
epidural	pertaining to the layer upon the dura mater (adjective)	infrapubic	below the pubic bone (adjective)

REVIEW ACTIVITIES

mammogram	breast x-ray film or x-ray picture
mammography	process of taking a breast x-ray
metacarpals	bones of the hand beyond the wrist bones (carpals)
metastasis (pl. metastases)	disease that spreads beyond its origin
metatarsals	bones of the foot beyond the ankle (tarsals)
pyrotoxin	toxin produced by fever or heat
septicemia	infection in the blood
septicopyemia	infection and pus in the blood
sterilization	process that kills all organisms
subdural	below the dura mater (adjective)
superciliary	pertaining to the eyebrow
superficial	on the surface (adjective)
superinfection	an infection on top of another infection
supracostal	above the ribs (adjective)
suprainguinal	above the groin
supralumbar	above the lumbar spine (adjective)
suprapubic	above the pubic bone (adjective)
suprarenal	above the kidney

suprarenopathy	disease of the suprarenal glands (adrenals)
symmetry	the same size and shape all around or on both sides
sympathetic	suffering along with, functional part of the autonomic nervous system
sympathoma	tumor of a sympathetic nerve
transcatheter	across a catheter
transfusion	transferring blood from one person to another
transillumination	use of light across a tube to view organs
transluminal	across the lumen of a vessel
transposition	placement of an organ on the opposite side
transsexual	a person who has changed sexes
transurethral	across the urethra
transvaginal	across the vagina
ultrasonography	use of ultrasound to make images from sound reflected through the body and computerized
ultrasound	high-frequency sound waves (inaudible)
ultraviolet	high-frequency light waves beyond the violet frequency

UNIT 12

Prefixes of Location and Medication Administration

12.1

Spirare is a Latin word meaning to breathe. Breathing is respiration. Breathing consists of the following two processes: expiration and inspiration. Think of the meaning as you analyze:

ex/pir/ation
eks spə **rā′** shun

expiration _____/_____/_____ (noun);

in/spir/ation
in spə rā′ shun

inspiration _____/_____/_____ (noun);

ex/cise
ek sīz′

excise _____/_____ (verb);

in/cise
in sīz′

incise _____/_____ (verb).

NOTE: The s is dropped from spire when preceded by ex.

12.2

inspiration
expiration

Look at the words in Frame 12.1. The word that means breathing in is _____ and breathing out is _____.

12.3

not

in- is a prefix that means in, into, or not. In/compatible drugs are drugs that do _____ mix well with each other.

12.4

not able

In/compet/ence occurs in an organ when it is *_____ to perform its function.

in/compet/ence
in **kom′** pə təns

Incompetence is a noun. When the ile/o/cec/al valve cannot perform its function, the result is ileocecal valve _____/_____/_____.

421

ANSWER COLUMN

	12.5
in/compet/ent in **kom**′ pə tent	In/compet/ent is an adjective. The _____ cervix could not help to maintain the pregnancy.
	12.6
incompetence	When blood seeps back through the aortic valves, aortic _____ or insufficiency occurs.
	12.7
incompetence incompetent	When a person is not able to think rationally enough to care for himself or herself, it may be called ment/al _____. You may even say the person is mentally _____ (adjective).
	12.8
in/continence in **kon**′ ti nəns in/continent in **kon**′ ti nent	Continence is the ability to control defecation and urination. Lack of control of waste removal is called _____/_____.The person who loses bladder control is _____/_____ (adjective).
	12.9

in/sane
in sān′
in/somnia
in **som**′ nē ə
in/coherent
in kō **hēr**′ ənt
	Build words meanings
	
	    not sane _____/_____;
	
	    unable to sleep _____/_____;
	
	    not coherent _____/_____.

	12.10
in/cision in **sizh**′ ən in/cis/ed in **siz**′ ′d	**in-** also means into. To in/cise (verb) is to cut into. The noun form of in/cise is _____/_____. The past tense verb form of incise is _____/_____/_____.
	12.11
ex/cise ek′ **sīz**′ ex/cis/ion ek **si**′ zhun	To cut into is to incise (verb). To cut out (remove) is to _____/_____ (verb). An _____/_____/_____ (noun) removes an organ or tissue.

ANSWER COLUMN

12.12

In/flamma/tion (noun) comes from a Latin term meaning "to set on fire". Our bodies are not literally set on fire, but, redness, swelling, pain, and heat occurs in irritated or infected tissues. The in/flamma/tory (adjective) response is part of our defense system. Tissues that are invaded by pathogens or receive physical injury become in/flamed (verb).

Complete the following statements:

in/flam/ed
in **flām**' 'd
in/flamma/tion
in flə **mā**' shun

The infected wound looked _____/_____ (verb).

_____/_____/_____ was one sign of an allergic reaction to the bee sting.

NOTE: Recall the suffix –itis means inflammation.

12.13

verb form of inject
one who (thing which)
  injects
procedure of injecting

In/ject means to introduce a substance into the body (usually through a needle).
Define the following

inject, injected *_____;

injector *_____

_____;

injection *_____.

**Intravenous (IV) infusion
using an infusion pump**
*(Photo by Marcia Butterfield,
Courtesy of Jackson Community College, Jackson, MI)*

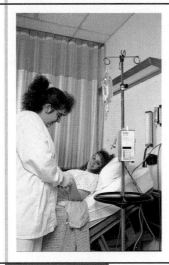

12.14

in/fusion
in **fyōō**' shən

Fluids such as normal (isotonic) saline with 5% dextrose may be introduced into a vein. This is an IV _____/_____.

12.15

infusion

The pump used to regulate the speed of flow of an IV is called
an _____ pump.

ANSWER COLUMN

12.16

In Latin *stillare* means to drip. In/stillation is putting medicated drops into an eye or body cavity. Medication (otic solution) dropped into an ear is an

in/still/ation
in stil ā′ shən

_____/_____/_____.

12.17

Recall that semen is a fluid substance that contains sperm. *Semin/o* is the combining form. Artificial in/semin/ation is a process of placing semen into the opening of the cervix using either husband (AIH) or donor (AID) sperm. Couples having difficulty with conception may be successful using artificial

in/semin/ation
in sem i nā′ shun

_____/_____/_____.

12.18

Use of a husband's sperm to fertilize an egg is called artificial

insemination

_____ by husband (AIH).

12.19

Now, see how many new vocabulary words you have just learned.
Build words that mean

ex/pire or ex/hale
ex/cision
in/spir/ation
in/cise

   to breath out (verb) _____/_____;
   cutting out (noun) _____/_____;
   breathing in (noun) _____/_____/_____;
   to cut into (verb) _____/_____.

12.20

Build words that mean

in/compentence
in/compatible
in/coherent
in/fusion
in/still/ation
in/flamed

   not competent (noun) _____/_____;
   not compatible _____/_____;
   not able to be understood _____/_____;
   solution introduced into a vein _____/_____;
   medication administration by drops _____/_____/_____;
   red, swollen, painful, warm _____/_____ (verb).

12.21

in, not, into

Remember that **in-** means _____, _____, or _____.

ANSWER COLUMN

TAKE A
CLOSER
LOOK

Use your dictionary
to find the answer.

12.22

Analyze the following **in-** words by writing their meaning and indicating the part of speech

	meaning	part of speech
injected	_____	(_____)
incision	_____	(_____)
inflamed	_____	(_____)
infusion	_____	(_____)
infested	_____	(_____)

12.23

bad

mal- is a French word that means bad. **mal-** is also a prefix that means bad or poor. Mal/odor/ous means having a _____ odor.

12.24

poorly formed or
  poor formation

Mal/aise (ma lāz′) means a general feeling of illness or feeling poorly.
Mal/formation means *_____
_____.

12.25

poor nutrition

poor absorption
  (as of nutrients)

Good nutrition is essential for good health. Mal/nutrition means
*_____.
Mal/absorption means
*_____.

12.26

mal/aise
ma **lāz**′
mal/nutrition
mal noō **tri**′ shun
mal/absorbtion
mal ab **sorb**′ shun
mal/formation
mal fôr **mā**′ shun

Build a "bad" word that means
feeling bad
_____/_____;
bad (poor) nutrition
_____/_____;
bad (poor) absorption
_____/_____;
bad (poor) formation
_____/_____.
Good!

ANSWER COLUMN

12.27

Mal/nutrition may take the form of overnutrition or undernutrition. Malnutrition may be caused by lack of nutrients, starvation, overeating, socioeconomic conditions, or emotional eating disorders. Hyper/phagia (overeating), anorexia nervosa (not eating), and bulimia (binging and purging) are all eating disorders. Look up the following terms in your dictionary and write more information about their meanings here.

hyperphagia _____

anorexia _____

anorexia nervosa _____

bulimia _____

compulsive overeating _____

Long term effects of anorexia nervosa (self-imposed malnutrition)

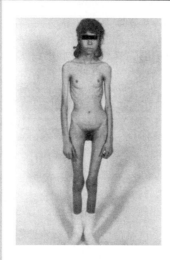

12.28

A person who is obsessed about being thin, and severely limits his or her food intake may have *_____.

an/o/rexia nervosa
an ôr **eks**′ ē ə ner **vō**′ sa

12.29

A person who may overeat and then take laxatives or force himself or herself to vomit to purge the stomach of the food may be suffering from

_____.

bul/imia
boo **lē**′ mē ə

ANSWER COLUMN

12.30

Look at the words in the next two frames. Now find the combining form for the disease malaria: _____/_____.

malari/o

12.31

Before people knew that mosquitoes carry the malaria parasite (*Plasmodium vivax*), they thought this disease was caused by "bad" night air. Analyze malaria (means bad air): _____/_____.

malari/a
mə **lair**′ ē ə

12.32

Analyze these words involving the disease malaria by drawing the diagonals and giving the part of speech:

		part of speech
malarial	_____	(_____)
malarious	_____	(_____)
malariology	_____	(_____)
malariotherapy	_____	(_____)

malari/al
malari/ous
malari/o/logy
malari/o/therapy
(You pronounce)

**Antagonistic muscle pair:
(A) extension–biceps
relaxed, triceps contracted;
(B) flexion–biceps
contracted, triceps relaxed**

Triceps contracted — Biceps relaxed   Triceps relaxed — Biceps contracted

(A)   (B)

12.33

uni- means one. bi- means two. tri- means three. The tri/ceps muscle has _____ heads. A tri/cuspid valve has _____ cusps. The tri/gemin/al nerve has _____ branches.

three
three
three

Look back to the numeric prefix table on page 350 to review Latin and Greek word parts.

ANSWER COLUMN

12.34

The three-headed muscle in the posterior upper arm is the

tri/ceps
trī′ seps

_____/_____.

12.35

Quintuplets are five infants born at the same time. Giving birth to three infants during the same pregnancy is having _____/_____.

tri/plets
trip′ letz

12.36

tri/gemin/al
trī **jem′** i nəl

The three-branched cranial nerve is the _____/_____/_____ nerve.

12.37

bi- means two. **furco-** means branching or dividing. To bi/furc/ate is to divide into two branches. When an artery divides into two, it

bi/furc/ates
bī′ fər kāts

_____/_____/_____ (verb) (e.g., carotid artery; see the illustration).

NOTE: The word root furc should make you think of "fork."

12.38

Bi/furcate is a verb. The noun is bi/furc/ation. When a nerve divides into two

bi/furc/ation
bī fer **kā′** shən

branches, a _____/_____/_____ (noun) is formed.

12.39

bifurcations

Various ducts in the body also form _____ (plural).

Blood vessels of the head and neck

Bifurcation of the carotid artery

12.40

two
two

The bi/ceps brachii is a muscle with _____ bellies.
A bi/cusp/id is a tooth with _____ cusps.

ANSWER COLUMN

two

two

Bi/foc/al glasses have _____ foci in one lens.

A bi/furc/ation has _____ branches.

12.41

Build words that mean

a tooth with two cusps

bi/cuspid

bī **kus**' pid

_____/_____;

lenses with two areas of focus

bi/focals

bī' fō kəlz

_____/_____;

one who is sexually attracted to both males and females

bi/sexual

bī **sex**' yōō əl

_____/_____;

the part of a structure that divides into two branches

bi/furcation

bī fer **kā**' shun

_____/_____;

a muscle with two heads

bi/ceps

bī' seps

_____/_____ brachii.

NOTE: Biceps is used both as a singular and as a plural form.

12.42

one

one

one

uni- means one. A uni/corn has _____ horn. Uni/ovular pertains to twins who develop from _____ ovum. Uni/vers/al means combined into _____ whole.

12.43

Later/al means pertaining to the side. Build words meaning pertaining to

one side

uni/later/al

yōō ni **lat**' er əl

_____/_____/_____;

bi/later/al

bī' lat er əl

two sides

_____/_____/_____;

tri/later/al

trī' lat er əl

three sides

_____/_____/_____.

12.44

multi- means many. Multi/cell/ular means made of many cells.

Build words meaning

made of two cells

bi/cell/ular

bī **sel**' yōō lar

_____/_____/_____;

uni/cell/ular or

yōō' nē **sel**' yōō lar

made of one cell only

_____/_____/_____.

mono/cell/ular

mon ō **sel**' yōō lar

ANSWER COLUMN

12.45

Some cells are multi/nucle/ar in nature. Build words meaning

    having one nucle/us (adjective)

uni/nucle/ar or
yōō ni **noo′** klē är   _____/_____/_____;

mono/nucle/ar   having two nucle/i

mon ō **noo′** klē är   _____/_____/_____.

bi/nucle/ar
bī′ noo klē ar   NOTE: Nucleus is singular, nuclei is plural, and nuclear is the adjectival form.

12.46

Bi/sexual has two meanings. It can indicate a person with physical characteristics of both males and females (hermaphrodite) or a person attracted to both males and females. A person with both male and female genitals may be said to be

bi/sexual   _____/_____ or a _____/_____.

bī **seks′** yōō əl

herm/aphrodite   NOTE: Refer back to Unit 11 Information Table of Sexuality Terms.

herm **af′** rō dīt

12.47

WORD ORIGINS

Hermaphrodites was the child of the god Hermes and the goddess Aphrodite. S/he exhibited characteristics of both the father and mother, male and female genders. Today the term hermaphrodite or intersexual means having both male and female characteristics.

12.48

Affective disorders are disturbances in emotional mood or mental state. Some people experience severe mood swings from a manic (excited) to a depressive

bi/polar   state. This experience of two polar extremes is called _____/_____

bī **pōl′** ar   affective disorder.

12.49

Build words that mean

    sexually attracted to both sexes

bi/sexual   _____/_____;

    having two poles (as in manic/depressive)

bi/polar   _____/_____.

12.50

Review

one   uni- means _____;

two   bi- means _____;

three   tri- means _____;

many   multi- means _____.

ANSWER COLUMN

12.51

Give the meaning of the following terms
bifurcation

dividing into two
  branches

*_____;

bisexual

attracted to both males
  and females

*_____;

bilateral

pertaining to both sides

*_____;

uninuclear

pertaining to having one
  nucleus

*_____;

hermaphrodite

individual possessing both
  male and female genitals

*_____.

PREFIX	MEANING	EXPLANATION
semi-	half	used with modern English words or words closer to modern English
hemi-	half	used more with medical terms

12.52

semi-
hemi-

There are two prefixes that mean half. They are _____ and _____.

12.53

Form words that mean

semi/circle
semi/conscious
semi/private

half circle _____/_____;
half conscious _____/_____;
half private (hospital room) _____/_____.

12.54

Build words meaning
  presence of only half a heart (noun)

hemi/cardi/a
hem ē **kär′** dē ə
hemi/gastr/ectomy
hem ē gast **rek′** tom ē
hemi/plegia or
hem ē **plē′** jē ə
hemi/paralys/is
hem ē par **al′** ə sis

_____/_____/____;
  removal of half the stomach
_____/_____/_____;
  paralysis of half the body (on one side)
_____/_____.

ANSWER COLUMN

12.55

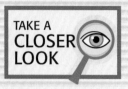

TAKE A CLOSER LOOK

Note the difference between these two words: hemiplegia (paralysis of one side of the body) and paraplegia (paralysis of the lower half of the body). Look up paraplegia, hemiplegia, and quadriplegia in your dictionary and read about these conditions.

12.56

semi/circul/ar
semi/norm/al
semi/coma/tose
(You pronounce)

Build words meaning
   half circular _____/_____/_____;
   half normal _____/_____/_____;
   half comatose _____/_____/_____.

12.57

hemi/plegia
hem′ē **plē**′ jē ə
hemi/sphere
hem′ i sfēr
hemi/an/esthesi/a
hem′ē an es **thēs**′ ē ə

Build words with the literal meaning of
   paralysis of half (one side) of the body
   _____/_____;
   half of a sphere (e.g., cerebral)
   _____/_____;
   anesthesia of half the body
   _____/_____/_____/____.

12.58

INFORMATION FRAME

genit/o comes from the Greek word *genesis,* meaning the beginning or formation. The reproductive system structures are called genit/als.

12.59

genit/al
jen′ i təl

A herpes simplex virus (HSV) infection in the area around the external genitalia is called _____/_____ herpes.

12.60

with

con- is a prefix that means with. Con/genit/al means born _____.

12.61

born with

A child with con/genit/al cataracts is *_____ cataracts.

ANSWER COLUMN

con/genit/al kon **jen**′ i təl	**12.62** There are many con/genit/al deformities. A child born with a lateral curvature of the spine has _____/_____/_____ scoliosis.
congenital	**12.63** Another way of saying a deformity with which one is born, is to say congenital anomaly. A child born with kyphosis (posterior curvature of the spine) has a _____ anomaly (abnormality).
congenital	**12.64** A child born with hydr/ophthalm/os has _____ glaucoma (increased fluid pressure condition of the eye).
congenital	**12.65** A child born with syphilis has _____ syphilis.

Child with Down syndrome—congenital anomaly

Abnormal curvatures of the spine: (A) kyphosis; (B) lordosis; (C) scoliosis

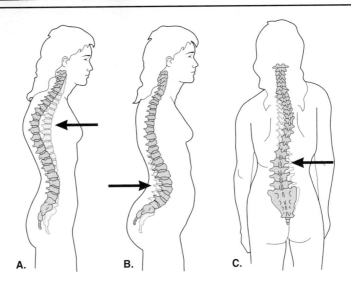

ANSWER COLUMN

12.66

con- prefix—with
sanguin/o combining form—blood
-ity noun suffix—quality
Using what you need of the above word parts, build a word meaning literally with blood or, in usage, blood relationship:

con/sanguin/ity
kon′ sang **gwin**′ i tē

_____/_____/_____.

12.67

consanguinity

Con/sanguin/ity is a relationship by descent from a common ancestor. The noun that expresses the relationship of cousins is _____.

12.68

sanguin/eous or
sang **gwin**′ ē us
sanguin/ous
sang′ gwin us

sanguin/o means bloody. Build a word meaning pertaining to bloody drainage on a dressing: _____/_____.

12.69

con/sanguin/ity
san/guin/ous or
 san/guin/eous
con/genit/al

Build words meaning
  having blood relationship _____/_____/_____;
  bloody _____/_____/_____;

  born with _____/_____/_____.

12.70

free of ease

dis- is a prefix that means to free of, to separate, or to undo. Dis/ease means, literally, *_____.

12.71

To dis/sect is to cut a tissue or to undo it (into parts) for purposes of study.
Write the following forms of the word dissect below
verb

dis/sect
dis **sekt**′
dis/section
dis **sek**′ shən
dis/sected
dis **sek**′ td

_____/_____;
noun
_____/_____;
past tense verb
_____/_____.

12.72

To dis/infect is to free of infective agents. Analyze the following terms and check definitions

dis/infect

dis/infect/ant

dis/infect/ion

dis/infect/ed

disinfect _____/_____;

disinfectant _____/_____/_____;

disinfection _____/_____/_____;

disinfected _____/_____/_____.

12.73

People with multiple personality disorder (MPD) dis/associate and experience various personas. Analyze and check definitions

dis/associate

dis/sociate

dis/sociated

dis/sociation

disassociate _____/_____;

dissociate _____/_____;

dissociated _____/_____;

dissociation _____/_____.

12.74

Recall that **dys-** means difficult or painful.

to free of, to undo

with

dis- is a prefix that means *_____.

con- is a prefix that means _____.

Use the following table to work Frames 12.75–12.84.

PREFIX	MEANING	LOOK UP MEANINGS
post-	behind	postnasal
	after	postmastectomy
ante-	before	antecubital
	forward	anteverted
pre-	before	premolar
	in front of	pretibial

12.75

post- means after.

after

after

after

behind

after

Post/prandial (pp) means _____ meals.

Post/cibum (pc) means _____ food.

Post/glucose (pg) means _____ ingesting glucose.

Post/esophageal means _____ the esophagus.

Post/menopausal means _____ menopause.

ANSWER COLUMN

12.76

pre- means before or in front of.

before

in front of

Pre/an/esthetic means _____ anesthesia.

Pre/hyoid means *_____ the hyoid bone.

12.77

ante- means before or forward.

before

forward

Ante/pyretic means _____ the fever.

Ante/flexion means _____ bending.

12.78

Peri/natal concerns events that are around birth. Nat/al means birth.

Think of the meaning while you analyze

postnatal

post/nat/al

pōst **nā**′ təl

_____/_____/_____;

pre/nat/al

prē **nā**′ təl

prenatal

_____/_____/_____;

ante/nat/al

an tē **nā**′ təl

antenatal

_____/_____/_____.

12.79

Febris in Latin means fever. Febr/ile means pertaining to fever.

Build words meaning

pertaining to after a fever

post/febr/ile

pōst′ **fē**′ brəl

_____/_____/_____;

ante/febr/ile

an′ tē **fē**′ brəl

pertaining to before a fever

_____/_____/_____.

NOTE: Natal refers to birth and terms related to the newborn baby.

Partum refers to delivery and terms related to the mother.

12.80

Build words meaning pertaining to

   after an operation

post/operative

pōst **op**′ er a tiv

_____/_____ (po);

post/coit/al

pōst **kō**′ it əl

   after coitus (intercourse)

_____/_____/_____;

post/part/um

pōst **par**′ tum

   after delivery (refers to the mother)

_____/_____/_____;

post/nat/al

pōst **nāt**′ al

   after delivery or birth (refers to the baby)

_____/_____/_____.

NOTE: Notice that most of the terms you are learning here start with prefixes and are adjectives.

ANSWER COLUMN

12.81

pre/operative
pre/mature
pre/scribe
pre/cancer/ous
(You pronounce)

pre- means before. Build a word (adjective) that means
before an operation _____/_____;
before maturity (readiness) _____/_____;
write before you can take (Rx) _____/_____;
before cancer develops _____/_____/_____.

12.82

SPELL
CHECK ✓

A prescription is written before a medication may be dispensed.
It is prescribed (Rx). "<u>Per</u>scription" it is <u>not</u> a word.

12.83

ante/version
an′ tē ver shən
ante/part/um
an tē **par**′ tum
ante/position
an tē pos **i**′ shən

Build terms that begin with **ante-**
turning forward
_____/_____;
before delivery
_____/_____/_____;
position in front
_____/_____.

12.84

after death
before death

Mortem means death (think of mortal). What do these terms mean?
postmortem *_____;
antemortem *_____.

NOTE: A.M. means **ante-** meridiem—before noon.
          P.M. means **post-** meridiem—after noon.

12.85

mort/ality
mor **tal**′ it ē
morbid/ity
mor **bid**′ it ē

In medicine mort/ality refers to the death rate and morbid/ity refers to the rate
of occurrence of disease. Statistics giving the ratio of deaths in a given population
is the _____/_____ rate. The ratio of disease in a given population
is the _____/_____ rate.

12.86

within the abdomen

Recall that **inter-** means between. **intra-** means within. Intra-abdominal
means *_____.

PROFESSIONAL PROFILES

A nurse is a health care professional who provides a wide variety of services including the most simple patient care tasks, sophisticated lifesaving procedures, management of health care teams, education, and research. The level of responsibility of each nurse is related to education, licensure, and experience. The following are descriptions of various levels and credentials.

Licensed practical nurse (LPN) is a graduate of a practical nursing program who has passed a state practical nursing licensing exam; most programs grant a certificate of completion.

Registered nurse (RN) is a graduate of a state board-approved school of nursing who has passed a state registered nurse exam; he or she may earn an associate degree, diploma, or bachelor's degree.

Nurse practitioner (NP) is an RN with advanced preparation for practice including clinical experience in diagnosis and treatment of illnesses. NPs may be allowed to practice independently depending upon state laws; this is a master's degree level.

Certified registered nurse anesthetist (CRNA) is an RN who administers anesthesia under the supervision of an anesthesiologist and receives specialized training and certification recognized by the American Association of Nurse Anesthetists.

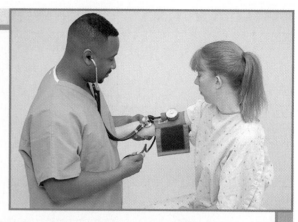

This nurse is assessing a young adult's blood pressure as part of a health program to enhance patient wellness

Clinical nurse specialist is an RN with a master's degree with a special competence in an area such as obstetrics, cardiology, or intensive care nursing.

Masters of Science in Nursing (MSN) is completion of a board-approved MSN program including clinical practicum and research. MSNs may work directly with patients, manage teams, or serve as administrators and educators in nursing programs.

RNs with Doctorate Degrees in Nursing (PhDs) work as educators and researchers in colleges and universities, or they may serve as hospital administrators.

ANSWER COLUMN

	12.87
within a cell	Intra/cellular means *_____.
within the uterus	Intra/uterine means *_____.

12.88

Using **intra-** and the adjectives ven/ous, spin/al, and lumb/ar, build words meaning

within a vein

intra/ven/ous
in' tra **vēn**' us

_____/_____/_____;

within the spine

intra/spin/al
in' tra **spīn**' əl

_____/_____/_____;

within the lumbar region

in'tra **lum**' bar

_____/_____/_____.

12.89

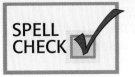

Intravenous ends in -ous, not -eous. Also watch the pronunciation: in' tra **vēn**' us.

Angle of injection for parenteral administration of medications

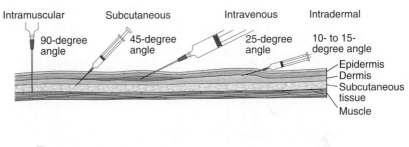

Intramuscular — 90-degree angle
Subcutaneous — 45-degree angle
Intravenous — 25-degree angle
Intradermal — 10- to 15-degree angle

Epidermis
Dermis
Subcutaneous tissue
Muscle

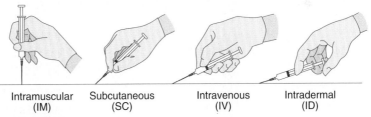

Intramuscular (IM)   Subcutaneous (SC)   Intravenous (IV)   Intradermal (ID)

12.90

Using **intra-** build adjectives meaning

within an artery

intra-/arteri/al
in' tra är **tēr**' ē əl

_____/-_____/_____;

within the cranium

intra/crani/al
in' tra **krā**' nē əl

_____/_____/_____;

within the bladder

intra/cyst/ic
in' tra **sis**' tik

_____/_____/_____;

within the aorta

intra-/aort/ic
in' tra ā **ôr**' tik

_____/-_____/_____.

NOTE: Take notice of the hyphen in intra-arterial and intra-aortic.

ANSWER COLUMN

intra/derm/al
intra/duoden/al
intra/thorac/ic
(You pronounce)

12.91

Build adjectives meaning
within the skin _____/_____/_____;
within the duodenum _____/_____/_____;
within the thoracic cavity _____/_____/_____.

ABBREVIATION	MEANING
ac	before meals (ante cibum)
ad lib	ad libetum as desired
AID	artificial insemination by donor's sperm
AIH	artificial insemination by husband's sperm
am, A.M.	ante meridiem (morning)
bid	bis in die, twice a day
caps	capsules
CRNA	certified registered nurse anesthetist
exc	excision
GNID	gram-negative intracellular diplococcus
gt/gtt, gtts	drop/drops
I&O	intake and output
IABP	intra-aortic balloon pump
ID	intradermal, identification
IM	intramuscular
inf	infusion
instill	instillation
IU	international unit
IUD	intrauterine device
IV	intravenous
LPN	licensed practical nurse
MSN	Masters of Science in Nursing
NP	nurse practitioner
pc	after meals (post cibum)
pm, P.M.	post meridiem (after noon)
PO	postoperative
po	by mouth (per os)
prn	pro renata, as needed or required
RN	registered nurse
sc, subcu, sq, subq	subcutaneous
tab	tablet(s)
tid	ter in die three times a day
ī, īī, īīī, īv, v̄	one, two, three, four, five (apothecary numbers)
†	death

ANSWER COLUMN

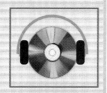

To complete your study of this unit, work the **Review Activities** on the following pages. Also listen to the audio CDs that accompany *Medical Terminology: A Programmed Systems Approach,* 9th edition, and practice your pronunciation.

Additional practice exercises for this unit are available on the Learner Practice CD-ROM found in the back of the textbook.

REVIEW ACTIVITIES

CIRCLE AND CORRECT

Circle the correct answer for each question. Then check your answers in Appendix A.

1. Which of the following means breathing out?
   a. excise
   b. incising
   c. exhale
   d. inspiration

2. If an organ does not function properly it may be said to be
   a. incontinent
   b. inflamed
   c. instilled
   d. incompetent

3. Which of the following is a noun form?
   a. inject
   b. injection
   c. injectable
   d. injecting

4. Which of the following prefixes does not mean bad or poor?
   a. mal-
   b. dys-
   c. mis-
   d. eu-

5. Anorexia literally means
   a. underweight
   b. starvation
   c. lack of appetite
   d. malnutrition

6. The three-bellied muscle of the back upper arm is the
   a. triangle
   b. deltoid
   c. tricuspid
   d. triceps

7. A person who switches from mania to depression and mood swings may have _____ disorder.
   a. multiple personality disorder
   b. hyperglycemia
   c. bipolar
   d. schizophrenia

8. Which of the following prefixes means with?
   a. con-
   b. contra-
   c. in-
   d. intra-

REVIEW ACTIVITIES

PREFIX AND WORD

Write the prefix that represents the direction. Then build a word using that prefix.

Prefix			Word
_____	1. out	breathe out (verb)	_____
_____	2. in	cut into (verb)	_____
_____	3. not	not competent	_____
_____	4. bad/poor	poor nutrition	_____
_____	5. three	three-branched nerve	_____
_____	6. two	two foci in one lens	_____
_____	7. one	one sided	_____
_____	8. half	half conscious	_____
_____	9. half	atrophy of half the body	_____
_____	10. with	born with	_____
_____	11. to free of	substance used to free of infective agents	_____
_____	12. after	after mastectomy	_____
_____	13. before	before surgery	_____
_____	14. in front of	in front of the frontal lobe	_____
_____	15. behind	behind the esophagus	_____
_____	16. before	before a fever	_____
_____	17. within	within the dermis	_____
_____	18. between	between the cells (review)	_____
_____	19. below	below the cutaneous (dermis) layer (review)	_____

SELECT AND CONSTRUCT

Select the correct word parts from the following list and construct medical terms that represent the given meaning.

ante	aria(l)	bi	cancer/ous	card/ia(o)	cell/ular
cibal	coit(us)(al)	comatose	con	continence(y)	febrile
fest(ed)(ing)	formation	fus(ed)(ion)	glucose	hemi	in
intra	ject(ion)(ed)	mal	natal	nuclear(us)	partum
plegia	post	pre	sane	semi	tri
uni					

1. before birth   _____

2. after delivery   _____

REVIEW ACTIVITIES

3. half of a heart   _____

4. partially (half) in a coma   _____

5. pertaining to one cell   _____

6. having one nucleus   _____

7. before the development of cancer   _____

8. put in using a needle (verb)   _____

9. not able to control urination   _____

10. not sane   _____

11. poor growth   _____

12. parasitic disease caused
    by *Plasmodium vivax*   _____

13. after intercourse   _____

14. before a fever   _____

15. after a meal   _____

16. before cancer develops   _____

DEFINE AND DISSECT

Give a brief definition and dissect each term listed into its word parts in the space provided. Check your answers by referring to the frame listed in parentheses and your medical dictionary. Then listen to the CDs to practice pronunciation.

1. expiration (12.1)   _____/_____/_____
                          pre   rt   suffix

    _____
                definition

2. incompetence (12.4)   _____/_____/_____
                            pre   rt   suffix

    _____

3. inflammation (12.12)   _____/_____/_____
                             pre   rt/suffix

    _____

4. malaise (12.24)   _____/_____
                         pre   rt/suffix

    _____

5. infusion (12.14)   _____/_____
                          pre   rt/suffix

    _____

REVIEW ACTIVITIES

6. malariology (12.32)

    _____/_____/_____

         rt   v   suffix

7. bicuspid (12.41)

    _____/_____

      pre   rt/suffix

8. uniovular (12.42)

    _____/_____

      pre   rt/suffix

9. bifurcation (12.38)

    _____/_____/_____

     pre   rt   suffix

10. semicomatose (12.56)

    _____/_____/_____

     pre   rt   suffix

11. hemigastrectomy (12.54)

    _____/_____/_____

     pre   rt   suffix

12. consanguinity (12.66)

    _____/_____/_____

     pre   rt   suffix

13. dissection (12.71)

    _____/_____

     pre   rt/suffix

14. postfebrile (12.79)

    _____/_____/_____

     pre   rt   suffix

15. precancerous (12.81)

    _____/_____/_____

     pre   rt   suffix

REVIEW ACTIVITIES

16. anteversion (12.83)

_____/_____

    pre   rt/suffix

17. intravenous (12.88)

_____/_____/_____

    pre   rt   suffix

18. incontinence (12.8)

_____/_____

    pre   rt/suffix

19. insemination (12.17)

_____/_____/_____

    pre   rt   suffix

20. bisexual (12.46)

_____/_____

    pre   rt/suffix

21. triplets (12.35)

_____/_____

    pre   rt/suffix

22. hemiplegia (12.54)

_____/_____

    pre   suffix

23. disassociate (12.73)

_____/_____

    pre   rt/suffix

24. perinatal (12.78)

_____/_____/_____

    pre   rt   suffix

25. intradermal (12.91)

_____/_____/_____

    pre   rt   suffix

REVIEW ACTIVITIES

ABBREVIATION MATCHING

Match the following abbreviations with their definition.

_____ 1. IUD   a. drops

_____ 2. IM   b. international units

_____ 3. PO   c. intravenous

_____ 4. IV   d. subcutaneous

_____ 5. ac   e. intake and output

_____ 6. bid   f. intramuscular

_____ 7. pc   g. intrauterine device

_____ 8. IU   h. before meals

                        i. postoperative

                        j. intradermal

                        k. twice a day

                        l. after meals

                        m. infusion

                        n. input and outtake

                        o. postprandial

ABBREVIATION FILL-INS

Fill in the blanks with the correct abbreviation.

9. excision _____

10. artificial insemination (husband) _____

11. intradermal _____

12. apothecary number three _____

13. before noon _____

14. infusion _____

15. as needed _____

CASE STUDIES

Write the term next to its meaning given on the following page. Then draw slashes to analyze the word parts. Note the use of medical abbreviations. Look these up in your dictionary or find them in Appendix B. If you have any questions about the answers, refer to your medical dictionary or check with your instructor for the answers in Appendix A.

REVIEW ACTIVITIES

CASE STUDY 12-1

Operative Report

Preoperative diagnosis: **Bilateral** adnexal masses, probable pelvic endometriosis, and **endometriomata**

Postoperative diagnosis: Bilateral adnexal masses, probable pelvic endometriosis, and endometriomata

Procedure: Total abdominal hysterectomy, bilateral **salpingo-oophorectomy,** lysis of **adhesions,** incidental **appendectomy**

Technique and findings: Under adequate general anesthesia the patient was prepped and draped in the usual sterile fashion placed in the supine position with an **intracystic** Foley catheter. A lower abdominal midline incision was made and the abdominal wall opened in the usual fashion. Upon entering the abdominal cavity, no unusual peritoneal fluid was noted. The upper abdomen was explored and found to be within normal limits. There were noted bilateral large ovarian endometriomata. The anterior cul-de-sac was free of adhesions, but the lower part of the sigmoid colon was adhered to the **posterior** wall of the cul-de-sac. The sigmoid adhesion was taken off the posterior wall of the uterus by sharp and blunt **dissection,** down past the uterosacral ligaments, freeing the cul-de-sac area. The bilateral endometriomata were ruptured, freeing the ovaries from the lateral pelvic walls. The round ligaments were bilaterally clamped, cut, and ligated with #1 chromic sutures. The **visceroperitoneum** between the round ligaments was **transversely incised** and the bladder bluntly **dissected** off the lower uterine segment of the cervix.

1. both sides _____
2. tumors of the endometrium _____
3. cut into (noun) _____
4. across (adverb) _____
5. the membrane on the abdominal organs _____
6. before surgery _____
7. cut apart (verb) _____
8. back _____
9. within the urinary bladder _____
10. excision of the appendix _____
11. excision of the ovaries and uterine tubes _____
12. tissues grown together _____
13. after surgery _____
14. cutting apart (noun) _____

REVIEW ACTIVITIES

CROSSWORD PUZZLE

Check your answers by going back through the frames or checking the solutions in Appendix C.

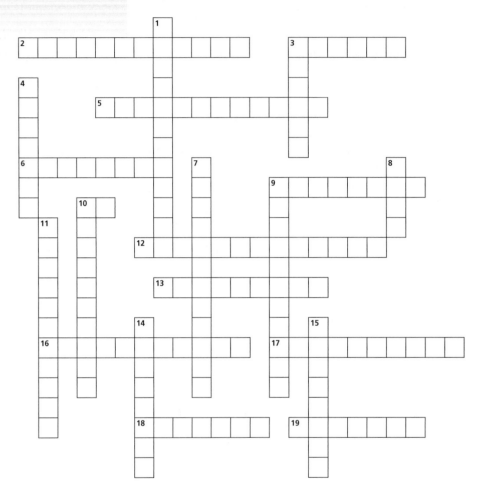

Across

2. subcu. means_____
3. two-headed muscle
5. poor nutritional status
6. a cut made into the body
9. synonym for antenatal
10. after meals (abbreviation)
12. partially conscious
13. involving both sides
16. medicines to fight bacteria (plural)
17. born with
18. three-headed muscle
19. to cut apart

Down

1. unable to control urination or defecation
3. sanguinous means___
4. generally poor feeling
7. process of administering medication using drops
8. hemiplegia is paralysis of _____ the body
9. before surgery
10. after delivery (the mother)
11. branched in two (noun)
14. at the site
15. introducing a substance into the body, such as through an IV

REVIEW ACTIVITIES

GLOSSARY

anorexia	lack of appetite or desire to eat
antefebrile	before a fever
anteflexion	bending forward
antemortem	before death
antenatal	before birth (prenatal)
antepartum	before delivery (mother)
anteposition	in front of
antepyretic	before a fever
anteversion	turning toward
bicellular	made of two cells
biceps	a two-bellied muscle (i.e., b. femoris, b. brachii)
bifocal	lens having two focus strengths
binuclear	having two nuclei
bipolar	having two poles
bisexual	attracted to two sexes
bulemia	condition of purging after eating
congenital	born with
consanguinity	with blood relationship
disassociate	to break apart
disinfect	to rid of infectious agents
dissect	to cut apart
excise	to take out
exhale	to breathe out
expiration	breathing out
genitals	reproductive system structures

hemianesthesia	anesthesia involving half the body
hemicardia	half a heart
hemigastrectomy	excision of half the stomach
hemiplegia	paralysis of one side of the body (right or left) (hemiparalysis)
incise	to cut into
incoherent	unable to be understood (speech)
incompatible	not compatible, does not associate well with
incompetency	not able to function properly
incontinence	inability to control urination or defecation
infested	organisms living within or on another organism
inflamed	act of being red, swollen, painful and warm (verb)
inflammation	condition with such symptoms as a red, swollen, and warm area (noun)
infusion	introducing a substance into a vein through a needle
inhale	to breathe in
injection	procedure of introducing a substance into the body through a needle
insane	not sane
insemination	process of introducing semen into the uterus or tubes
insomnia	unable to fall asleep
inspiration	breathing in

REVIEW ACTIVITIES

instillation	applying drops
intercellular	between the cells
intra-abdominal	within the abdomen
intra-aortic	within the aorta
intra-arterial	within the artery
intracranial	within the cranium
intracystic	within the urinary bladder
intradermal	within the dermal layer
intraduodenal	within the duodenum
intrathoracic	within the thorax (thoracic cavity, chest)
malaise	generally poor feeling, not feeling well
malformation	poor formation
malnutrition	poor nutrition, missing essential nutrients
malodorous	smelling bad
morbidity	related to illness
mortality	related to death
postcibal	after meals
postcoital	after intercourse
postesophageal	in back of the esophagus
postfebrile	after a fever
postglucose	after glucose is administered
postmastectomy	after mastectomy surgery
postmenopausal	after menopause is complete

postmortem	after death
postnatal	after birth (baby)
postoperative	after surgery
postpartum	after delivery (mother)
postprandial	after meals
preanesthetic	before anesthesia
precancerous	condition that may lead to cancer
prefrontal	in front of the frontal bone
preoperative	before surgery
prescribe	write an order for before it can be done
sanguineous	bloody (also, sanguinous)
semicircle	half of a circle
semicomatose	partially in a coma
semiconscious	partially conscious (half)
semiprivate	situation in which half a room is shared
subcutaneous	the layer below the dermis of the skin
triceps	a three-bellied muscle (i.e., t. femoris, t. brachii)
unicellular	of one cell (also, monocellular)
unilateral	one sided
uninuclear	having one nucleus (also, mononuclear)

UNIT 13

Respiratory System and Pulmonology

Notice how these word parts about breathing and lungs were built from **pne**.

Combining Form	Meaning	Medical Term
pne/o	breathing	**pne/o**/pne/ic
pneum/o	air (lung)	**pneum/o**/thorax
pneumon/o	lung	**pneumon**/ectomy
-pnea (suffix)	fast/breathing	tachy/**pnea**

13.1

Pneumon/o is used in medical words concerning lungs.

excision of part or all of a lung

Pneumon/ectomy means *_____.

pneumon/o/tomy

Incision into the lung is a _____/_____/_____.

noō′ mə **nôt**′ ə mē

13.2

any disease of the lungs

Pneumon/o/pathy means *_____.

Form a word meaning hemorrhage of a lung

pneumon/o/rrhagia

_____/_____/_____.

noō′ mə nō **rā**′ jē ə

13.3

INFORMATION FRAME

Pneumon/ia is an acute inflammation of the lungs caused by a variety of bacteria, fungi, and viruses. Often antibiotics are used to treat pneumonia. Another word for pneumon/ia is pneumon/itis.

ANSWER COLUMN

Lung x-ray PA view showing pneumonia

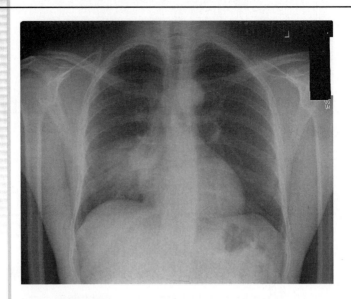

13.4

Form words meaning surgical puncture of a lung to remove fluid

pneumon/o/centesis
nōō mə nō sen **tē**′ sis
thorac/o/centesis
thôr′ ə kō sen **tē**′ sis

_____/_____/_____.

Surgical puncture of the chest to remove fluid is

_____/_____/_____.

13.5

The two words meaning inflammation of the lungs are

pneumon/ia
nōō **mōn**′ yə
pneumon/itis
nōō mə **nī**′ tis

_____/_____ and

_____/_____.

13.6

lungs

Pneumocystis carinii pneumonia is an infection caused by a protozoan-like organism. People debilitated by immunodeficiency disease, such as AIDS, are particularly susceptible to this disease, which affects the _____.

13.7

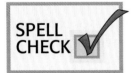

Think of the "pn" rule for pronunciation when saying words such as pneumonia. The p is silent when pn begins the word. Also, remember eu makes the "ū" sound. The e is written in front of the u.

ANSWER COLUMN

WORD ORIGINS

atel/ectasis
at əl **ek**′ ta sis

13.8

In Greek *ateles* means imperfect and *ektasis* means expand or dilate. **-ectasia** and **-ectasis** are suffixes used to mean dilation or expansion. Atel/ectasis is the imperfect expansion of the lungs, more commonly known as a collapsed lung. Trauma to the chest that causes a lung to collapse
is _____/_____.

---

collapsed

13.9

A congenital lung defect may cause atel/ectasis or a _____ lung.

---

pneumon/o/pexy
nōō′ mə nō pek′ sē

13.10

Prolapsed lung tissue can be surgically attached (fixated) by a procedure called
_____/_____/_____.

---

melan

13.11

Recall that **melan/o** means black. Pneumon/o/melan/osis is a lung disease often found in coal miners in which lung tissue becomes black due to breathing black dust. The word root for black is _____.

---

pneumon/o
melan
osis

13.12

Pneumon/o/melan/osis literally means a condition of black lungs.
Analyze this word
_____/_____ combining form for lung
_____ word root for black
_____ suffix—condition

---

pneumonomelanosis
nōō′ mə nō mel′ ə **nō**′ sis
pneumonomelanosis

13.13

The inhalation (breathing) of black dust over time results in
_____.
The inhalation of soot or black smoke for extended periods can also cause
_____.

---

myc

13.14

Pneumon/o/myc/osis means a fungal disease of the lungs. The word root that means fungus is _____.

ANSWER COLUMN

13.15

fungus (singular)   or
fung′ gəs
fungi (plural)
fun′ jī, **fung′** gī

Myces is a Greek word meaning mushroom or fungus. **myc/o** seen any place in a word should make you think of _____.

13.16

fungi or fungus

In high school biology, you read about and/or learned the words mycelium and mycelial. myc is the word root for *_____.

13.17

pneumon/o/myc/osis
nōō **mon′** ō mī kō′ sis

A myc/osis is any condition caused by a fungus. A condition of lung fungus is _____/_____/_____/_____.

13.18

myc/oid
mī′ koid
myc/o/logy
mī **kol′** ə jē

Build words meaning resembling fungi _____/_____; science

and study of fungi _____/_____/_____.

13.19

pharyng/o/myc/osis
fair in′ gō mī **kō′** sis
rhin/o/myc/osis
rī′ nō mī **kō′** sis
dermat/o/myc/osis
der mat′ tō mī **kō′** sis
myc/o/dermat/itis
mī kō der ma **tī′** tis

Build words meaning fungal disease (condition) of the pharynx (throat) _____/_____; fungal disease (condition) of the nose

_____/_____/_____/_____; fungal disease of the skin

_____/_____/_____/_____; inflammation of the skin

caused by a fungus _____/_____/_____/_____.

13.20

INFORMATION FRAME

pneum/o and **pneumon/o** can both refer to the lung. **pneum/o** is derived from the Greek word *pneuma* (for wind or breath). **pneum/o** is also used in words to mean air.

13.21

lung or lungs

pneumon/o comes from the Greek word *pneumon* (lung). **pneumon/o** is used in words that refer to the *_____. The lungs are shown on page 459.

ANSWER COLUMN

13.22

air

pneum/o is used in most words to mean _____, as in pneumatic drill, but it can also be used to mean lung.

13.23

Thorax is a noun and suffix for chest cavity. Your use of **pneum/o** will be in words about air. Pneum/o/derm/a means a collection of air under the skin. A collection of air in the chest cavity (thorax) is a

pneum/o/thorax
noo mō **thôr**′ aks

_____/_____/_____.

13.24

Hydrotherapy means treatment with water. Treatment with compressed air

pneum/o/therapy
noo mō **ther**′ ə pē

is called _____/_____/_____.

13.25

The tach/o/meter in cars measures the number of revolutions per minute of the drive shaft. An instrument that measures air volume in respiration

pneum/o/meter
noo **mom**′ ə tər

is a _____/_____/_____.

13.26

A collection of air and serum (**ser/o**) in the chest cavity is pneum/o/ser/o/thorax. A collection of air and pus in the thoracic cavity

pneum/o/py/o/thorax
noo mō pī ō **thôr**′ aks
pneum/o/hem/o/thorax
noo mō hē′ mō **thôr**′ aks
pneum/o/thorax
noo mō **thôr**′ aks

is a _____/_____/_____/_____/_____,
while a collection of air and blood in this same cavity is a

_____/_____/_____/_____/_____.

Air forced into the chest is a _____/_____/_____.

13.27

pulmon/o is another combining form for lung used in only a few words. Pulmonary and pulmonic are both used as adjectives meaning pertaining to the lungs. The heart valve through which blood travels to the lungs is the

pulmon/ary
pul′ mon air ē

_____/_____ valve.

13.28

Blood flows from the heart to the lungs via the

pulmon/ary or pulmon/ic
pul **mon**′ ik
lungs

_____/_____ artery.
Cardi/o/pulmonary refers to the heart
and the _____ (CPR = cardiopulmonary resuscitation).

Heart with pulmonary arteries and veins

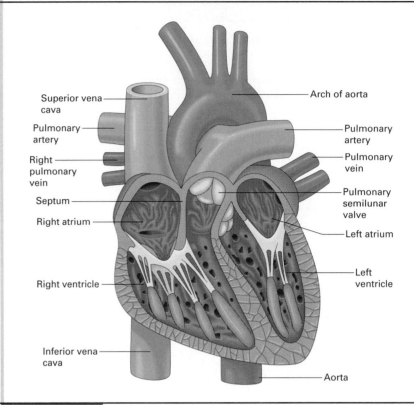

Superior vena cava

Pulmonary artery

Right pulmonary vein

Septum

Right atrium

Right ventricle

Inferior vena cava

Arch of aorta

Pulmonary artery

Pulmonary vein

Pulmonary semilunar valve

Left atrium

Left ventricle

Aorta

13.29

Look up embolus in your dictionary. An embolus is a thrombus (clot) that moves. A blood clot moving to the lung is called a

* _____.

pulmonary embolus
pul′ mon air ē **em**′ bol us

Study the following table of respiratory symptoms:

Term	Symptom
a/pnea	absence of breathing
dys/pnea	difficult breathing
hyper/pnea	increased rate and depth of breathing
tachy/pnea	rapid breathing
brady/pnea	slow breathing
ortho/pnea	able to breathe only when sitting up or standing
hem/o/pty/sis	expectorating (coughing up) blood
hyper/ventil/ation	excessive movement of air in and out of lungs, sighing respirations
hyp/oxia	low oxygen levels in organs and tissues
cyan/osis	bluish color due to hypoxia

13.30

INFORMATION FRAME

pne/o is the combining form for breathing or breath. It is used most often in its suffix form, **-pnea**, to form words about breathing. Normal breathing has a regular rhythm and rate, about 12 to 16 breaths per minute (bpm) for adults. The rates increase with activity and body temperature increases.

13.31

a/pnea
ap′ nē ə
brady/pnea
brad ip **nē**′ ə
orth/o/pnea
ôr **thop**′ nē′ ə
hem/o/pty/sis
hēm **op**′ tə sis

Build breathing words that mean
   absence of breathing
   _____/_____;
   slow breathing
   _____/_____;
   able to breathe only when sitting up
   _____/____/_____;
   coughing up blood
   _____/____/_____/_____.

13.32

orth/o/pnea
ör **thop**′ nē ə

Recall that **orth/o** means straight. Orth/o/pnea is difficulty breathing if laying straight in a horizontal position. For the patient with orthopnea to breath well, it may be necessary to elevate a patient's head and shoulders by propping them up with two or three pillows. This is referred to as two or three pillow
_____/____/_____.

13.33

INFORMATION FRAME

Recall that **hem/o** refers to blood. Sputum is a combination of mucus and other fluids and substances that have entered the respiratory tract. **ptyal/o** is used to refer to either saliva or sputum. Hem/o/pty/sis is a condition of bloody sputum. Ptyal/o/rrhea is a flow of saliva.

13.34

hem/o/pty/sis
hēm **op**′ tə sis

If a patient is coughing up sputum containing blood this is called
_____/____/_____/_____.

13.35

pytal/o/rrhea
tī ə lō **rē**′ ə

Someone who drools because of excess saliva may be said to have
_____/____/_____ or ptyalism.

ANSWER COLUMN

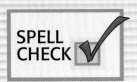

SPELL CHECK ✓

tī′ əl izm

hēm op′ tə sis

13.36

pt as a consonant combination is another Greek origin spelling. Watch the pronunciation and spelling. The *p* is silent when at the beginning of the word as when using *pt, ps,* and *pn.*

EXAMPLE: ptyal/ism.
The p is pronounced if it occurs in the middle of the word.
EXAMPLE: hem/o/pty/sis.
Try the following words on your own.
psych/o/logy
pneumon/ia
ptyal/o/rrhea

13.37

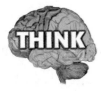

THINK

Use the following information to work Frames 13.37–13.68. If you have forgotten a word part, remember, you may look back. The respiratory system is illustrated in the figure on page 459. Seeing the parts as you work will make your work more interesting.

Air enters the nose and nasal cavity—**nas/o** (Remember **rhin/o**? Use **nas/o** in this work.)
   goes to the pharynx—**pharyng/o**
   to the larynx—**laryng/o**
   to the trachea—**trache/o**
   to the bronchi (us)—**bronch/o**
   to the alveoli (us)—**alveol/o** (oxygen enters the bloodstream here and carbon dioxide is exhaled).
The lungs
   are covered by the pleura—**pleur/o**.
The diaphragm (**phren/o**) is a muscle that assists with inhalation and exhalation. The phrenic nerve innervates the diaphragm.

13.38

nasal cavity

nas/o is used in words about the nasal cavity. Nas/o/antr/itis means inflammation of the antrum (maxillary sinus) and the *_____.

13.39

chin

Taken from the Latin *mentum*, **ment/o** is the combining form for chin. Nas/o/ment/al means pertaining to the nasal cavity and _____.

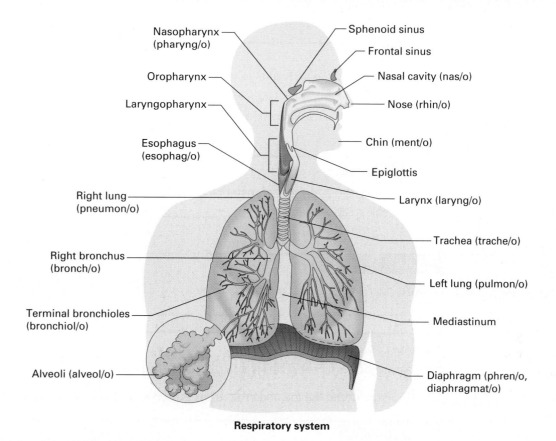

Nasopharynx (pharyng/o)

Oropharynx

Laryngopharynx

Esophagus (esophag/o)

Right lung (pneumon/o)

Right bronchus (bronch/o)

Terminal bronchioles (bronchiol/o)

Alveoli (alveol/o)

Sphenoid sinus

Frontal sinus

Nasal cavity (nas/o)

Nose (rhin/o)

Chin (ment/o)

Epiglottis

Larynx (laryng/o)

Trachea (trache/o)

Left lung (pulmon/o)

Mediastinum

Diaphragm (phren/o, diaphragmat/o)

Respiratory system

ANSWER COLUMN

13.40

Build words meaning
  pertaining to the nose (cavity)
  _____/_____;
  inflammation of the nose (cavity)
  _____/_____;
  instrument to examine the nose (cavity)
  _____/____/_____.

nas/al
nā′ zəl
nas/itis
nā **zī′** tis
nas/o/scope
nā′ zō skōp

13.41

Build words (you may use your dictionary if necessary) meaning
  inflammation of nose and pharynx
  _____/____/_____/_____;
  pertaining to the nasal and frontal bone
  _____/____/_____/_____;
  pertaining to the nose and lacrimal duct
  _____/____/_____/_____.

nas/o/pharyng/itis
nās′ ō far in **jī′** tis
nas/o/front/al
nās′ ō **front′** əl
nas/o/lacrim/al
nās′ ō **lak′** rim əl

ANSWER COLUMN

<table>
<tr><td>WORD ORIGINS</td><td>

13.42

Epi/staxis is a Greek term built from the prefix **epi-**, which means upon, and staxis meaning dripping or oozing. Although there is no mention of blood in the term, epi/staxis is the medical term for nosebleed or hemorrhage from the nose.

</td></tr>
<tr><td>

epi/staxis
e pē **staks**′ is

</td><td>

13.43

Hypertension, stress, dryness of membranes, and/or sinusitis may all lead to a nosebleed also called _____/_____.

</td></tr>
<tr><td>

nose and pharynx (throat)

</td><td>

13.44

Nas/o/pharyng/eal means pertaining to the
* _____.

</td></tr>
<tr><td>

pharynx
far′ inks

</td><td>

13.45

A pharyng/o/lith (far ing′ ō lith) is a calculus in the wall of the _____.

NOTE: Pronounced like *fair* and *inks*. Larynx is pronounced like *lair* and *inks*.

</td></tr>
<tr><td>

pharynx (work on the pronunciation)

</td><td>

13.46

A pharyng/o/myc/osis (far ing′ ō mī **kō**′ sis) is a fungus disease of the _____.

</td></tr>
<tr><td>

pharyng/itis
far′ in **jī**′ tis
pharyng/o/cele
fə **ring**′ gō sēl
pharyng/o/tomy
far′ ing **got**′ ə mē

</td><td>

13.47

Build words meaning
  inflammation of the pharynx
  _____/_____;
  herniation of the pharynx
  _____/_____/_____;
  incision of the pharynx
  _____/_____/_____.

</td></tr>
</table>

Pharyngitis *(Courtesy of the Centers for Disease Control and Prevention [CDC])*

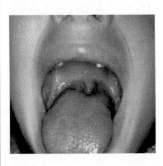

ANSWER COLUMN

	13.48
	The pharynx is the throat. Build words meaning (you put in slashes): disease of the pharynx
pharyng/o/pathy	_____;
	surgical repair of the pharynx
pharyng/o/plasty	_____;
	instrument to examine the pharynx
pharyng/o/scope (You pronounce)	_____.

	13.49
laryng/o (You pronounce)	**laryng/o** is used to build words that refer to the larynx. The larynx contains the vocal cords. When referring to the organ of sound, use _____/_____.
	NOTE: Musical notes make up a chords. Ligaments in the body are cords.

	13.50
	Form a word that means inflammation of the larynx
laryng/itis lar′ in **jī**′ tis	_____/_____.
	NOTE: **laryng/o** is also used to indicate throat, as in otorhinolaryngologist (ENT).

	13.51
	After a bad cold, a patient may have laryngitis with accompanying pain. Pain in
laryng/algia lar′ in gal′ jē ə	the larynx is called _____/_____.

	13.52
	Anything that obstructs the flow of air from the nose to the larynx may call
laryng/o/stomy	for creating a new opening, or a _____/_____/_____.

	13.53
	When a temporary opening is wanted into the larynx, the surgical procedure is a laryng/o/tomy. An incision into the larynx is called a
laryng/o/tomy lar′ ing **got**′ ə mē	_____/_____/_____.
	Remember the "g" rule for pronunciation in Frames 13.44–13.55.

	13.54
herniation of the larynx	A laryng/o/cele is a *_____.

ANSWER COLUMN

13.55

Build words meaning
  any disease of the larynx

laryng/o/pathy

_____/_____/_____;

  instrument used to examine the larynx

laryng/o/scope

_____/_____/_____;

  spasm of the larynx

laryng/o/spasm
(You pronounce)

_____/_____/_____.

13.56

a condition of the trachea
  with pus formation

The trachea (**trache/o**) is the windpipe. Trache/o/py/osis means
*_____
_____.

13.57

hemorrhage from the
trachea

Trache/o/rrhagia means
*_____
_____.

13.58

Build words meaning
  pain in the trachea

trache/algia
trā′ kē **al**′ jē ə
trache/o/tomy
trā′ kē **ot**′ ə mē
trache/o/cele
trā′ kē ō sēl

_____/_____;

  incision into the trachea

_____/_____/_____;

  herniation of the trachea

_____/_____/_____.

13.59

Build words meaning
  examination of the trachea

trache/o/scopy
trā′ kē **os**′ kō pē
trache/al
trā′ kē ə l
trache/o/laryng/o/tomy

_____/_____/_____;

  pertaining to the trachea

_____/_____;

  incision of trachea and larynx

_____/_____/_____/_____/_____;

ANSWER COLUMN

trā′ kē ō lär′ in go′ tō mē
trache/ostomy
trā′ kē **os**′ tō mē
endo/trache/al
en′dō **trā**′ kē əl

surgical creation of a new opening in the trachea

_____/_____;

within the trachea

_____/_____/_____.

13.60

inflammation of the
  bronchi

an instrument to
  examine the bronchi

use of a flexible
  bronchofiberscope to
  examine the
  tracheobronchial tree

Bronch/itis means *_____
_____.

A bronch/o/scope is *_____
_____.

Bronch/o/fiber/o/scopy is *_____
_____.

13.61

Build words meaning
  calculus in a bronchus

bronch/o/lith
bron′ kō lith
bronch/o/scopy
bron **kos**′ kə pē
bronch/o/rrhagia
bron′ kô **rā**′ jē ə

  _____/_____/_____;
  examination of a bronchus (with instrument)
  _____/_____/_____;
  bronchial hemorrhage
  _____/_____/_____.

13.62

Build words meaning
  formation of a new opening into a bronchus

bronch/o/stomy
bron **kos**′ tō mē
bronch/o/spasm
bron′ kō spazm
bronch/o/rrhaphy
bron **kôr**′ ə fē

  _____/_____/_____;
  spasm of a bronchus
  _____/_____/_____;
  suturing of a bronchus
  _____/_____/_____.

13.63

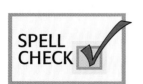

SPELL CHECK ✓

Plural means more than one; pleural refers to the membrane around the lungs.
The plural of pleura is pleurae.

ANSWER COLUMN

13.64

pertaining to the pleura
inflammation of the
pleura

Pleur/al means *_____.
Pleur/itis means *_____
_____.

Build words meaning

pleur/algia
ploo **ral**′ jē ə
pleur/o/dynia
ploor′ **din**′ ē ə
pleur/o/centesis
ploor′ ō sen **tē**′ sis

pain in the pleura _____/_____
or
_____/_____/_____;
surgical puncturing of the pleura
_____/_____/_____.

13.65

Build words meaning
pertaining to the membrane attached to the lung

viscer/o/pleural
vis′ er ō **ploo**′ rəl
pleur/o/lith
ploor rō lith
pleur/ectomy
ploor **ek**′ tō mē

_____/_____/_____;
calculus in the pleura
_____/_____/_____;
excision of part of the pleura
_____/_____.

13.66

TAKE A
CLOSER
LOOK

Look up the word pleurisy. Read all your dictionary has to say about this disease.
Its synonym is pleuritis. Write the treatment described here:

_____
_____
_____

13.67

pleur/isy
ploor′ ri sē

Inflammation of the pleura is pleuritis or _____/_____.

13.68

phren/o/plegia
fren ō **plē**′ jē ə

The phrenic nerve controls the diaphragm. The combining form for diaphragm
is **phren/o**. **-plegia** is the suffix for paralysis.
Paralysis of the diaphragm is _____/_____/_____.

PROFESSIONAL PROFILES

Respiratory therapists (RRTs or CRTs) perform physiologic (i.e., arterial blood gases) and pulmonary (i.e., breathing) tests to determine respiratory health or impairment. They administer breathing treatment and other respiratory procedures to maintain or improve ventilatory function to patients in hospital and ambulatory care settings. It is also possible for the respiratory therapist to specialize in pulmonary function testing or to be cross-trained to perform cardiopulmonary testing such as stress tests. The National Board for Respiratory Care (NBRC) sets standards for education and credentialing of registered respiratory therapists (minimum two years) and certified respiratory therapists (minimum one year).

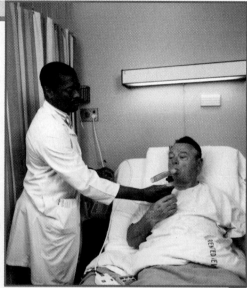

Respiratory therapist (RT) administering nebulizing mist treatment (NMT)

ANSWER COLUMN

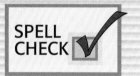

SPELL CHECK ✓

13.69

Watch your spelling of the word diaphragm. It has a silent *g*.

13.70

phren/ectomy
fren **ek**′ tō mē
phren/ic/ectomy
fren i **sek**′ tō mē

Removal of a portion of the phrenic nerve is a _____ / _____

or

_____ / _____ / _____.

13.71

left

In medicine we go back to the original meaning of sinister to find the combining form **sinistr/o**, which means _____.

13.72

left

ad- as a prefix or **-ad** as a suffix means toward. Sinistr/ad means toward the _____.

ANSWER COLUMN

13.73

Using **sinistr/o**, build words meaning

pertaining to the left

_____/_____;

sinistr/al
sin′ is trəl

displacement of the heart to the left

_____/____/_____/___;

sinistr/o/cardi/a
sin′ is trō **kär**′ dē ə

pertaining to the left half of the cerebrum

_____/____/_____/_____.

sinistr/o/cerebr/al
sin′ is trō **ser**′ ə brəl

13.74

Using manual (hand) and pedal (foot), build words meaning

left-handed

_____/____/_____/_____;

sinistr/o/man/ual
sin′ is trō **man**′ yōō əl

left-footed

_____/____/_____/_____.

sinistr/o/ped/al
sin′ is trō **pē**′ dəl

13.75

right

The opposite of **sinistr/o** is **dextr/o**. **dextr/o** means _____.

13.76

right

Dextr/ad means toward the _____.

13.77

Build words meaning

pertaining to the right

_____/_____;

dextr/al
dek′ strəl

displacement of the heart to the right

_____/____/_____/___;

dextr/o/cardi/a
dek′ strō **kär**′ dē ə

displacement of the stomach to the right

_____/____/_____/_____.

dextr/o/gastr/ia
dek′ strō **gas**′ trē ə

13.78

Refer to Frame 13.74 if necessary and build words meaning

right-handed _____/____/_____/_____;

right-footed _____/____/_____/_____.

dextr/o/man/ual
dextr/o/ped/al
(You pronounce)

ANSWER COLUMN

	13.79
ped/i/algia ped ē **al′** jē ə pod/algia pod **al′** jē ə	**pod/o** (Greek) and **ped/i** (Latin) are both combining forms for foot. Two terms for foot pain are _____/_____/_____ and _____/_____ .
	13.80
ped/i pod/o	The two combining forms for foot are _____/_____ and _____/_____ .
	13.81
pod/iatrist pō **dī′** ə trist	Suffixes **-iatrist** (noun) and **-iatric** (adjective) are used to indicate medical professionals or physicians. A health professional responsible for care of conditions of the feet is a _____/_____ (DPM). The specialty is called podiatry.
	13.82
pod/iatric pō dē **a′** trik	A hammertoe operation is a type of _____/_____ (adjective) treatment.
	13.83
spasm of the hand chir/o	*Cheir* is a Greek word for hand. Look up chir/o/spasm; it means _____ . The combining form for hand is _____/____ .
	13.84
hands	Chir/o/practors (doctor of chiropractic [DC]) use their hands to manipulate the body for therapy. In the adjective chir/o/practic, the word root **chir/o** means _____ .
	13.85
chir/o/practic kī′ rō **prak′** tik	Spinal manipulation is a form of _____/_____/_____ (adjective) treatment.
	13.86
chir/o/plasty **kī′** rō plas tē	Surgical repair of the hand is called _____/_____/_____ .

ANSWER COLUMN

13.87

pedi/a is a combining form that comes from the Greek word *pedias*, meaning child. A physician specialist who treats children

is a _____/_____/_____.

pedi/a/trician
pē′ dē a **tri**′ shən

Pediatrician assisting a child with listening to her own heart sounds

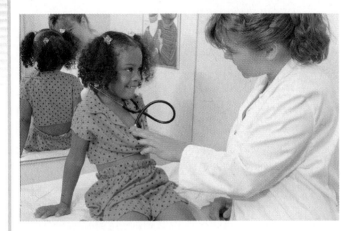

13.88

Recall **-iatric** is a suffix meaning medical or physician. The medical specialty for treatment of diseases of children is _____/_____/_____.

pedi/a/trics
pē′ dē a′ triks

13.89

A psych/iatrist is a medical doctor who specializes in the study of diagnosing and treating mental disorders. _____ is the suffix used to indicate a medical professional.

-iatrist

13.90

A psychiatrist provides _____/_____/_____ treatment.

psych/i/atric
sī′ kē **a**′ trik

13.91

ger/i means old age. Ger/ont/o/logy is the study of treatment of aging and the elderly. The medical specialty involving treating diseases related to old age is

_____/_____/_____.

ger/i/atrics
jer′ ē **a**′ triks
ger/ont/o/logy
jer′ on **tol**′ ō jē

The study of aging is

_____/_____/_____/_____.

NOTE: Ontology is the study of a developmental process, i.e. embryology or gerontology.

PROFESSIONAL PROFILES

Registered Health Information Administrators (RHIAs) manage health information departments in hospitals to ensure accurate, complete, orderly, and timely record keeping. They help plan hospital systems for better patient care and provide statistics for research, accreditation, and assistance with financial management.

Registered Health Information Technicians (RHITs) complete, index, code, file, and abstract statistical information and prepare medical records for release. In many institutions they also perform management functions. The American Health Information Management Association (AHIMA) sets standards for education programs (ranging from correspondence courses to bachelor's degrees), registration, and accreditation of medical records professionals.

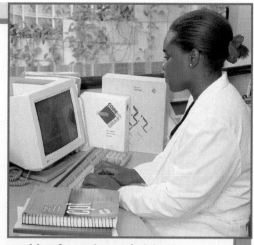

Health Information technician

Abbreviation	Meaning	Abbreviation	Meaning
ABG	arterial blood gases	NBRC	National Board for Respiratory Care
AD	right ear (auris dexter)		
AHIMA	American Health Information Management Association	NMT	nebulizing mist treatment
		O_2	oxygen
RHIT	registered health information technician	PD	pulmonary disease
		PE	pulmonary edema, physical exam, pulmonary embolism
AS	left ear (auris sinister)		
CO_2	carbon dioxide	Peds	pediatrics
COLD	chronic obstructive lung disease	PFT	pulmonary function test
		PND	paroxysmal nocturnal dyspnea, postnasal drip
COPD	chronic obstructive pulmonary disease		
		R	respiration (rate)
CPR	cardiopulmonary resuscitation	RHIA	registered health information administrator
CRT	certified respiratory therapist		
DC	doctor of chiropractic medicine	RRT	registered respiratory therapist
DPM	doctor of podiatric medicine	RT	respiratory therapist
HIPAA	Health Insurance Portability and Accountability Act of 1996	TB	tuberculosis
		TC & DB	turn, cough, and deep breathe
ICU	intensive care unit	URI	upper respiratory infection
IS	incentive spirometer		

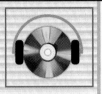

To complete your study of this unit, work the **Review Activities** on the following pages. Also listen to the audio CDs that accompany *Medical Terminology: A Programmed Systems Approach,* 9th edition, and practice your pronunciation.

Additional practice exercises for this unit are available on the Learner Practice CD-ROM found in the back of the textbook.

REVIEW ACTIVITIES

CIRCLE AND CORRECT

Circle the correct answer for each question. Then, check your answers in Appendix A.

1. Word root for lung
   a. pnea
   b. pneumonia
   c. pneumon
   d. pulmonary

2. Combining form for fungus
   a. monilo
   b. myo
   c. myco
   d. mycelio

3. Noun for throat
   a. pharynx
   b. trachea
   c. esophagus
   d. phalanx

4. Adjective for kidney
   a. nephriac
   b. nephroc
   c. cystic
   d. renal

5. Which of the following does *not* refer to the lung?
   a. thoraco
   b. pulmonary
   c. pneumono
   d. pneumo

6. Combining form for air:
   a. pneumono
   b. pneumo
   c. pnea
   d. pulmono

7. Combining form for nasal cavity
   a. rhin
   b. mento
   c. naso
   d. antro

8. Singular of pharynges
   a. pharynx
   b. pharyngos
   c. pharyno
   d. pharynge

9. Sound made by the g in laryngocele
   a. s
   b. k
   c. j as in job
   d. g as in goat

10. Combining form for right
    a. dextro
    b. dextrose
    c. dextrous
    d. dexter

11. Combining form for the windpipe
    a. esphago
    b. laryngo
    c. pharyngo
    d. tracheo

12. Epistaxis refers to
    a. upon the stomach
    b. after dinner
    c. difficulty breathing
    d. nose bleed

REVIEW ACTIVITIES

ART LABELING

Label the structures of the respiratory system by matching them with their correct combining form.

_____1.   a. alveol/o

_____2.   b. bronch/o

_____3.   c. trache/o

_____4.   d. laryng/o

_____5.   e. rhin/o

_____6.   f. pharyng/o

_____7.   g. phren/o

                 h. pulmon/o

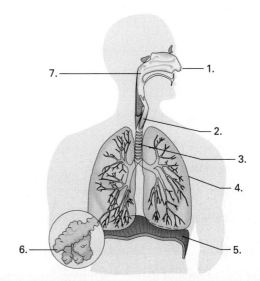

SELECT AND CONSTRUCT

Select the correct word parts from the following list and construct medical terms that represent the given meaning.

al	algia	ary	atrician	blast	bronch(o)(i)
centesis	chir(o)	constriction	dermat/o	dextr(o)	dilatation
dilation	dynia	ectasis	ectomy	embol	fungi
hist(o)	iatrist	ic	ism	itis	laryn(x)(g)(o)
lith	(o)logy	lysis	manual	melan(o)	mental
myc(o)	nas(o)	oma	osis	pathy	pedal
pedi	pharynx(go)	phren(o)	plegia	pleur(o)(a)	pneumon/o
practor	psych	pulmon/o	rrhagia	scope (y)	sinistr/o
stomy	thorac/o	trache(o)	us		

1. adjective for lung

   _____

2. black lung disease

   _____

3. fungal infection of the skin

   _____

4. a moving blood clot

   _____

5. the study of fungi

   _____

6. pertaining to the nose and chin

   _____

7. instrument used to look at the throat

   _____

REVIEW ACTIVITIES

8. surgical puncture of the membrane around the lung   _____

9. right-footed   _____

10. left-handed   _____

11. physician specialist for children   _____

12. destruction of tissue   _____

13. inflammation of the bronchi   _____

14. pain in the voice box   _____

15. paralysis of the diaphragm   _____

16. dilatation of the bronchi   _____

17. physician specialist in mental disorders   _____

18. making a new opening in the trachea   _____

19. doctor using hands to manipulate the spine   _____

DEFINE AND DISSECT

Give a brief definition and dissect each term listed into its word parts in the space provided. Check your answers by referring to the frame listed in parentheses and your medical dictionary. Then listen to the CDs to practice pronunciation.

1. pneumonocentesis (13.4)   _____/_____/_____
                                    rt   v   suffix

   _____
                          definition

2. pneumonomelanosis (13.13)   _____/_____/_____/_____
                                      rt   v   rt   suffix

   _____

3. pharyngomycosis (13.19)   _____/_____/_____/_____
                                    rt   v   rt   suffix

   _____

4. pneumothorax (13.23)   _____/_____/_____
                                rt   v   rt

   _____

5. pulmonic (13.28)   _____/_____
                             rt   suffix

   _____

6. pneumopyothorax (13.26)   _____/_____/_____/_____/_____
                                   rt   v   rt   v   rt

   _____

REVIEW ACTIVITIES

7. pneumohemothorax (13.26)

_____/_____/_____/_____/_____
rt　　　v　　　rt　　　v　　　　rt

8. pulmonary (13.27)

_____/_____
rt　　　　suffix

9. embolus (13.29)

_____/_____
rt　　　suffix

10. pneumonia (13.5)

_____/_____
rt　　　suffix

11. mycology (13.18)

_____/_____/_____
rt　　　v　　　suffix

12. dermatomycosis (13.19)

_____/_____/_____/_____
rt　　　v　　　rt　　　　suffix

13. nasitis (13.40)

_____/_____
rt　　　suffix

14. pharyngomycosis (13.46)

_____/_____/_____/_____
rt　　　v　　　rt　　　　suffix

15. nasoantritis (13.38)

_____/_____/_____/_____
rt　　　v　　　rt　　　　suffix

16. nasopharyngitis (13.41)

_____/_____/_____/_____
rt　　　v　　　rt　　　　suffix

17. tracheolaryngotomy (13.59)

_____/_____/_____/_____/_____
rt　　　v　　　rt　　　v　　　suffix

18. pleurisy (13.67)

_____/_____
rt　　　suffix

REVIEW ACTIVITIES

19. bronchorrhaphy (13.62)

_____/____/_____
rt　　　v　　　suffix

_____

20. phrenectomy (13.70)

_____/_____
rt　　　suffix

_____

21. sinistrocardia (13.73)

_____/____/_____/____
rt　　　v　　　rt　　suffix

_____

22. dextromanual (13.78)

_____/____/____/_____
rt　　　v　　rt　　suffix

_____

23. podiatric (13.82)

_____/_____
rt　　suffix

_____

24. pediatrician (13.87)

_____/____/_____
rt　　　v　　　suffix

_____

25. chiropractor (13.84)

_____/____/_____
rt　　　v　　　rt/suffix

_____

26. laryngotomy (13.53)

_____/____/_____
rt　　　v　　　suffix

_____

27. bronchoscopy (13.61)

_____/____/_____
rt　　　v　　　suffix

_____

28. pleurocentesis (13.64)

_____/____/_____
rt　　　v　　　suffix

_____

29. psychiatrist (13.89)

_____/_____
rt　　　suffix

_____

30. gerontology (13.91)

_____/_____/____/_____
rt　　　rt　　　v　　suffix

_____

REVIEW ACTIVITIES

31. cardiopulmonary (13.28)

_____/_____/_____/_____
     rt   v   rt   suffix

_____

32. atelectasis (13.8)

_____/_____
       rt   suffix

_____

ABBREVIATION MATCHING

Match the following abbreviations with their definition.

_____ 1. PND

_____ 2. RT

_____ 3. ICU

_____ 4. AS

_____ 5. URI

_____ 6. ABG

_____ 7. DC

_____ 8. NMT

_____ 9. RRT

_____10. CPR

a. intensive care unit

b. partial pressure of oxygen

c. registered respiratory therapist

d. tuberculosis

e. current procedures in respiratory therapy

f. postnasal drip

g. urinary tract infection

h. doctor of chiropractic

i. right ear

j. nebulizing mist treatment

k. arterial blood gases

l. left ear

m. upper respiratory infection

n. respiratory therapy (department)

o. arteriobiogram

p. cardiopulmonary resuscitation

q. dentist

ABBREVIATION FILL-INS

Fill in the blanks with the correct abbreviation.

11. pulmonary edema _____

12. pulmonary function test _____

13. carbon dioxide _____

14. respiration (rate) _____

15. chronic obstructive pulmonary disease _____

16. registered health information administrator _____

REVIEW ACTIVITIES

MATCHING

Match the breathing term on the left with its description on the right.

_____ 1. apnea   a. difficult (painful) breathing

_____ 2. hemoptysis   b. fast breathing

_____ 3. dyspnea   c. slow breathing

_____ 4. orthopnea   d. bloody sputum

_____ 5. bradypnea   e. absence of breathing

_____ 6. tachypnea   f. breathing best when sitting up

_____ 7. atelectasis g. collapsed lung

CASE STUDIES

Write the term next to its meaning given below. Then draw slashes to analyze the word parts. Note the use of medical abbreviations. Look these up in your dictionary or find them in Appendix B. If you have any questions about the answers, refer to your medical dictionary or check with your instructor for the answers in Appendix A.

CASE STUDY 13-1

Postop Visit

Pt: Male, age 11

Dx: 1. Status **asthmaticus**

2. Probable **viral syndrome**

Peter Puffer is an eleven-year-old boy with no known history of asthma, although he does have a history of **bronchitis** during which he has had episodes of wheezing. Peter has had **respiratory symptoms** and fever since Monday morning and now has increasing respiratory distress on the day of admission. He was seen in the office of Dr. Neumo who reported tightness in the chest. **Pulse oximetry** revealed an O_2 saturation of 83%. Peter was therefore sent to the hospital, treated overnight with **oxygen, intravenous** aminophylline and Bronkosol, as well as **IV** Zinacef. He appears to be more comfortable at this point with less **tachypnea** and better oxygen saturation.

1. inflammation of the bronchi   _____

2. heart rate   _____

3. fast breathing   _____

4. within a vein   _____

5. measurement of oxygen   _____

6. oxygen symbol   _____

7. percent symbol   _____

8. pertaining to breathing   _____

9. spasms of the bronchi   _____

10. pertaining to a virus   _____

REVIEW ACTIVITIES

11. O_2 _____

12. intravenous _____

13. feelings and experiences _____

14. series of symptoms that form a disease _____

CROSSWORD PUZZLE

Check your answers by going back through the frames or checking the solutions in Appendix C.

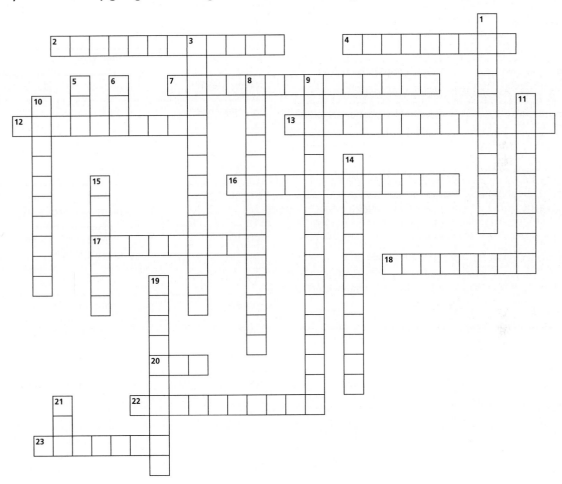

Across

2. instrument to look at the voice box
4. sit up straight to breathe
7. cancer-fighting drugs
12. synonym for gerontology
13. condition known as athlete's foot
16. DC
17. pertaining to lung
18. synonym for pleuritis
20. arterial blood gases (abbreviation)
22. inflamed bronchi
23. moving clot

Down

1. right-footed
3. left-handed
5. upper respiratory infection
6. pulmonary function test (abbreviation)
8. back of the throat up near the nose (adj.)
9. black lung disease
10. coughing up blood (bloody sputum)
11. study of tissues
14. new permanent opening in the windpipe
15. difficulty breathing
19. foot doctor
21. podiatrist (abbreviation)

REVIEW ACTIVITIES

GLOSSARY

apnea	absence of breathing
atelectasis	collapsed lung
bradypnea	slow breathing
bronchitis	inflammation of the bronchi
broncholith	bronchial stone
bronchorrhagia	hemorrhage of the bronchi
bronchorrhaphy	suture of the bronchi
bronchoscopy	examination of the bronchi with a bronchoscope
bronchospasm	uncontrolled contraction of the bronchial muscles
cardiopulmonary	pertaining to heart and lungs
chiroplasty	surgical repair of the hand
chiropractic	practice of using hands for therapeutic spinal and skull manipulation, a philosophy of medicine based on musculoskeletal alignment and holistic health practices
chiropractor	doctor of chiropractic (DC)
dermatomycosis	fungal infection of the skin (mycodermatitis)
dextral	pertaining to the right
dextrocardia	heart displaced to the right
dextrogastria	stomach displaced to the right
dyspnea	difficulty (painful) breathing
embolus	a moving blood clot (embolism)
endotracheal	inside the trachea
epistaxis	nosebleed
hemoptysis	bloody sputum
fungi	plural of fungus

geriatrics	medical specialty studying aging and related diseases (gerontology)
hyperpnea	increase in depth and rate of breathing
laryngalgia	larynx pain (laryngodynia)
laryngitis	inflammation of the voice box (larynx)
laryngocele	herniation of the larynx
laryngopathy	any disease of the larynx
laryngoscope	an instrument used to examine the larynx
laryngospasm	uncontrolled contraction of the vocal cords
laryngostomy	making a new, permanent opening in the larynx
laryngotomy	making a temporary incision into the larynx
larynx	the voice box
manual	pertaining to the hands
mycoid	resembling a fungus
mycology	the science and study of fungi
nasoantritis	inflammation of the nose and antrum
nasofrontal	pertaining to the nasal and frontal bones
nasolacrimal	pertaining to the nose and lacrimal ducts
nasomental	pertaining to the nose and chin
nasopharyngeal	pertaining to the nasopharynx (nose and pharynx)
nasopharyngitis	inflammation of the nose and pharynx

REVIEW ACTIVITIES

nasoscope	instrument used to examine the nose
orthopnea	dyspnea when lying down (straight) or any position other than sitting or standing upright
otorhinolaryngologist	physician specialist in diseases of the ear, nose, and throat
pedal	pertaining to the foot
pedialgia	foot pain (podalgia)
pediatrician	physician specialist in children's diseases and development
pharyngocele	herniation (weakening of the wall) of the throat
pharyngomycosis	fungal infection of the throat
pharyngoplasty	surgical repair of the throat
pharyngoscope	instrument used to examine the throat
pharynx	throat
phrenectomy	excision of part of the phrenic nerve (phrenicectomy)
phrenoplegia	paralysis of the diaphragm
pleural	pertaining to the pleura
pleuralgia	pleural membrane pain (pleurodynia)
pleurectomy	excision of part of the pleura
pleurisy	inflammation of the pleura (pleuritis)
pleurocentesis	surgical puncture of the pleura to remove fluid
pleurolith	stone in the pleural cavity
pneumohemothorax	air and blood in the thoracic cavity
pneumometer	instrument for measuring air volume
pneumonectomy	excision of the lung

pneumonia	inflammation of the lung
pneumonocentesis	surgical puncture of the lung to remove fluid (pneumocentesis)
pneumonomelanosis	black lung disease
pneumonomycosis	fungal infection of the lung
pneumonopathy	any lung disease
pneumonopexy	surgical fixation of a prolapsed lung (pneumonoplasty)
pneumonorrhagia	hemorrhage of the lung
pneumonotomy	incision into the lung
pneumotherapy	treatment using air
pneumothorax	air in the thoracic cavity
podiatrist	specialist in care of conditions of the feet; may also perform surgery of the foot
psychiatrist	physician specialist in mental disorders
ptyalorrhea	flow of saliva
pulmonary	pertaining to the lung (pulmonic)
rhinomycosis	fungal infection in the nose
sinistral	pertaining to the left
tachypnea	fast breathing
trachea	windpipe
trachealgia	tracheal pain
tracheocele	herniation of the tracheal wall
tracheopyosis	condition of pus in the trachea
tracheorrhagia	hemorrhage of the trachea
tracheoscopy	process of inspecting the trachea
tracheostomy	surgical creation of an opening in the trachea
tracheotomy	incision into the trachea

UNIT 14

Word Parts for Night, Sleep, Split, Skeletal System, and Orthopedics

ANSWER COLUMN	
	14.1 There are two combining forms that mean night. One is Latin, **noct/i**, the other is Greek, **nyct/o**. Noct/i/luca are microscopic marine animals that make the ocean glow during the _____.
night	
	14.2 Those of you who have studied music know that a noct/urne is dreamy music, sometimes called _____ music.
night	
WORD ORIGINS	**14.3** In Greek mythology sleep and death were related to night. Somnus (Sleep) and Thanatos (Death) were the sons of Nox (Night).
	14.4 ambul, from the Latin *ambulare,* is a word root meaning walk. Look up the meaning of these terms about walking ambul/atory *_____; ambul/ance *_____.

able to walk
a vehicle for transporting
  the sick (who
  cannot walk)	

	14.5 ambul is the word root for walk. Noct/ambul/ism literally means walking at night. Sleepwalking is what you mean when you use the word _____/_____/_____.
noct/ambul/ism nokt **am′** byoo lizm	

480

ANSWER COLUMN

	14.6
somn/ambul/ism som **nam**′ byoo lizm	somn is the word root for sleep. A common term for sleepwalking is _____/_____/_____.
	14.7
somnambulism	Sleepwalking can occur at any age, but childhood is the most common age for _____.
	14.8
somnambulism	People are not really asleep when they sleepwalk. They appear to be asleep but are really suppressing the memory of what they do. They are indulging in _____.
	14.9
night	**nyct/o** is another combining form for night. It comes from the Greek word *nyx*. Nyct/algia means pain during the _____.
	14.10
night	Nyct/albumin/uria means the presence of albumin in the urine only during the _____.
	14.11
nyct/al/opia nik′ tə **lō**′ pē ə	Nyct/al/opia means night blindness or difficulty in seeing at night. Vitamin A is associated with night vision. Lack of vitamin A in the diet is one cause of _____/_____/_____.
WORD ORIGINS	**14.12** al comes from the Greek *alaos,* meaning blind. Nyctalopia literally means night blind vision.
	14.13
nyctalopia	Nyct/al/opia has several causes. Retinal fatigue from exposure to very bright light is a cause of _____.
	14.14
nyctalopia	Retinitis pigmentosa is another cause of _____.

ANSWER COLUMN

14.15

Using **nyct/o** and **noct/i** build two words that mean
abnormal fear of night

nyct/o/phobia
nik′ tō **fō**′ bē ə
noct/i/phobia
nok′ ti **fō**′ bē ə

_____/_____/_____

_____/_____/_____ ;

unusual attraction to the night

nyct/o/philia
nik′ tō **fil**′ ē ə
noct/i/philia
nok′ ti **fil**′ ē ə

_____/_____/_____

_____/_____/_____ .

14.16

Noct/uria means excessive urination during the night. Another word that means the same as nocturia is _____/_____ .

nyct/uria
nikt **yōōr**′ ē ə

14.17

Two words that mean excessive urination during the night are
_____/_____ and
_____/_____ .

nyct/uria
noct/uria

14.18

ankyl/o means immovable or fixed. Ankylosed means stiffened.
Ankyl/o/blephar/on means adhesions resulting in
* _____ .

immovable eyelids

14.19

Ankyl/osis, such as in ankylosing spondylitis, is a condition of
_____ of the spine.

immobility

Use the following table to build words for Frames 14.20–14.22.

Combining Form	Noun or Suffix
aden/o (gland)	aden/ia
cardi/o (heart)	cardi/a
cheil/o (lips)	cheil/ia
dactyl/o (digits)	dactyl/ia
dent/o (teeth)	dent/ia

Combining Form	Noun or Suffix
derm/o (skin)	derm/a
	-derm/ia
gastr/o (stomach)	gastr/ia
gloss/o (tongue)	gloss/ia
onych/o (nails)[a]	onych/ia
ophthalm/o (eyes)[a]	ophthalm/ia
ot/o (ears)	ot/ia
phag/o (eat)	**-phag/ia**
pneumon/o (lung)	pneumon/ia
proct/o (anus + rectum)	proct/ia
urethr/o (urethra)	urethr/ia
[a]new in Unit 15	

NOTE: The **-ia** suffix means conditon.

14.20

Ankyl/o/stoma means lockjaw (stiff mouth). Build words meaning (remember, you may look back) adhesions of lips (immovable lips)

ankyl/o/cheilia
ang′ ki lō **kī**′ lē ə

_____/_____/_____;

closure (immobility) of the anus and rectum

ankyl/o/proctia
ang′ ki lō **prok**′ shē ə

_____/_____/_____;

abnormal fear of ankylosis

ankyl/o/phobia
ang′ ki lō **fō**′ bē ə

_____/_____/_____.

14.21

Build words meaning
   tongue tied (stiff tongue)

ankyl/o/glossia
ang′ ki lō **glos**′ ē ə

_____/_____/_____;

ankyl/o/dactylia
ang′ ki lō dak **til**′ ē ə

adhesions of fingers (immovable fingers) or toes

_____/_____/_____.

14.22

noun
condition

-ia is a (choose one) _____ (noun/adjective/verb) suffix meaning

_____.

ANSWER COLUMN

-stasis
viscer/o/stasis
vi′ ser **os**′ tə sis

14.23

-stasis is used as a suffix and means stopping or controlling. To say that you control an organ or what that organ produces, use the combining form for organ (**viscer/o**) plus the suffix _____ to form
_____/_____/_____.

---

stopped or controlled

14.24

Fung/i/stasis is a condition in which the growth of fungi is
*_____.

---

control or stopping
  bile flow

14.25

Chol/e/stasis means
*_____.

---

enter/o/stasis
en′ tə **ros**′ tə sis
py/o/stasis
pī **os**′ tə sis

14.26

Read Frame 14.23 again. Build words meaning
  controlling the small intestine
  _____/_____/_____;
  stopping the formation of pus
  _____/_____/_____.

TAKE A
CLOSER
LOOK

14.27

Acceptable alternative pronunciations of terms with **-stasis** as a suffix include
arteri/o/stasis   ar tēr ē ō **stā**′ sis;
enter/o/stasis   en ter ō **stā**′ sis;
hem/o/stasis   hēm ō **stā**′ sis.

---

hem/o/stasis
hē **mos**′ tə sis
phleb/o/stasis or
fleb **os**′ tə sis
ven/o/stasis
vēn **os**′ tə sis
arteri/o/stasis
är tir′ ē **os**′ tə sis

14.28

Build words meaning
  controlling the flow of blood
  _____/_____/_____;
  checking flow in the veins
  _____/_____/_____;
  checking flow in the arteries
  _____/_____/_____.

ANSWER COLUMN

14.29

schizo- (prefix), schisto- (prefix), and -schisis (suffix) have a complicated evolution from the Greek language. They mean split, cleft, or fissure. Build words meaning split speech (incomprehensible speech)

schizo/phas/ia
skit′ zō **fā**′ sē ə

_____/_____/_____;

nails (**onych/o**)—condition

schiz/onych/ia
skit′ zō **nik**′ ē ə

_____/_____/_____.

NOTE: schizo- and schisto- are combining forms used as prefixes.

14.30

Schiz/o/phren/ia literally means split mind. It is actually a group of severe mental disorders in which thinking, emotions, and behavior are disturbed. A person with delusions of persecution, jealousy, and hallucinations may suffer from paranoid

schizo/phren/ia
skit′ zō **fre**′ nē ə

_____/_____/_____.

14.31

schizophrenia

Anti/psych/otic medications and psych/o/therapy are treatments used for those with _____.

Cleft palate (Courtesy of Dr. Joseph Konzelman, School of Dentistry, Medical College of Georgia)

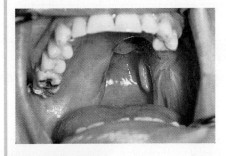

14.32

A fissure is a troughlike cleft in a structure.
Build words using **schisto-**:

split tongue

schisto/gloss/ia
shis′ tō **glos**′ ē ə

_____/_____/_____;

split cell (cell with a fissure)

schist/o/cyte
shis′ tō sīt

_____/_____/_____;

split chest (fissure)

schist/o/thorax
shis′ tō **thôr**′ aks

_____/_____/_____.

ANSWER COLUMN

14.33

Build words using **-schisis** as a suffix:
cleft palate (**palat/o**)

palat/o/schisis
pal ə **tos**′ ki sis
uran/ō/schisis
yōor ə **nos**′ ki sis
rach/i/schisis
rā **kis**′ ki sis

_____/_____/_____ ;
cleft palate (**uran/o**)
_____/_____/_____ ;
split spine (**rach/i**)
_____/_____/_____ .

14.34

TAKE A CLOSER LOOK

Look up spina bifida in your dictionary. This condition is synonymous with rachischisis. Read about the two types and write notes here.

_____

_____

14.35

schisto/som/iasis
shis′ tō sō **mī**′ ə sis

In your dictionary, read about the disease schistosomiasis and _Schistosoma japonicum._ Schistosomiasis is an important disease in terms of world health. Because of increased worldwide travel, all people should be concerned with the disease _____/_____/_____ .

14.36

split

Learn the words involving the combining forms used as prefixes and suffixes for "split". Schizophrenia will be one of them. **schizo-**, **schisto-**, and **-schisis** mean _____ .

14.37

carpi
kär′ pī

Carpos is a Greek word meaning wrist. Locate the carpal bones. The plural of carpus is _____ .

14.38

carp

From carpus and carpi, derive a word root that refers to the wrist. It is _____ .

14.39

carp/al
kär′ pəl

Carpal tunnel syndrome is an occupational hazard to those who perform repetitive hand movement, for example, medical transcriptionists. The adjectival form for carpus is _____/_____ .

ANSWER COLUMN

14.40

Look at the words (in your medical dictionary) that begin with carp. The combining form that is used in words about the wrist is _____/_____.

carp/o

14.41

Close your dictionary. Build words meaning

    pertaining to the wrist (adjective)

carp/al
kär′ pəl

    _____/_____;

    pertaining to the wrist and metacarpals

carp/o/meta/carp/al
kär′ pō **met′** ə kär pəl

    _____/_____/_____/_____/_____;

    excision of all or part of the wrist

carp/ectomy
kär **pek′** tə mē

    _____/_____.

14.42

wrist

carp/o in a word refers to the _____.

Bones of the left hand

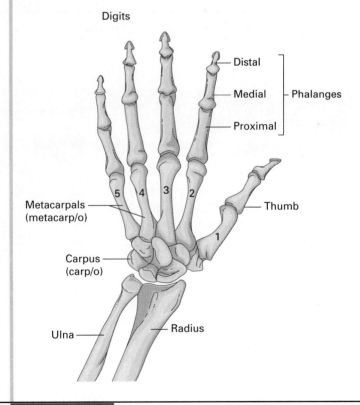

Digits

Distal

Medial — Phalanges

Proximal

Metacarpals
(metacarp/o)

Thumb

Carpus
(carp/o)

Ulna

Radius

14.43

meta/carp/als
met′ ə **kär′** palz

Recall that **meta-** means beyond. The bones in the hand "beyond" the carpals are called the _____/_____/_____.

ANSWER COLUMN

14.44

Refer to the illustration of the foot on page 489. **tars/o** is the combining form for the tarsal bones in the ankle. From what you already know about the prefix **meta-**, name the bones that are located beyond the tarsals:

_____/_____.

meta/tarsals
met′ ə **tar**′ salz

14.45

Locate the following bones

    carpals _____;

    tarsals _____.

wrist

ankle

14.46

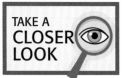

The bones that protrude from the ankles on both the inside and outside are really parts of two bones. Look at the illustration of the bones of the foot. The lateral malleolus is a protrusion on the fibula bone. The medial malleolus is a protrusion on the distal end of the tibia.

PROFESSIONAL PROFILES

Registered occupational therapists (OTR)—The American Occupational Therapy Association (AOTA) information brochure defines occupational therapy as "the use of purposeful activity with individuals who are limited by physical injury or illness, psychosocial dysfunction, developmental or learning disabilities, poverty and cultural differences, or the aging process to maximize independence, prevent disability, and maintain health. The practice encompasses evaluation, treatment, and consultation." Preparation for this profession requires completion of a baccalaureate degree from an approved college including an internship experience. An occupational therapist may specialize in a particular area of expertise such as hand therapy or substance abuse rehabilitation.

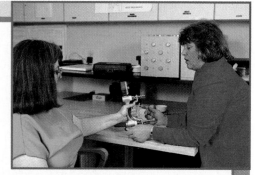

Occupational therapist assisting patient with grip strength test *(Photo by Marcia Butterfield, courtesy of Foote Memorial Hospital, Jackson, MI)*

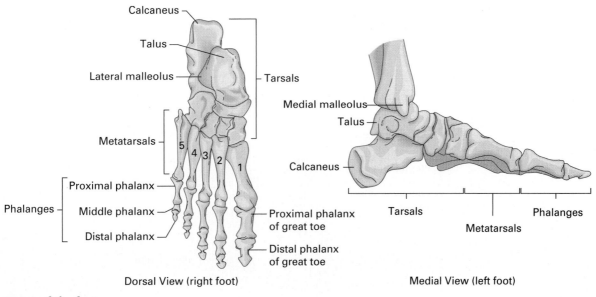

Dorsal View (right foot)   Medial View (left foot)

Bones of the foot

ANSWER COLUMN

	14.47
bones of the fingers and/or toes	Locate the phalang/es. They are the *_____ _____.
	14.48
phalang phalanx	The word root for phalanges is _____. The singular form of phalanges is _____.
	14.49
phalang/itis fal′ an **ji**′ tis phalang/ectomy fal′ an **jek**′ tə mē	Build words meaning inflammation of phalanges _____/_____; excision of a phalanx (singular) _____/_____.
	14.50
scapula	Locate the acromi/on process. It is a projection of the _____ (check a dictionary if necessary). **acromi/o** is the combining form.
	14.51
acromi/o	The combining form for the acromion is _____/_____.

Skeletal system

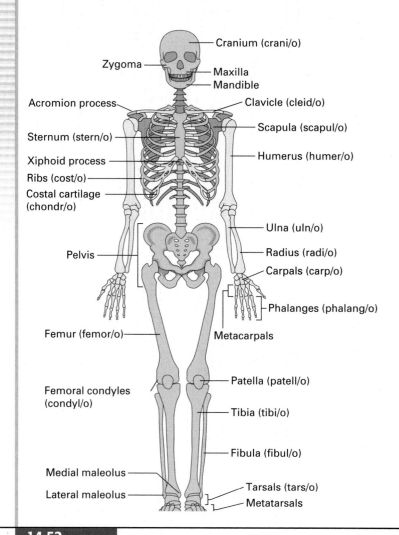

- Cranium (crani/o)
- Zygoma
- Maxilla
- Mandible
- Acromion process
- Clavicle (cleid/o)
- Sternum (stern/o)
- Scapula (scapul/o)
- Xiphoid process
- Humerus (humer/o)
- Ribs (cost/o)
- Costal cartilage (chondr/o)
- Ulna (uln/o)
- Pelvis
- Radius (radi/o)
- Carpals (carp/o)
- Phalanges (phalang/o)
- Femur (femor/o)
- Metacarpals
- Patella (patell/o)
- Femoral condyles (condyl/o)
- Tibia (tibi/o)
- Fibula (fibul/o)
- Medial maleolus
- Lateral maleolus
- Tarsals (tars/o)
- Metatarsals

14.52

Find words in your dictionary meaning
pertaining to the acromion
acromi/al _____/_____;
ə **krō**′ mē əl
acromi/o/humer/al pertaining to the acromion and humerus
ə krō′ mē ō **hyōō**′ mər əl _____/_____/humer/al;
acromi/o/clavicul/ar pertaining to the acromion and the clavicle
ə krō′ mē ō kla **vik**′ yōō lar _____/_____/_____/_____.

14.53

Look at Frame 14.52. Can it start you looking for another combining form?
humer/o Try. It is _____/_____.

ANSWER COLUMN

humerus	**14.54** **humer/o** is used in words to refer to the bone of the upper arm, which is named the _____.

14.55

(pick three of four)
humeral
humeroradial
humeroscapular
humeroulnar

Find three words in your dictionary that begin with humer or **humer/o**. They are

_____;

_____;

_____.

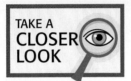

TAKE A
CLOSER
LOOK

14.56

Look up the term fracture in your medical dictionary. You should find at least ten different types of fractures described. Read about them and study the illustration of fractures. Notice that some are closed, some open, some complete, incomplete, displaced, and some not. Write the terms of interest in your notebook and then take a "break."

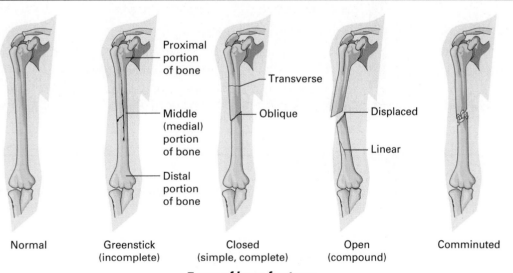

Proximal portion of bone

Transverse

Middle (medial) portion of bone

Oblique

Displaced

Linear

Distal portion of bone

Normal

Greenstick (incomplete)

Closed (simple, complete)

Open (compound)

Comminuted

Types of bone fractures

radi/o/ulnar
rā′ dē ō **ul**′ nar

14.57

The radius (**radi/o**) and ulna (**uln/o**) are located in the forearm.
If both are fractured, it would be described as a
_____/_____/_____ fracture.
(Abbreviation: FxBB, fracture of both bones.)

ANSWER COLUMN

14.58

Refer back to the drawing of the skeleton. Locate a condyle. A condyle is a rounded process that occurs on many bones. The word root for condyle

condyl

is _____.

14.59

INFORMATION FRAME

Falls, bumps, crashes, and disease that put stress on bones often cause cracks and breaks called fractures. Study the following table to learn about how these fractures are described. Then compare them to your notebook, dictionary research, and the illustration on page 491.

Fracture Facts	
complete	break through the width of the bone
incomplete	break not through the width of the bone
closed	[simple fracture] skin is not broken
open	[compound fracture] bone ends protrude through the skin
pathologic fracture	diseased area that weakens the bone
fracture reduction and fixation	
closed manipulation	movement of body part to cause bone ends to align without surgery
internal fixation	screws or nails in bone under the skin (ORIF)
external fixation	screws attached to an external bar (OREF)

14.60

Two rounded processes at the medial and lateral distal ends of the femur are

condyles
kon′ dīlz

the femoral _____.

14.61

In Latin *femur* means thigh. **femor/o** is the combining form for the longest bone in the body, the femur (thigh bone—notice the spelling). Look at the illustration

femur
fē′ mer
femor/al
fem′ er əl

of the skeleton. The proximal end of the _____ is part of the hip joint. The artery that supplies blood to the leg is called
the _____/_____ artery.

ANSWER COLUMN

SPELL CHECK ✓

14.62

Watch the spelling of fem*ur* as it changes to **femor/o** to make the combining form.

14.63

The tibia is the shin bone. Use **tibi/o** as the combining form. The fibula is a thin, long bone lateral to the tibia. Use **fibul/o** for the fibula. If both bones are broken in the same injury, it would be a _____/_____/_____ fracture.

tibi/o/fibular
ti′ bē ō **fib**′ yōo lär

14.64

One way to remember the location of the tibia and fibula is to think of the tibia aligned with the big toe (both start with t). The fibula is aligned with the little toe, and a little lie is a fib. In any case, the thicker shin bone on the big toe side is the _____ and the thinner, lower leg bone on the little toe side

is the _____.

tibia
ti′ bē ə
fibula
fib′ yōo la

14.65

A rounded bony process on any bone is a condyle.
Build words meaning
    excision of a condyle
    _____/_____;
    resembling a condyle
    _____/_____;
    upon a condyle
    _____/_____.

condyl/ectomy
kon′ di **lek**′ tə mē
condyl/oid
kon′ di loid
epi/condyle
ep i **kon**′ dil

14.66

Condyl/ar is an adjective meaning pertaining to a _____. The femoral _____ is a rounded end of the bone.

condyle
condyle

14.67

Locate the calcaneus bone (also calcaneum). The plural of calcaneus is _____.

calcanea
kal **kā**′ nē ə

14.68

calcane

From calcaneus and calcanea, derive the word root for the heel _____.

14.69

In your medical dictionary, look at the words beginning with calcane.
Derive the combining form that is used in words that refer to the heel:

calcane/o

_____/_____.

14.70

Close your dictionary. Now build words meaning
  pertaining to the heel

calcane/al
kal **kā**′ nē əl
calcane/o/dynia
kal kā′ nē ō **din**′ ē ə or
calcane/algia
kal kā nē **al**′ jē ə

_____/_____;

  pain in the heel

_____/_____/_____

  or

_____/_____.

14.71

The bones of the pelvis include the ischium, ilium, and pubis. Locate them
and their combining forms in the illustration below.
Write the combining forms below.

ischi/o
ili/o
pub/o

  ischium _____/_____
  ilium _____/_____
  pubis _____/_____

**Anterior view of bones of
the pelvis**

Sacrum (sacr/o) —
Sacroiliac joint
Iliac crest (ili/o)
Ilium (ili/o) —
Anterior superior
iliac spine
Coccyx (coccyg/o)
Acetabulum
Ischial spine (ischi/o) —
Obturator foramen
Ischium (ischi/o) —
Symphysis pubis (pub/o)

ANSWER COLUMN

14.72

It is easy to confuse ilium with ileum because they are pronounced the same and differ [in spelling] by only one letter. Remember i-l-**e**-um is part of the small intestine of the digestive system and the e reminds us of eat. The combining forms are also spelled differently, **ile/o** for ileum (small intestine) and **ili/o** for ilium (pelvic bone).

14.73

From what you have just learned, try this question. In which body system would you find the ile/o/cecal valve?

digestive system

_____

In which body system would you find the iliac crest?

skeletal system

_____

Good!

14.74

CONGRATULATIONS!

You are now finding your own combining forms. Feels good, doesn't it?
Let's do some more.

14.75

ischia
is′ kē ə

Locate the ischium. The plural of ischium is _____. Refer to the illustration of the pelvis.

14.76

ischi
ischi/o

From ischium and ischia, derive a word root that refers to the part of the hip bone on which the body rests when sitting. The word root is _____; the combining form is _____/_____.

14.77

In your dictionary, find words meaning
    pertaining to ischium and rectum

ischi/o/rect/al
is′ kē ō **rek**′ təl
ischi/o/neuralgia
is′ kē ō nōō **ral**′ jē ə
ischi/o/pub/ic
is′ kē ō **pyōō**′ bik

    _____/_____/_____/_____;
    neuralgic pain in the hip (synonym is sciatica)
    _____/_____/_____/_____;
    pertaining to the ischium and pubis
    _____/_____/_____/_____.

SPELL
CHECK ✓

14.78

Close your dictionary. Build words meaning
   pertaining to the ischium

ischi/al
is′ kē əl
ischi/o/cele
is′ kē ō sēl

   _____/_____;
herniation through the ischium
   _____/_____/_____.

14.79

ischi/o in a word refers to the part of the hip bone known as the

ischium
is′ kē ə m

   _____.

14.80

pubes
pyōo′ bēz
pub/o
supra/pub/ic
sōo pra **pyoo′** bik

Locate the pubis in the illustration of the pelvis. The plural of
pubis is _____.
The combining form is _____/_____.
A _____/_____/_____ incision is made above the pubis.

**Types of abdominal
incisions**

Subcostal

Epigastric;
midline

Paramedian

Transverse

Umbilical cord
incision for
scopes

Mc Burney

Suprapubic

Pfannnenstiel

14.81

Close your dictionary. Recall that **femor/o** is the combining form for femur. Using
pub/o and **femor/o**, build a word meaning pertaining to the pubis and femur:

pub/o/femor/al
pyōo bō **fem′** ər əl

   _____/_____/_____/_____.

ANSWER COLUMN

14.82

stern/o

Using the previous illustration of the skeletal system, locate the sternum.
The combining form for sternum is _____/_____.

14.83

With your dictionary open, find words meaning
   pertaining to the sternum and pericardium

stern/o/peri/cardi/al
stûr′ nō per i **kärd**′ ē əl
_____/_____/_____/_____/_____;
stern/o/cost/al
stûr′ nō **kos**′ təl
   pertaining to the sternum and ribs
_____/_____/_____/_____.

14.84

Close the dictionary. Build words meaning
   pertaining to the sternum

stern/al
_____/_____;
   pain in the sternum

stern/algia
_____/_____ or
stern/o/dynia
_____/_____/_____.
(You pronounce)

14.85

sternum
breastbone

stern/o in a word makes you think of the _____, which is the
_____.

14.86

Recall **cost/o** refers to ribs. The xiphoid (from the Greek *xiphos,* meaning sword)
process is the projection at the inferior end of the sternum. **xiph/o** is the
combining form. A word meaning pertaining to the xiphoid process and the ribs is

xiph/o/cost/al
zi′ fō **kos**′ təl
_____/_____/_____/_____.

14.87

The plural of gangli/on is gangli/a. A gangli/on is a collection of nerve cell bodies.
Now that you have a system, form the word root/combining form for ganglion:

gangli/o
_____/_____.

14.88

ganglia

The main cerebral nerve centers are called the cerebral _____.

ANSWER COLUMN

14.89

Any one of three neural masses found in the cervical region is called a cervical
_____/_____, whereas all three are referred to as the cervical
_____/____.

gangli/on
gangli/a

14.90

You are now ready to find word roots and their combining forms by another
method. Look up spine in your dictionary. A synonym for spine is
_____.

backbone

14.91

Look in your dictionary for words beginning with rach. rach is the word root for
_____.

spine

14.92

There are two word roots that mean spine. One is rach (**rachi/o**), the other is
spondyl (**spondyl/o**). Build a word that means inflammation of the spine:
_____/_____.

rach/itis
rə **kī**′ tis or
spondyl/itis
spon di **lī**′ tis

14.93

Words beginning with the combining forms **rachi/o** or **spondyl/o** refer to the
_____.

spine

14.94

Using **rachi/o**, build words meaning
   spine pain
   _____/_____;
   incision into the spine
   _____/____/_____.

rachi/algia
rā′ kē **al**′ jē ə
rachi/o/tomy
rā′ kē **ot**′ ō mē

14.95

Using **rachi/o**, build words meaning
   a synonym for rachialgia
   _____/____/_____;
   instrument to measure spinal curvature
   _____/____/_____;
   spinal paralysis
   _____/____/_____.

rachi/o/dynia
rā′ kē ō **din**′ ē ə
rachi/o/meter
rā′ kē **om**′ ə tər
rachi/o/plegia
rā′ kē ō **plē**′ jē ə

ANSWER COLUMN

Spinal column

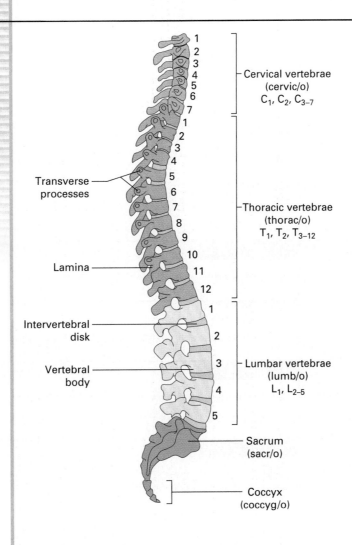

Cervical vertebrae
(cervic/o)
C_1, C_2, C_{3-7}

Transverse processes

Thoracic vertebrae
(thorac/o)
T_1, T_2, T_{3-12}

Lamina

Intervertebral disk

Vertebral body

Lumbar vertebrae
(lumb/o)
L_1, L_{2-5}

Sacrum
(sacr/o)

Coccyx
(coccyg/o)

14.96

In the same manner, using **rach/i**, build words meaning
   fissure of the spine (split spine)

rachi/schisis
rā **kis**′ kis is
rach/itis
rā **kī**′ tis

_____ / _____;
inflammation of the spine

_____ / _____.

14.97

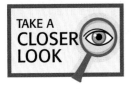

TAKE A
CLOSER
LOOK

The three basic types of spinal curvature are kyphosis (posterior curvature), lordosis (anterior curvature), and scoliosis (lateral curvature). Refer back to the illustration in Unit 12, on p. 433.

ANSWER COLUMN

The following word parts refer to regions of the spine.

Combining Form	Adjective
cervic/o	cervical
thorac/o	thoracic
lumb/o	lumbar
sacr/o	sacral
coccyg/o	coccygeal

14.98

cervical

A device used to immobilize the neck is a _____ collar.

14.99

neck

Cervic/al traction is applied as a treatment for an injured _____.

14.100

Recall that the cervix is the neck of the uterus. The plural of cervix is

cervices

_____.

14.101

cervic/o
sûr′ vi kō

Build a combining form for cervix. The combining form takes **o**.
The combining form is _____/_____.

14.102

Build words meaning
  excision of the cervix

cervic/ectomy
sûr′ vi **sek′** tō mē
cervic/itis
sûr′ vi **sī′** tis
cervic/al
sûr′ vi kəl

_____/_____;
  inflammation of the cervix
_____/_____;
  pertaining to the cervix
_____/_____.

14.103

INFORMATION
FRAME

cervic/o can mean the neck, the neck of the uterus as well as several other types of anatomic necks. In usage you are not likely to confuse them. The next frame will make the point. Refer to the previous illustration of the spinal column.

ANSWER COLUMN

	14.104
neck	Cervic/o/faci/al means pertaining to the face and _____.
neck	Cervic/o/brachi/al means pertaining to the arm and _____.
neck	Cervic/o/thoracic means pertaining to the chest and _____.

14.105

Study these phrases that refer to a necklike structure.
cervix of the axon—constriction between the cell body and the axon
cervix dentis—neck of the tooth
cervix uteri—neck of the uterus
cervix vesicae urinariae—neck of the urinary bladder

14.106

cervix
ser′ viks

In the previous phrases, the term that means neck is _____.

14.107

brachi/o is the combining form for arm. It is used to describe bones and blood
vessels in the arm. The biceps brachii is a muscle in the _____.

arm
arm

The brachial artery is an artery in the _____.

14.108

The muscle that extends from the upper arm to the radial bone is the
brachi/o/radi/alis
brā′ kē ō rā dē **al′** is   _____/____/_____/_____ muscle.

14.109

Build words that mean pertaining to the
   artery of the arm

brachi/al
brā′ kē əl   _____/_____;
brachi/o/radi/alis   arm and radius muscle
brā′ kē ō rā dē **al′** is   _____/____/_____/_____;
brachi/o/cephal/ic   arm and head
brā′ kē ō se **fal′** ik   _____/____/_____/_____.

14.110

The joint between the sacrum and the ilium is the
sacr/o/ili/ac   _____/____/_____/_____ joint.
sak rō **il′** ē ak

14.111

Build terms meaning
pertaining to the thorax and lumbar spines

thorac/o/lumbar
thôr′ ə kō **lum**′ bär

_____/_____/_____;
pertaining to the sacrum and the sciatic nerve

sacr/o/sciat/ic
sak′ rō sī **a**′ tik

_____/_____/_____/_____;
removal of the coccyx

coccyg/ectomy
kok′ si **jek**′ tō mē

_____/_____.

14.112

Provide the adjectival forms for

cervic/al
thorac/ic
sacr/al
coccyg/eal

cervix _____/_____;
thorax _____/_____;
sacrum _____/_____;
coccyx _____/_____.

14.113

A lamina (**lamin/o**) is a thin, flat sheet, plate, or membrane. A lamin/ectomy is the removal of the lamina of the vertebral posterior arch that has been ruptured (ruptured disk). One treatment to repair an intervertebral disk herniation may be

lamin/ectomy
lam′ in **ek**′ tō mē

_____/_____.

14.114

disk is the word root for intervertebral disk. A myel/o/gram (spinal x-ray) is used to diagnose disk herniation. Removal of a herniated disk is called a

disk/ectomy
dis **kek**′ tō mē
myel/o/gram
mī′ el ō gram

_____/_____ after which a spinal fusion may be performed. The x-ray that can be used to view the spine is a

_____/_____/_____.

***Herniated disk* with nerve root and spinal cord displaced by bulging disk** *(transverse section)*

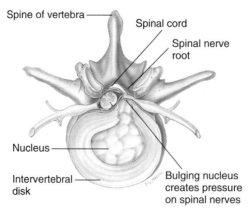

Spine of vertebra

Spinal cord

Spinal nerve root

Nucleus

Intervertebral disk

Bulging nucleus creates pressure on spinal nerves

ANSWER COLUMN

Abbreviation	Meaning
AMB	ambulate, ambulatory
AOTA	American Occupational Therapy Association
C_1, C_2, C_{3-7}	cervical vertebrae 1–7
DPM	podiatrist (doctor of podiatric medicine)
Fx	fracture
FxBB	fracture of both bones
hs	hour of sleep (*hora somni*), at bedtime
L_1, L_2, L_{3-5}	lumbar vertebrae 1–5
LP	lumbar puncture
lt, L	left
OREF	open reduction external fixation
ORIF	open reduction internal fixation
ORTH	orthopedist, orthopedics
OTR	registered occupational therapist
rt, R	right
T_1, T_2, T_{3-12}	thoracic vertebrae 1–12
y/o, yr	year(s) old, year(s)

To complete your study of this unit, work the **Review Activities** on the following pages. Also listen to the audio CDs that accompany *Medical Terminology: A Programmed Systems Approach,* 9th edition, and practice your pronunciation.

Additional practice exercises for this unit are available on the Learner Practice CD-ROM found in the back of the textbook.

REVIEW ACTIVITIES

CIRCLE AND CORRECT

Circle the correct answer for each question. Then, check your answers in Appendix A.

1. Combining form for night
   a. narco
   b. necro
   c. nycto
   d. noct

2. Suffix meaning in the urine
   a. -uro
   b. -uremia
   c. -urine
   d. -uria

REVIEW ACTIVITIES

3. Word root for immovable or fixed
   a. syn
   b. ankyl
   c. stasis
   d. spondyl

4. Noun ending
   a. -ia
   b. -ic
   c. -ous
   d. -ed

5. Prefix for inward
   a. exo-
   b. meso-
   c. inner-
   d. eso-

6. Suffix for split
   a. -stasis
   b. -schiz
   c. -schisis
   d. -schist

7. Adjectival form for wrist bones
   a. carpi
   b. carpal
   c. carpus
   d. metacarpal

8. Combining form for one of the pelvic bones
   a. ischium
   b. ileo
   c. ilio
   d. ishci

9. Word root for walk
   a. somn
   b. duct
   c. kines
   d. ambul

10. Suffix for control or stopping
    a. -rrhexis
    b. -stasis
    c. -schisis
    d. -ectasis

11. Bony process at the end of the sternum
    a. amnion
    b. acromion
    c. xiphoid
    d. phalanx

12. Combining form for spine
    a. rachi/o
    b. spondyl
    c. myel/o
    d. ischi/o

SELECT AND CONSTRUCT

Select the correct word parts from the following list and construct medical terms that represent the given meaning.

acromi/o(on)	al	algia	ambul/o/ism	ankylo	ar
arteri/o	ate	brachi/o(al)	calcane/o	carp(o)(al)	cephalic
cervic/o(al)	choudr/o	clavicul/o(ar)	condyl/o(ar)	cost/o(al)	dactyl/ia/o
dynia	ectomy	femor/o	fibul/o	fungi	humer/o(al)
ili/o	ischi/o	ism	itis	meta	myco
noct/i	nyct/o	opia	palat/o	patell/o	phasi/o(ia)
pub(o)(is)(ic)	rachi/o	scapul/o(ar)	schisis	schizo	som n/o/ia
stasis	stern/o(al)	tars/o	tomy	urano	uria
xiph/o(oid)					

1. breast bone pain _____

2. pertaining to the arm and head _____

3. control of fungal growth _____

4. including the ischium and pubis _____

5. excision of a rounded bony process _____

6. split spine (spina bifida) _____

7. cleft palate _____

8. pertaining to the cartilage end of the sternum and the ribs _____

REVIEW ACTIVITIES

9. the bones of the hand beyond the wrist   _____

10. split speech (incomprehensible)   _____

11. sleepwalking   _____

12. night blindness   _____

13. excessive urination at night   _____

14. stiffened fingers   _____

15. pertaining to the ilium   _____

16. pertaining to the pubis   _____

17. pertaining to the thighbone   _____

18. pertaining to the kneecap   _____

19. pertaining to the fibula   _____

20. the bones of the ankle   _____

21. the bones of the foot (not toes)   _____

22. the heel bone   _____

23. the ribs   _____

24. pertaining to cartilage   _____

FIND THE FORM

Give the correct combining form and adjectival form for each of the following bones.

	Combining Form	Adjectival Form
skull	1. _____	_____
first seven vertebrae	2. _____	_____
clavicle	3. _____	_____
scapula	4. _____	_____
acromion process	5. _____	_____
humerus	6. _____	_____
sternum	7. _____	_____
xiphoid process	8. _____	_____
ulna	9. _____	_____
radius	10. _____	_____
carpus	11. _____	_____
metacarpus	12. _____	_____
phalanx	13. _____	_____
ischium	14. _____	_____
ilium	15. _____	_____

REVIEW ACTIVITIES

	Combining Form	Adjectival Form
pubis	16. _____	_____
femur	17. _____	_____
patella	18. _____	_____
tibia	19. _____	_____
fibula	20. _____	_____
tarsus	21. _____	_____
metatarsus	22. _____	_____
calcaneus	23. _____	_____
ribs	24. _____	_____
cartilage	25. _____	_____

DEFINE AND DISSECT

Give a brief definition, and dissect each term listed into its word parts in the space provided. Check your answers by referring to the frame listed in parentheses and your medical dictionary. Then listen to the CDs to practice pronunciation.

1. noctambulism (14.5)

_____ / _____ / _____
rt   rt   suffix

_____
definition

2. nyctalopia (14.11)

_____ / _____ / _____
rt   rt   suffix

_____

3. somnambulism (14.6)

_____ / _____ / _____
rt   rt   suffix

_____

4. ankylodactylia (14.21)

_____ / _____ / _____ / _____
rt   v   rt   suffix

_____

5. nycturia (14.16)

_____ / _____ / _____
rt   rt   suffix

_____

6. enterostasis (14.26)

_____ / _____ / _____
rt   v   suffix

_____

REVIEW ACTIVITIES

7. schizophrenia (14.30)

_____/_____/_____

       pre   rt   suffix

8. schistosomiasis (14.35)

_____/____/_____

       pre   rt   suffix

9. palatoschisis (14.33)

_____/____/_____

     rt   v   suffix

10. calcaneodynia (14.70)

_____/____/_____

     rt   v   suffix

11. carpometacarpal (14.41)

_____/____/_____/____/____

     rt   v   pre   rt suffix

12. ischioneuralgia (14.77)

_____/____/____/____

     rt   v   rt   suffix

13. sternopericardial (14.83)

_____/____/_____/_____/____

   rt   v   pre   rt   suffix

14. acromiohumeral (14.52)

_____/____/_____/____

     rt   v   rt   suffix

15. epicondyle (14.65)

____/_____

     pre   rt/suffix

16. ganglion (14.87)

_____/____

        rt   suffix

17. xiphocostal (14.86)

_____/____/_____/____

     rt   v   rt   suffix

REVIEW ACTIVITIES

18. laminectomy (14.113)

_____/_____
rt   suffix

_____

19. diskectomy (14.114)

_____/_____
rt   suffix

_____

20. fungistasis (14.24)

_____/_____/_____
rt   v   suffix

_____

21. rachischisis (14.96)

_____/_____
rt   suffix

_____

22. antipsychotic (14.31)

_____/_____/_____
pre   rt   suffix

_____

23. metatarsal (14.44)

_____/_____/_____
pre   rt   suffix

_____

24. radioulnar (14.57)

_____/_____/_____/_____
rt   v   rt   suffix

_____

25. pubofemoral (14.81)

_____/_____/_____/_____
rt   v   rt   suffix

_____

26. cervicobrachial (14.104)

_____/_____/_____/_____
rt   v   rt   suffix

_____

27. tibiofibular (14.63)

_____/_____/_____/_____
rt   v   rt   suffix

_____

REVIEW ACTIVITIES

ART LABELING

Label the structures of the skeleton by writing the number in front of the correct word part and write the body part indicated.

_____	xiph/o	_____
_____	condyl/o	_____
_____	femor/o	_____
_____	cleid/o	_____
_____	phalang/o	_____
_____	carp/o	_____
_____	radi/o	_____
_____	humer/o	_____
_____	cost/o	_____
_____	scapul/o	_____
_____	uln/o	_____
_____	metatars/o	_____
_____	tibi/o	_____
_____	fibul/o	_____
_____	vertebr/o	_____
_____	stern/o	_____
_____	crani/o	_____
_____	ili/o	_____
_____	ischi/o	_____
_____	patell/o	_____

REVIEW ACTIVITIES

ABBREVIATION MATCHING

Match the following abbreviations with their definition.

_____ 1. ORTH   a. noctambulism

_____ 2. FxBB   b. first thoracic vertebra

_____ 3. hs   c. fracture

_____ 4. AMB   d. orthodontist

_____ 5. LP   e. bedtime

_____ 6. L_1 f. fracture of both bones

_____ 7. Fx   g. ambulate

_____ 8. T_3 h. first lumbar vertebra

       i. twice a night

       j. long-playing record

       k. lumbar puncture

       l. orthopedist

       m. third thoracic vertebra

ABBREVIATION FILL-INS

Fill in the blanks with the correct abbreviation.

9. third cervical vertebra _____

10. fracture of both bones _____

11. registered occupational therapist _____

12. American Occupational Therapy Association _____

13. right _____

14. years old _____

15. open reduction internal fixation _____

CASE STUDIES

Write the term next to its meaning given below. Then draw slashes to analyze the word parts. Note the use of medical abbreviations. Look these up in your dictionary or find them in Appendix B. If you have any questions about the answers, refer to your medical dictionary or check with your instructor for the answers in Appendix A.

REVIEW ACTIVITIES

CASE STUDY 14-1

Operative Report

Pt: **M**, 15 **y/o**

Dx: **Fracture lateral** condyle, **right** elbow

Procedure: Open **reduction, internal fixation** of fracture. Carl Cracken was **anesthetized**; the skin was prepped with Betadine, **sterile** drapes were applied, and the **pneumatic** tourniquet inflated around the right arm. An **incision** was made around the area of the lateral **epicondyle** through a Steri-drape, and this was carried through **subcutaneous** tissue, and the fracture site was easily exposed. **Inspection** revealed the fragment to be rotated in two planes about 90 degrees. It was possible to **manually** reduce this quite easily, judicious manipulation resulted in an almost **anatomic** reduction. This was fixed with two pins driven across the **humerus**. These pins were cut off below skin level. The wound was closed with some plain catgut subcutaneously and 5-0 nylon in the skin. Dressings were applied to Mr. Cracken and the tourniquet released. A long arm cast was applied. The patient was transfered to **PAR** in good condition.

1. looking _____

2. using the hands _____

3. toward the side _____

4. cut into _____

5. free of microorganisms _____

6. below the skin _____

7. pertaining to body structures _____

8. inside _____

9. Fx _____

10. uses air (adjective) _____

11. made to have no sensation _____

12. surgery to restore position _____

13. hold in place _____

14. upon the condyle _____

15. upper arm bone _____

16. male _____

17. years old _____

18. Rt _____

19. Post Anesthesia Recovery _____

REVIEW ACTIVITIES

CROSSWORD PUZZLE

Check your answers by going back through the frames or checking the solutions in Appendix C.

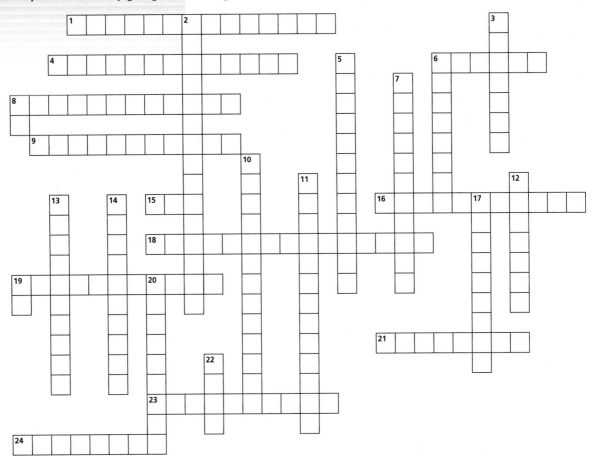

Across

1. including the upper arm bone and the shoulder blades
4. severe mental disorder with hallucinations
6. __ tunnel syndrome
8. synonym for spina bifida cystica
9. excision of herniated lamina of a disk
15. podiatrist (abbreviation)
16. foot bones beyond the tarsals
18. muscle from upper arm to radius bone
19. synonym for mycostasis
21. group of nerve cell bodies
23. night blindness
24. walk (verb)

Down

2. sleeping sickness caused by a liver fluke
3. process at the end of the sternum
5. sleepwalking
6. plural for heel bone
7. physician specialist in skeletal disorders
8. right (abbreviation)
10. pertaining to neck and face
11. cleft palate
12. bone you sit on
13. pain in the breast bone
14. stop blood flow
17. condition of stiffening
19. fracture (abbreviation)
20. vehicle for emergency transport
22. orthopedist (abbreviation)

REVIEW ACTIVITIES

GLOSSARY

acromioclavicular	joint between the collar bone and the acromion process	cervical	pertaining to the neck, neck of the uterus, other necklike structure
acromiohumeral	joint between the acromion process and the humerus	cervicectomy	excision of the cervix of the uterus
acromion	the bony projection on the scapula at the humeroscapular joint	cervicitis	inflammation of the cervix of the uterus
ambulance	vehicle used to transport patients	cervicobrachial	pertaining to the neck and arm
ambulatory	able to walk, walking (ambulate)	cervicofacial	pertaining to the neck and the face
ankyloblepharon	stiffened, adhered eyelids	cholestasis	control of bile flow
ankylocheilia	stiffened lips	condyle, condylar	a rounded process on a bone end
ankylodactylia	stiff, immovable fingers and toes	condylectomy	excision of a condyle
ankyloglossia	tongue tied (stiff tongue)	condyloid	resembling a condyle
ankylophobia	abnormal fear of ankylosis	diskectomy	excision of herniated intervertebral disk (discectomy)
ankyloproctia	closure (immobility) of the anus and rectum	enterostasis	control of intestinal flow
ankylosis	condition of stiffening, loss of mobility	epicondyle	upon a condyle
arteriostasis	control of arterial flow	femur, femoral	the thigh bone
brachial	pertaining to the arm	fibula	small, long bone in lower leg lateral to tibia
brachiocephalic	pertaining to the arm and head	fungistasis	control or stop growth of a fungus (mycostasis)
brachioradialis	muscle that extends from the upper arm to the radial bone	ganglion	a collection of nerve cell bodies
calcaneodynia	heel pain (calcanealgia)	hemostasis	control of blood flow (hematostasis)
calcaneum, calcaneus, calcanea	heel bone	humeroradial	pertaining to the humerus and the radius
carpi, carpus, carpal	wrist bones	humeroscapular	pertaining to the humerus and the scapula

REVIEW ACTIVITIES

humeroulnar	pertaining to the humerus and the ulna
ileum	third part of the small intestine
ilium	upper pelvic bone
ischiocele	herniation through the ischial bone
ischioneuralgia	pain in the nerves near the ischium (sciatica)
ischiopubic	pertaining to the ischium and the pubis
ischiorectal	pertaining to the ischium and the rectum
laminectomy	excision of the lamina of the vertebral posterior arch
metacarpi	hand bones distal to the carpi
metatarsals	foot bones distal to the tarsals
noctambulism	sleepwalking (somnambulism)
nyctalbuminuria	excretion of albumin in urine at night
nyctalgia	pain during the night
nyctalopia	night blindness
nyctophobia	abnormal fear of the night (noctiphobia)
nycturia	excessive urination during the night (nocturia)
palatoschisis	cleft palate (uranoschisis)
phlebostasis	control of venous flow
pubofemoral	pertaining to the pubic bone and the femur
pyostasis	control of pus formation
rachialgia	spinal pain (rachiodynia)
rachiometer	instrument to measure spinal curvature

rachioplegia	spinal paralysis
rachischisis	split spine (spina bifida cystica)
rachitis	inflammation of the spine (spondylitis)
radioulnar	pertaining to the radius and the ulna
scapula	shoulder blade
schistoglossia	split tongue (fissure)
schistosomiasis	infestation with *Schistosoma* (*mansoni, japonicum, haematobium*) flukes
schizonychia	split finger nails or toenails
schizophasia	split speech (incomprehensible)
schizophrenia	severe mental disorder in which thinking, emotions, and behavior are disturbed (includes paranoia, hallucination, delusion, persecution, and jealousy)
sternalgia	sternal pain (sternodynia)
sternopericardial	pertaining to the sternum and the pericardium
tarsi, tarsus, tarsal	bones of the ankle (not including the tibia)
tibia	shin bone, medial to fibula
tibiofibular	pertaining to the tibia and fibula
viscerostasis	control of an organ
xiphocostal	pertaining to the xiphoid process and the ribs
xiphoid (process)	cartilage bony projection on the distal end of the sternum

UNIT 15

Ophthalmology, Endocrinology, and Medical Specialties

ANSWER COLUMN	
	15.1
inflammation of the eye pertaining to the eye	**ophthalm/o** is used in words to mean eye. Ophthalm/itis means * _____. Ophthalm/ic means * _____. NOTE: Ocular also means pertaining to the eye.
	15.2
pain in the eye	Ophthalm/algia and ophthalm/o/dynia both mean * _____.
	15.3
SPELL CHECK ✓ ophthalmic off **thal**′ mik	Watch your spelling on this one. Before building words with this root, be sure you have the phth order of **ophthalm/o** straight. Pronounce it: off **thal**′ mō
	15.4
ophthalm/o/ptosis or off thal′ mop **tō**′ sis exophthalmos eks of **thal**′ mōs ophthalm/o/meter of′ thal **mom**′ ə ter	Build words meaning herniation of an eye (abnormal herniation or protrusion) _____/_____/_____; instrument for measuring the eye (curvature of the cornea) _____/_____/_____.

515

ANSWER COLUMN

Lateral view of eyeball interior

Ciliary body and muscle (cycl/o)
Suspensory ligament
Conjunctiva (conjunctiv/o)
Iris (irid/o)
Pupil (core/o)
Path of light
Anterior chamber (aqueous humor)
Cornea (corne/o) (kerat/o)
Lens (phac/o)
Posterior chamber (vitreous humor)

Retina (retin/o)
Retinal arteries and veins
Fovea centralis (fone/o)
Optic nerve
Choroid coat
Sclera (scler/o)

15.5

Build words meaning
   any ocular disease

opthalm/o/pathy
of' thal **mop**' ə thē

_____/_____/_____;

ophthalm/o/plasty
of **thal**' mō plas tē

plastic surgery of the eye

_____/_____/_____;

ophthalm/o/plegia
of' thal mō **plē**' jē ə

paralysis of the eye (muscles)

_____/_____/_____.

15.6

Ophthalm/o/logy is the medical specialty studying eye disease and surgery of the eye. We call the physician who practices this specialty an

ophthalm/o/logist
of' thal **mol**' ō jist

_____/_____/_____.

15.7

Ophthalm/o/scopy is the examination of the interior of the eye.
The instrument used for this examination is an

ophthalm/o/scope
of **thal**' mō skōp
ophthalm/o/scopy
of' thal **mos**' kō pē

_____/_____/_____.

The process of performing an examination of the eye with a scope is

_____/_____/_____.

ANSWER COLUMN

The following table analyzes word parts pertaining to the eye and vision.

Word Part	Use
op/ia	suffix for vision
opt/ic	adjective—pertaining to vision
opt/o	combining form for vision
ophthalm/o	combining form for eye
ophthalm/ic	adjective—pertaining to eye

15.8

opt/o refers to vision. Use **opt/o** to build words meaning

one who measures visual acuity

_____/_____/_____;

the cranial nerve for vision (adjective)

_____/_____;

the measurement of vision (practice of assessing vision disorders)

_____/_____/_____.

NOTE: In some areas optometrists are licensed to treat eye disease and prescribe medications.

opt/o/metrist
op′ **tom**′ ə trist
opt/ic
op′ tik
opt/o/metry
op **tom**′ e trē

PROFESSIONAL PROFILES

Certified **ophthalmic assistants (COAs)**, **technicians (COTs)**, and **medical technologists (COMTs)** play an important role in assisting ophthalmologists by assessing visual acuity, performing diagnostic tests (e.g., glaucoma screening), assisting with minor and major ophthalmic surgical procedures, and providing patient education. The Joint Commission on Allied Health Personnel in Ophthalmology (JCAHPO) is the certifying agency for ophthalmic medical personnel.

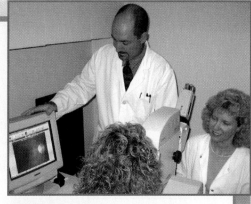

Ophthalmic technician preparing patient for exam

ANSWER COLUMN

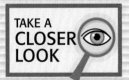

TAKE A
CLOSER
LOOK

15.9

Notice the difference between the following
ophthalmologist—physician (MD or DO) specialist in treating diseases of the eye
and performing surgery; and
optometrist—licensed practitioner (OD) limited to eye examinations and
prescribing corrective lenses.
Both are called doctor, having received doctorate degrees from schools of
medicine or optometry.

15.10

ophthalm/ic
of **thal**′ mik

A special technician who assists ophthalmologists with eye exams and helps fit
corrective lenses is called a certified _____/_____ technician
(COT).

15.11

Recall word roots indicating colors. **-opia** is a suffix denoting vision.
Cyan/opia is a defect in vision that causes objects to appear blue.
Form words meaning
   yellow vision

xanth/opia
zan **thō**′ pē ə
chlor/opia
klor **ō**′ pē ə
erythr/opia
er i **thrō**′ pē ə

_____/_____ ;
   green vision
_____/_____ ;
   red vision
_____/_____ .

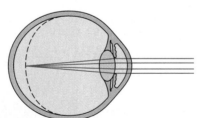

Myopia (nearsightedness)
Light rays focus in front
of the retina

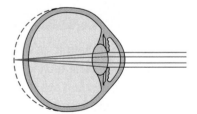

Hyperopia (farsightedness)
Light rays focus beyond
the retina

15.12

nearsightedness
farsightedness
loss of accommodation
double vision

Look up the following terms and note the type of vision they describe.
my/opia _____;
hyper/opia _____;
presby/opia *_____;
dipl/opia *_____.

ANSWER COLUMN

15.13

heart
double
double

diplo- means double. Diplo/cardia means having a double _____.
Diplo/genesis means production of _____ parts
or _____ substances.

15.14

dipl/opia
dip **lō′** pē ə

-opia is an involved form that we can use as a suffix. **-opia** means vision.
Build a word meaning double vision: _____/_____.

15.15

diplopia

There are many kinds of diplopia. Crossed eyes causes one kind of
_____.

15.16

diplopia

When both eyes fail to record the same image on the brain,
_____ occurs.

15.17

-opia

If you can see close objects but not distant ones, you may have my/opia or close
vision. Presby/opia is experienced by older people as a loss of accommodation by
the lens. The word literally means old vision. In each of these terms the suffix for
vision is _____.

15.18

both

ambi- means both or both sides. Ambi/later/al means pertaining to
_____ sides.

15.19

both

An ambi/dextr/ous person can work well with _____ hands.

15.20

ambi/opia
am bē **ō′** pē ə

A word that means both eyes (OU—both eyes) forming separate images (vision)
is _____/_____.
NOTE: Ambiopia is a term not commonly used in optometry.

15.21

dipl/opia
(You pronounce)

dipl- and **diplo-** are prefixes meaning double. The result of separate vision from
both eyes is a double image or double vision. Medically, double vision can be
expressed as _____/_____.

NOTE: **diplo-** and **ambi-** are combining forms used as prefixes.

ANSWER COLUMN

my/opia
mī **ō**′ pē ə

15.22

Hyper/opia means farsightedness (able to focus on objects at a distance). The opposite of hyperopia is nearsightedness, or _____/_____.

ambi/valence
am **biv**′ ə ləns
ambi/valent
am **biv**′ ə lənt

15.23

Look up ambivalence in any dictionary. Read its meaning. Analyze this word and the word ambivalent.

_____/_____

_____/_____

diplo/coccus
dip lō **kok**′ əs

15.24

Recall that a diplo/bacillus is a bacillus that occurs in pairs. A coccus that grows in pairs is a _____/_____.

TAKE A CLOSER LOOK

15.25

Light travels through the lens of the eye, it is refracted, and an image is focused on the retina. **-opter** is a suffix meaning visible. A di/opter (Greek: *dia*, meaning through, and *optos*, meaning that which sees) is a unit of measurement of refraction in the eye.

di/opter
dī′ op ter

15.26

Glasses or contact lenses are used to correct myopia, hyperopia, or presbyopia. A prescription written for corrective lenses that reads OS + 1 D means left eye one _____/_____.

dia/scope
dī′ ə skōp

15.27

A micr/o/scope is an instrument for examining something small. An instrument used for examining (looking) through is a _____/_____.

dia-

15.28

A diascope is a glass plate held against the skin. The skin is examined through the diascope to see superficial lesions (erythematous and others). The prefix for through is _____.

ANSWER COLUMN

15.29

WORD ORIGINS

Tropia is from the Greek *tropē* meaning turning. In ophthalmology, when the eyes appear to be turned in an abnormal position while open, it is referred to as a strabismus or squint. The medical terms used indicating the eye position include exo/tropia, eso/tropia, hyper/tropia, hypo/tropia, and cyclo/tropia.

15.30

exo/tropia
eks ō **trō**′ pē ə
eso/tropia
es ō **trō**′ pē ə
hyper/tropia
hī per **trō**′ pē ə
hypo/tropia
hī pō **trō**′ pē ə

exo- means outward. **eso-** means toward. **hypo-** means downward. **hyper-** means upward. From what you have just learned, build words that mean

eyes pointing outward

_____/_____;

eyes pointing inward

_____/_____;

eyes pointing upward

_____/_____;

eyes pointing downward

_____/_____.

Good!

15.31

upward
downward
inward
outward

Write the abnormal direction of the eye positions indicated below

hypertropia _____

hypotropia _____

esotropia _____

exotropia _____

15.32

hypo/tropia
hī pō **trō**′ pē ə

Hyper/tropia results when an eye muscle moves one eye upward. When one eye turns downward, we call it _____/_____.

15.33

strabismus
stra **bis**′ mus
or squint

Another term for exotropia, esotropia, hypertropia, and hypotropia is

_____.

15.34

eu/phoria
yoō **fôr**′ ē ə

phor(ia) means to carry or bear. Dys/phoria means a feeling of depression—you carry with you an ill (bad) feeling. The word that means feeling of well-being is

_____/_____.

ANSWER COLUMN

15.35

euphoria

When your diet is good, you have enough rest, and the world is a wonderful place in which to be, you are enjoying a state of _____.

OD right eye   OS left eye

Esotropia   **Exotropia**

15.36

phor/opt/er
for **op**′ ter
phor/o/meter
fôr **om**′ ə tər
di/opter
dī **op**′ ter

A phor/opt/er is an instrument used to determine the prescription strength needed for corrective lenses. An optometrist may use a
_____/_____/_____.
The instrument that measures the tone and pull of the eye-moving (bearing) muscles is a _____/_____/_____.

The unit measure for vision is the _____/_____.

15.37

blephar/o

Blephar/o/ptosis means prolapse of an eyelid. The combining form for eyelid is
_____/_____.

15.38

eyelid
eyelid

Edema is swelling due to fluid retention. Blepharedema means swelling of the _____. blephar/o seen anywhere makes you think of the _____.

15.39

WORD ORIGINS

The word edema is related to the name of the Greek tragic hero Oedipus the king. Oedipus comes from the Greek verb *oidein* (to become swollen) and literally translated means swollen foot. After a bizarre series of events, Oedipus kills his father and marries his own mother. Freud named his Oedipus complex theory after this story. The oe in Oedipus was later changed to e, and the modern English medical term became edema: Edema/tous is the adjectival form.

15.40

blephar/itis
blef′ ə **rī**′ tis

Blephar/edema means swelling of the eyelid. Build words that mean
  inflammation of an eyelid
  _____/_____;

ANSWER COLUMN

blephar/otomy
blef′ ə **rot**′ ə mē

incision of an eyelid

_____/_____.

15.41

Build words that mean
excision of lesions on the eyelid

_____/_____;

blephar/ectomy
blef′ ər **ek**′ tō mē

surgical repair of an eyelid

_____/_____/_____;

blephar/o/plasty
blef′ ə rō plas tē

twitching of an eyelid

_____/_____/_____;

blephar/o/spasm
blef′ ə rō spaz əm

prolapse of an eyelid (droopy eyelid)

_____/_____/_____;

blephar/o/ptosis
blef′ ər op **tō**′ sis

suture of the eyelid

_____/_____/_____.

blephar/o/rrhaphy
blef′ ər **or**′ ə fē

15.42

The conjunctiva is the membrane that lines the eyelids (palpebral conjunctiva) and the sclera (ocular conjunctiva). Look up conjunctivitis in your dictionary. There are over thirty types of inflammation of the conjunctiva or

conjunctiv/itis
kon junk′ ti **vī**′ tis

_____/_____.

15.43

Look up cornea in your dictionary. Look at the words that begin with corne.

corne/o

A combining form for cornea is _____/_____. Look at the illustration of the eye on page 516.

Write the meaning and analyze by inserting the slashes for the following terms:
corneal

corne/al, cornea
kôr′ nē əl

_____/_____, _____;
                                        meaning

corneoiritis

corne/o/ir/itis, pertaining
to the cornea and iris,
kôr′ nē ō ī **rī**′ tis

_____/_____/_____/_____, _____;
                                              meaning

corneoscleral

corne/o/scler/al, pertaining
to the cornea and sclera
kôr′ nē ō **sklir**′ əl

_____/_____/_____/_____, _____.
                                              meaning

15.44

From the preceding frame identify two word roots that mean iris and sclera.
They are _____ and _____.

ir, scler

15.45

Locate the lens. **phac/o** is the combining form for the crystalline lens of the eye.
Recall that **-cele** is used for herniation or dislocation. Build a word that means
dislocation of the lens: _____/_____/_____.

phac/o/cele
fā′ kō sēl

15.46

WORD
ORIGINS

The lens is shaped like a lentil. In Greek, *phacos* means lentil. Lentils have a
biconvex shape just like the crystalline lens of the eye.

15.47

Cataracts are opacities of the lens of the eye. Cataracts can be treated with an
ultrasonic device to emulsify the lens for removal.
This procedure is called _____/_____ emulsification.

phac/o
fā′ kō

NOTE: Phacoemulsification is part of a lens implant surgical procedure.

15.48

TAKE A
CLOSER
LOOK

Look up the first word in your dictionary beginning with scler.
It is _____. Read about the sclera.
Does the word root plus the Greek word *scleras*,
meaning hard, from which it is derived, suggest an already
familiar combining form to you?
It is _____/_____/_____, which means
*_____.
(Remember sclerosis.)

sclera
sklir′ ə
scler/o/sis
condition of hardness

15.49

The sclera of the eye is the white, "hard" outer coat of the eye.
Build words meaning
   pertaining to the sclera (adjective)
   _____/_____;
   excision of the sclera (or part)
   _____/_____;

scler/al
sklair′ əl
scler/ectomy
sklair **ek′** tə mē

ANSWER COLUMN

scler/o/stomy
sklair **os**′ tə mē
scler/itis
sklair **ī**′ tis

formation of an opening into the sclera

_____ / _____ / _____ ;

inflammation of the sclera

_____ / _____ .

15.50

Look at the diagram of the eye on page 527. The colored part of the eye is the

iris
ī′ ris

_____ .

15.51

TAKE A CLOSER LOOK

Look up iris in your dictionary. ir and irid are word roots for the iris. **ir/o** and **irid/o** are both combining forms for iris. ir has limited use, usually with **-itis**, indicating inflammation of the iris. Also, look up the plural form of iris.

15.52

With the information in Frame 15.51 and the word root you found,
build words meaning

    inflammation of the iris

ir/itis

_____ / _____ ;

    inflammation of the cornea and iris

corne/o/ir/itis

_____ / ____ / _____ / _____ ;

    inflammation of the sclera and iris

scler/o/ir/itis
(You pronounce)

_____ / ____ / _____ / _____ .

15.53

You may have found in your dictionary the plural of iris.

ir/ides
ir′ i dēz, **ī**′ ri dēz
irid/o

It is _____ / _____ .

The combining form for iris is _____ / _____ .

15.54

Using **irid/o**, build words meaning

    protrusion of the iris (dislocation)

irid/o/cele
i **rid**′ ō sēl (ī **rid**′ ō sel)
irid/algia
ir′ i **dal**′ jē ə (ī ri **dal**′ jē ə)
irid/ectomy
ir′ i **dek**′ tə mē
(ī′ ri **dek**′ tə mē)

_____ / ____ / _____ ;

    pain in the iris

_____ / _____ ;

    excision of part or all of the iris

_____ / _____ .

15.55

Build words meaning (you insert the slashes)
  prolapse of the iris

irid/o/ptosis
ī′ rid op **tō**′ sis
    _____;

irid/o/malacia
ī′ rid ō mal **ā**′ shə
  softening of the iris

    _____;

irid/o/rrhexis
ī′ rid ō **rek**′ sis
  rupture of the iris

    _____.

15.56

The two words to express paralysis of the iris are

irid/o/plegia
ī rid ō **plē**′ jē ə
    _____/_____/_____ and

irid/o/paralysis
ī rid ō pə **ral**′ ə sis
    _____/_____/_____.

15.57

The following forms make you think of

iris   ir _____
iris   **irid/o** _____
sclera (hard) **scler/o** _____
cornea   **corne/o** _____

15.58

Look up retina in your dictionary. Read about the retina and look at the words beginning with retin in your dictionary. The combining form for words about the

retin/o   retina is _____/_____.

15.59

Build words meaning
  pertaining to the retina

retin/al
ret′ i nəl
    _____/_____;

retin/itis
ret i **nī**′ tis
  inflammation of the retina

    _____/_____;

retin/o/pexy or
ret′ i nō pek sē
  fixation of a detached retina (repair)

retin/o/plasty
ret′ i nō **plas**′ tē
    _____/_____/_____.

ANSWER COLUMN

15.60

The instrument used to examine the refractive error of the eye (retina) is the
_____/_____/_____.

retin/o/scope
ret′ i nō skōp
retin/o/scopy
ret i **nos**′ kə pē

The process of using a
retinoscope is _____/_____/_____.

NOTE: The proper term for retinoscopy is skiascopy. Look it up!

15.61

INFORMATION FRAME

Glaucoma is disease of the eye in which the intraocular pressure is increased.
If glaucoma is not treated, the person will become blind. The three basic types
of glaucoma are open angle, angle closure, and congenital.

15.62

One part of a complete eye exam includes checking the intraocular pressure.
This is done to look for signs of _____.

glaucoma
glou **cō**′ ma

External structures of the right eye

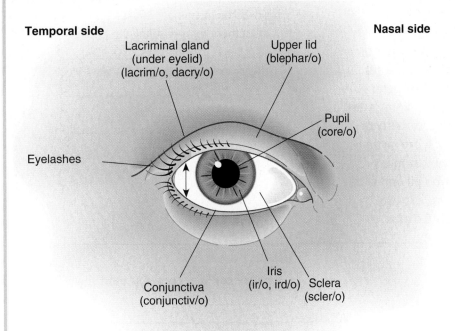

Temporal side   Nasal side

Lacriminal gland
(under eyelid)
(lacrim/o, dacry/o)

Upper lid
(blephar/o)

Pupil
(core/o)

Eyelashes

Conjunctiva
(conjunctiv/o)

Iris
(ir/o, ird/o)

Sclera
(scler/o)

RIGHT EYE

ANSWER COLUMN

<table>
<tr><td></td><td></td></tr>
</table>

INFORMATION
FRAME

15.63

The pupil in the eye is the opening in the iris through which light passes.
Identify the pupil in the illustration of the eye on page 527. The word root
for pupil is cor.

15.64

One combining form for pupil is **cor/e**.
  Build words meaning
    pupil out of place

cor/ectopia   _____/_____;
kôr′ ek tō′ pē ə
cor/e/lysis   destruction of the pupil
kôr′ el′ ə sis   _____/_____/_____;
cor/ectasia (is)   dilatation (stretching) of the pupil
kôr′ ek tā′ zhə   _____/_____;
anis/o/coria   unequal pupil size
an ī′ sō **kôr′** ē ə   _____/_____/_____.

15.65

core/o is used also as a combining form for pupil. Using **core/o**,
build words meaning
    instrument for measuring the pupil

core/o/meter or   _____/_____/_____;
kôr ē **om′** ə ter   measurement of the pupil
pupil/o/meter   _____/_____/_____;
pyoo pil om′ ə ter   plastic surgery of the pupil
core/o/metry or   _____/_____/_____.
kôr ē **om′** ə trē
pupil/o/metry
pyoo pil om′ ə trē
core/o/plasty
kôr ē ō **plas′** tē

15.66

Whether **cor/e** or **core/o** is used, the word root for pupil of the eye is

cor   _____.

15.67

corne   You have already learned one word root for cornea. It is _____. Another word
                             root for cornea is kerat, and it is the more commonly used form.
                             (Think of kerats [carrots] and corn.)

ANSWER COLUMN

15.68

kerat
kerat/o

The word root most commonly used for cornea is _____. The combining form is _____/_____.

15.69

Using **kerat/o**, build words meaning
    forward bulging (dilatation) of the cornea

kerat/ectasia (is)
ker ə tek **tā**′ zhə
kerat/o/cele
ker′ ə tō sēl
kerat/o/plasty
ker′ ə tō plas tē

    _____/_____;
    herniation of the cornea (protrusion of the cornea)
    _____/_____/_____;
    plastic operation of the cornea (corneal transplant)
    _____/_____/_____.

15.70

Again using **kerat/o**, build words meaning
    incision of the cornea

kerat/o/tomy
ker ə **to**′ tō mē
kerat/o/rrhexis
ker′ ə tō **rek**′ sis
kerat/o/scler/itis
ker′ ə tō skler **ī** tis

    _____/_____/_____;
    corneal rupture
    _____/_____/_____;
    inflammation of cornea and sclera
    _____/_____/_____/_____.

15.71

kerat/o/tomy

Making small incisions into the cornea to improve vision for those with myopia is called radial _____/_____/_____.

15.72

TAKE A CLOSER LOOK

The combining form for ciliary body is **cycl/o**. Look up the ciliary body in your dictionary or an anatomy book and understand what it is. Turn to **cycl/o** words in your dictionary. *Cyclos* is Greek for circle. The ciliary body encircles the inside of the iris.

15.73

Find words meaning
    paralysis of the ciliary body (noun)

cycl/o/plegia
sī klō **plē**′ jē ə
cycl/o/pleg/ic
sī klō **plē**′ jik
cycl/o/keratitis
sī klō ker ə **tī**′ tis

    _____/_____/_____;
    paralysis of the ciliary body (adjective)
    _____/_____/_____/_____;
    ciliary body and cornea inflammation
    _____/_____/_____.

ANSWER COLUMN

15.74

The following combining forms make you think of

iris	**irid/o** _____
retina	**retin/o** _____
pupil	**cor/e** _____
pupil	**core/o** _____
cornea	**kerat/o** _____
cornea	**corne/o** _____
ciliary body	**cycl/o** _____

15.75

tears

tearing

Look up lacrim/al in your dictionary. Lacrimal means pertaining to _____.
Lacrim/ation is _____.

15.76

lacrim/al
lak′ ri məl

The gland that secretes tears is the _____/_____ gland.

15.77

lacrimal

The sac that collects lacrimal fluid is the _____ sac.

15.78

nas/o/lacrim/al
nā zō **lak′** ri məl

Lacrimal fluid is drained away by means of the
_____/_____/_____/_____ duct.

15.79

Lacrimal fluid keeps the surface of the eye moistened. It is continually forming
and being drained. When there is more formed than can be drained through a
duct, you say the person is

crying or tearing

* _____.

15.80

dacry
-rrhea

Lacrimation means crying. Excessive lacrimation is called dacry/o/rrhea. This word
gives you another word root for tear. It is _____, and the suffix for flow is
_____.

15.81

lacrimation
lak ri **ma′** shun
dacry/o/rrhea
da′krē ō **rē′** ə

Flow of tears is either _____ or

_____/_____/_____.

ANSWER COLUMN

15.82

Analyze (you insert the slashes and define)
dacryocystitis

dacry/o/cyst/itis
dak′ rē ō sis **tī**′ tis
tear sac inflammation

_____ ,

* _____ ;

dacryoadenalgia

dacry/o/aden/algia
dak′ rē ō ad′ ə **nal**′ jē ə
pain in a tear gland

_____ ,

* _____ ;

dacry/oma
dak′ rē **ō**′ mə
tumor of the tear duct
or gland

dacryoma

_____ ,

* _____ .

15.83

Define and insert the slashes
dacryopyorrhea

dacry/o/py/o/rrhea
discharge of pus from
 tear gland

_____ ,

* _____ ;

dacry/o/cyst/o/cele
hernia of the tear sac

dacryocystocele

_____ ,

* _____ ;

dacry/o/lith
stone in the tear sac
(You pronounce)

dacryolith

_____ ,

* _____ .

15.84

If necessary you may use your dictionary to complete the following
dacryorrhea means

excessive flow of tears

* _____ .

dacryocystoptosis means

prolapse of the tear sac

* _____ .

a dacryocystotome is

an instrument for cutting
 (incising) the tear sac

* _____ .

15.85

Look in your dictionary for words beginning with **onych**. These words refer to

nails

the _____ .

ANSWER COLUMN

15.86

onych/o

By studying words beginning with onych, you can find its combining form. The combining form that refers to nail is _____/_____.

15.87

SPELL CHECK ✓

Watch your spelling and pronunciation. The y is pronounced with a short "i" sound and the ch like a "k": o-n-y-c-h.

15.88

onych/oid
on' i koid
onych/oma
on i **kō'** mə
onych/osis
on i **kō'** sis

Build words meaning
   resembling a fingernail
   _____/_____;
   tumor of the nail (or nail bed)
   _____/_____;
   any nail condition
   _____/_____.

15.89

onych/o/malac/ia
on' i kō ma **lā'** shə
onych/o/myc/osis
on' i kō mī **kō'** sis
onych/o/phagia
on' i kō **fā'** jē ə

Build words meaning
   softening of the nails
   _____/_____/_____/_____;
   fungus infection (condition) of the nails
   _____/_____/_____/_____;
   nail biting (eating)
   _____/_____/_____.

15.90

hidden nail or condition
  of nail being hidden

Recall that crypt means hidden. Onych/o/crypt/osis means literally
*_____.

15.91

ingrown nail (usually a
  toenail)

Look up onychocryptosis (on' i k⁻o krip tō' sis) in your dictionary. It refers to an
*_____.

15.92

Par/onych/ia is a condition of infection in the tissues around the nail. If the cuticle around the nail is infected, this is called _____/_____/_____, also known as a "run around." To see this condition look at the pictures below.

par/onych/ia
par' ō **nik**' ē ə

15.93

trich/o is used in words to mean hair. A trich/o/genous substance promotes the growth of _____.

hair

(A) Paronychia, infection of tissues around the nail

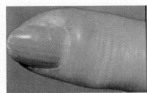

(B) Onychomycosis, caused by parasitic fungus

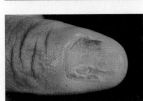

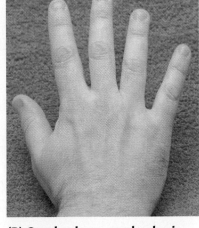

(C) Onychocryptosis, ingrown nail

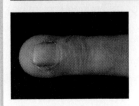

(D) Onychophagy, onychophagia, bitten nails

15.94

Lith/iasis is the formation of calculi. Trich/iasis is the formation of _____ (in the wrong places).

hair

15.95

Using **trich/o**, build words meaning
  hairy tongue (noun)
  _____/____/_____;
  resembling hair
  _____/_____;
  abnormal fear of hair
  _____/____/_____;
  any hair disease
  _____/____/_____.

trich/o/glossia
trik' ō **glos**' ē ə
trich/oid
trik' oid
trich/o/phobia
trik' ō **fō**' bē ə
trich/o/pathy
trik **op**' ə thē

ANSWER COLUMN

15.96

eat or swallow
eating or swallowing

Recall that **phag/o** means *_____, and
phagia is a condition of *_____.

15.97

eats (or ingests)
eating (or ingesting)

A phag/o/cyte is a cell that _____ microorganisms.
Phag/o/cyt/osis is the process of the cells _____
microorganisms.

15.98

phag/o/cyte
phag/o/cyt/osis
(You pronounce)

A cell that eats cells is a _____/_____/_____.
The process is _____/_____/_____/_____.

15.99

the ingestion of cells by
   phagocytes or
   phagocytosis

Cyt/o/phagy is another way of saying *_____
_____.

15.100

cyt/o/meter
sī **tom**′ ə tər
cyt′/ō/metry
sī **tom**′ ə trē

Recall that an instrument for measuring (counting) cells is a
_____/_____/_____, and the process of measuring (counting)

cells is _____/_____/_____.

15.101

cyt/o/stasis
sī **tos**′ tə sis
cyt/o/scopy
sī **tos**′ kə pē

Stopping or controlling cells is called
_____/_____/_____.
Examination of cells is
_____/_____/_____.

15.102

micr/o/phage
mī′ krō fāj

A large phagocyte is called a macr/o/phage. A small phagocyte is called a
_____/_____/_____.

15.103

trich/o/phagy (ia)
tri **kof**′ ə jē

Onych/o/phagy (onychophagia) is nail biting. A word that means hair swallowing
is _____/_____/_____.

ANSWER COLUMN

aer/o/phagy (ia)
air **of**′ ə jē

Air swallowing is
_____/_____/_____.

15.104

Recall the prefix **endo-** means inside. Endo/crine literally means to secrete inside. Hormones are secreted from the _____/_____ glands.

endo/crine
en′ dō krin

15.105

The medical specialty studying the endocrine system is called
_____/_____/_____.
The specialist (physician) in the study of the endocrine system is called an
_____/_____/_____/_____.

endo/crin/ology
en′ dō krin **o**′ lō jē
endo/crin/o/logist
en′ dō krin **ol**′ ō jist

The following table analyzes word parts related to the endocrine system. Refer to the illustration on page 536.

Combining Form	Meaning	Example
thyroid/o, thyr/o	thyroid gland	thyroidectomy
thym/o	thymus gland	thymosin
adren/o	adrenal gland	adrenalin
pancreat/o	pancreas	pancreatitis
oophor/o	ovary	oophoroma
testic/, orchid/o, orchi/o testis		testicular

Review the male and female reproductive systems, in Unit 5.

15.106

Analyzing the following hormones, name the gland by which they are produced
adren/o/corticoid (cortisone)

adrenal gland (adrenal cortex)
thyroid gland

* _____ ;
thyr/o/xine, or thyr/o/xin
* _____ ;
test/o/sterone

testes

_____.

See how much you have learned about word building!

Endocrine system structures

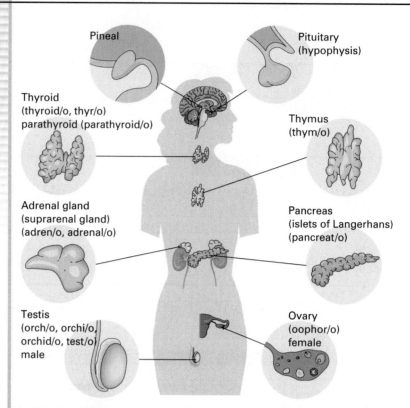

Pineal

Pituitary
(hypophysis)

Thyroid
(thyroid/o, thyr/o)
parathyroid (parathyroid/o)

Thymus
(thym/o)

Adrenal gland
(suprarenal gland)
(adren/o, adrenal/o)

Pancreas
(islets of Langerhans)
(pancreat/o)

Testis
(orch/o, orchi/o,
orchid/o, test/o)
male

Ovary
(oophor/o)
female

15.107

Hyper/thyroid/ism is an overactive thyroid. An underactive (slow-acting) thyroid
condition is called_____/_____/_____.

hypo/thyroid/ism
hī pō **thī′** roid izm

15.108

Build terms meaning
   any disease condition of the adrenal glands
   _____/_____/_____;
   enlargement of the adrenal glands
   _____/_____/_____;
   destruction of adrenal tissue
   _____/_____/_____.

adren/o/pathy
ad′ rēn **op′** ath ē
adren/o/megaly
ad′ rēn ō **meg′** əl ē
adren/o/lysis
ad′ rēn **ol′** ə sis

15.109

The adrenal glands are also called the supra/renal glands because they are above
the kidneys. Epi/nephr/ine is a hormone produced by the supra/renal glands.
Define these two terms
supra/renal
*_____;

above the kidneys
   (adrenal)

ANSWER COLUMN

a hormone produced upon the kidney	epi/nephr/ine * _____.

15.110

There are many hormones produced by the pituitary gland. Look up pituitary in your dictionary and read about its function. The pituitary gland (hypophysis) has

anterior
posterior

front and back lobes. These are called the _____ lobe and the _____ lobe.

15.111

For another review recall that **-emia** is a suffix that means

condition of the blood
  or in the blood

* _____.

15.112

Isch/emia (is kē' mē ə) is a condition in which blood flow is interrupted. Blood cancer (a sign being abnormally increased leukocyte count) is called

leuk/emia
lōō **kē**' mē ə

_____/_____.

15.113

blood

A transient isch/emic attack (TIA) is a temporary interruption of _____ flow, usually occurring in the brain.

15.114

Build words meaning
  reduction in red blood cells

an/emia
e **nē**' mē ə
hyper/emia
hī pər **ē**' mē ə
ur/emia
yōō **rē**' mē ə

_____/_____;
too much blood (in one part)
_____/_____;
urine constituents in the blood
_____/_____.

15.115

-emia is used as a suffix meaning in the blood. **hemat/o** is a combining form used as a prefix meaning blood. Build words meaning
  blood in the urine

hemat/ur/ia
hēm at **yōō** rē ə
ur/emia
yōō **rē**' mē ə

_____/_____/_____;
urine in the blood
_____/_____.

PROFESSIONAL PROFILES

Emergency medical technicians (EMTs) provide basic emergency medical care including first aid, CPR, immobilizing injuries, extricating accident victims from unsafe environments, and providing transportation. They may work directly in the field or in emergency departments. **Paramedics (EMT-Ps)** provide advanced life support such as using monitors and defibrillators, administering intravenous medications, as well as basic emergency care. Licensure requirements vary greatly throughout North America, and education ranges from private short course instruction to college-based programs offering associate degrees.

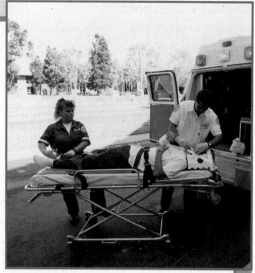

Emergency medical personnel aiding a patient

ANSWER COLUMN

15.116

You now know many prefixes, suffixes, and combining forms. You even know how to find combining forms and form singular and plural forms of a word. You also know several ways to find combining forms in your dictionary.

TAKE A CLOSER LOOK

15.117

To prove it again, look up trauma in your dictionary. It means a

wound or injury

* _____ .

15.118

Traumat/o/logy is the study of wound care. The combining form for trauma is

traumat/o

_____ / _____ .

15.119

The study of caring for wounds is called

traumat/o/logy
trô mə **tol**′ ə jē
traumat/ic
trô **ma**′ tik

_____ / _____ / _____ .
Pertaining to wounds or woundedness is
_____ / _____ .

ANSWER COLUMN

wounds or injuries

trauma

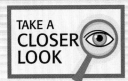

TAKE A
CLOSER
LOOK

15.120

A trauma center may provide 24-hour care for treatment of
*_____. Physicians can specialize in
treatment of emergency cases including _____.

15.121

A trauma can produce many injuries. Look up the following in the dictionary
and write their definitions
abrasion *_____;
contusion *_____;
evulsion *_____;
puncture *_____;
fracture *_____;
laceration *_____.
These are all types of wounds. Getting wounded is traumat/ic.

As a final review, notice that each of these medical specialties uses medical
terminology. Use your knowledge of word-building systems to fill in the blanks in
the following table. Check your answers on the next page.

Specialty	Specialist	Limits of Field
pathology	(15.122)	diseases—nature and causes
(15.123)	dermatologist	(15.124)
neurology	(15.125)	nervous system diseases
(15.126)	gynecologist	female diseases
urology	(15.127)	male diseases and all urinary diseases
(15.128)	endocrinologist	glands of internal secretion
oncology	(15.129)	neoplasms (new growths)
(15.130)	(15.131)	heart
ophthalmology	(15.132)	eye
(15.133)	otorhinolaryngologist	(15.134)
obstetrics	(15.135)	pregnancy, childbirth, and puerperium
(15.136)	geriatrician	old age
pediatrics	(15.137)	children
(15.138)	orthopedist	bones and muscles
psychiatry	(15.139)	mental disorders
(15.140)	audiologist	hearing function
radiology	(15.141)	diagnostic imaging therapeutic x-ray
(15.142)	chiropractor	(15.143)
(15.144)	podiatrist	diseases of the foot

Specialty	Specialist	Limits of Field
	pathologist (15.122)	
dermatology (15.123)		skin (15.124)
	neurologist (15.125)	
gynecology (15.126)		
	urologist (15.127)	
endocrinology (15.128)		
	oncologist (15.129)	
cardiology (15.130)	cardiologist (15.131)	
	ophthalmologist (15.132)	
otorhinolaryngology (15.133)		ear-nose-throat (15.134)
	obstetrician (15.135)	
geriatrics (15.136)		
	pediatrician (15.137)	
orthopedics (15.138)		
	psychiatrist (15.139)	
audiology (15.140)		
	radiologist (15.141)	
chiropractic (15.142)		manipulation therapy (15.143)
podiatry (15.144)		

ANSWER COLUMN

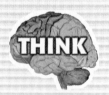

15.122

Great!
See, you really are competent in the study of systematic medical terminology.

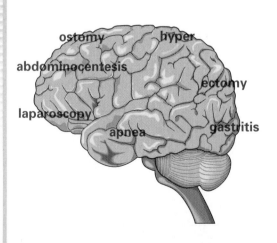

Abbreviation	Meaning
ACTH	adrenocorticotropic hormone
AOA	American Optometric Association
COA	certified ophthalmic assistant
COMT	certified ophthalmic medical technologist
COT	certified ophthalmic technician
d, D	diopter
EMT	emergency medical technician
EMT-P	EMT—paramedic
ENT	ear, nose, throat specialist
EOMI	extraocular movement intact (muscles)
FSH	follicle-stimulating hormone
Fx	fracture
HCG	human chorionic gonadotropin
L&A	light and accommodation
Laser	light amplification by stimulated emission of radiation
mg	milligram(s) (0.001 gram)
mm	millimeter(s) (0.001 meter)
OAG	open-angle glaucoma
OB	obstetrician, obstetrics
OD	right eye (oculus dexter)
OD	doctor of optometry
OS	left eye (oculus sinister)
OU	both eyes (oculus uterque)
PERRLA	pupils equal, round, reactive to light and accommodation
T_3, T_4	triiodothyronine, tetraiodothyronine (thyroid function tests)
TIA	transient ischemic attack
TSH	thyroid-stimulating hormone

ANSWER COLUMN

Now work the last **Review Activities** on the following pages and listen to the audio CDs that accompany *Medical Terminology: A Programmed Systems Approach,* 9th Edition, and practice your pronunciation.

Additional practice exercises for this unit are available on the Learner Practice CD-ROM found in the back of the textbook.

Congratulations on your completion of this programmed study of medical terminology! May what you have learned in this course of study sustain you throughout your experiences in the health care field. Do not forget to celebrate your success!

REVIEW ACTIVITIES

CIRCLE AND CORRECT

Circle the correct answer for each question. Then check your answers in Appendix A.

1. Prefix meaning inward
   a. inter-   b. exo-
   c. infra-   d. eso-

2. Suffix for vision
   a. -ophthalmic   b. -metry
   c. -opia   d. -ophthic

3. Combining form for yellow
   a. jaundice   b. xantho
   c. chloro   d. yello

4. Which of the following means nearsightedness?
   a. myopia   b. hyperopia
   c. presbyopia   d. exophoria

5. Combining form for eye
   a. optalmo   b. opthalmo
   c. optic   d. ophthalmo

6. Word root for lens
   a. lens   b. phac
   c. kerat   d. corne

7. Combining form for nail
   a. onycho   b. omphalo
   c. optic   d. onchyo

8. Word root for suprarenal glands
   a. aden   b. glandul
   c. genit   d. adren

9. Prefix meaning overactive
   a. hyper-   b. ultra-
   c. supra-   d. meta-

10. Combining form for eyelid
    a. maculo   b. cyclo
    c. lacrimo   d. blepharo

11. Which of the following does not have to do with tearing?
    a. lacrimation   b. cycloplegia
    c. dacryorrhea   d. dacryocystitis

12. Word root for hair
    a. omphal   b. trich
    c. cyclo   d. onycho

13. Combining form for double
    a. onycho   b. bi
    c. diplo   d. di

14. One combining form for cornea
    a. kerato   b. irido
    c. cyclo   d. coreo

REVIEW ACTIVITIES

SELECT AND CONSTRUCT

Select the correct word parts from the list below and construct medical terms that represent the given meaning.

adren	al	aniso	blephar	cardia
cele	cor(ne)(ia)	crypt	cyclo	dacry/o
diplo	disk	ectas(ia)(is)	ectomy	emia
emulsification	epi	eso	hyper	hypo
in(e)	ir	irid/o	itis	kerat (core)
lacrim	lamin/o	(o)logy	lysis	malacia
megaly	metry	my	myco	naso
nephrine	onych/o	oophoro	ophthalmo	opia
opt(ic)(o)	orchid	osis	otomy	pathy
phac/o	phobia	phoria	plasty	plegia
presby/o	ptosis	retin(o)	rrhea	rrhexia
scope	thym/o	thyro(oid)	tomy	traumat/o
trich/o	trop/ia			

1. specialty measuring vision _____

2. paralysis of the ciliary body _____

3. softening of the nails _____

4. inflammation of the iris _____

5. excessive flow of tears _____

6. removal of the lens through a
   destruction procedure _____

7. hormone produced by the
   glands above the kidneys _____

8. farsightedness _____

9. instrument to examine the retina _____

10. study of wounds _____

11. surgical repair of the eye _____

12. dilatation of the pupil _____

13. prolapse of the eyelid _____

14. incision into the cornea _____

15. enlargement of the thyroid _____

16. unequal pupil size _____

REVIEW ACTIVITIES

17. inward crossed eyes

_____

18. old eye (vision)

_____

19. ingrown (hidden) nail

_____

20. surgical repair of the retina

_____

DEFINE AND DISSECT

Give a brief definition and dissect each term listed into its word parts in the space provided. Check your answers by referring to the frame listed in parentheses and your medical dictionary. Then listen to the CDs to practice pronunciation.

1. exotropia (15.30)

_____/_____
pre   rt/suffix

_____
definition

2. phoropter (15.36)

_____/_____/_____
rt   rt   suffix

_____

3. paronychia (15.92)

_____/_____/_____
pre   rt   suffix

_____

4. ophthalmologist (15.6)

_____/____/_____
rt   v   suffix

_____

5. myopia (15.12)

_____/_____
rt   suffix

_____

6. optometrist (15.8)

_____/____/_____
rt   v   rt/suffix

_____

7. blepharoplasty (15.41)

_____/____/_____
rt   v   suffix

_____

8. corneoiritis (15.43)

_____/____/____/_____
rt   v   rt   suffix

_____

9. phacocele (15.45)

_____/____/_____
rt   v   suffix

_____

REVIEW ACTIVITIES

10. retinoscopy (15.60)

_____/_____/_____
rt   v   suffix

11. corelysis (15.64)

_____/_____/_____
rt   v   suffix

12. keratoscleritis (15.70)

_____/_____/_____/_____
rt   v   rt   suffix

13. nasolacrimal (15.78)

_____/_____/_____/_____
rt   v   rt   suffix

14. dacryocystocele (15.83)

_____/_____/_____/_____/_____
rt   v   rt   v   suffix

15. onychophagia (15.89)

_____/_____/_____
rt   v   suffix

16. trichopathy (15.95)

_____/_____/_____
rt   v   suffix

17. phagocytosis (15.98)

_____/_____/_____/_____
rt   v   rt   suffix

18. endocrinologist (15.105)

_____/_____/_____/_____
pre   rt   v   suffix

19. adrenocorticoid (15.106)

_____/_____/_____
rt   v   rt/suffix

20. hypothyroidism (15.107)

_____/_____/_____
pre   rt   suffix

21. adrenomegaly (15.108)

_____/_____/_____
rt   v   suffix

REVIEW ACTIVITIES

22. uremia (15.114)

_____/_____

rt   rt/suffix

23. pathologist (table)

_____/_____/_____

rt   v   suffix

24. oncology (table)

_____/_____/_____

rt   v   suffix

25. otorhinolaryngologist (table)

_____/_____/_____/_____/_____/_____/_____

rt   v   rt   v   rt   v   suffix

26. orthopedist (table)

_____/_____/_____/_____

rt   v   rt   suffix

27. radiology (table)

_____/_____/_____

rt   v   suffix

28. chiropractor (table)

_____/_____/_____

rt   v   rt/suffix

29. podiatry (table)

_____/_____

rt   suffix

30. audiology (table)

_____/_____/_____

rt   v   suffix

REVIEW ACTIVITIES

ART LABELING

Label the structures of the eye by matching the number with the combining form. Then write the structure name in the blank.

_____	corne/o, kerat/o	_____
_____	retin/o	_____
_____	scler/o	_____
_____	cycl/o	_____
_____	core/o	_____
_____	phac/o	_____
_____	irid/o	_____
_____	blephar/o	_____
_____	conjunctiv/o	_____
_____	lacrim/o, dacry/o	_____

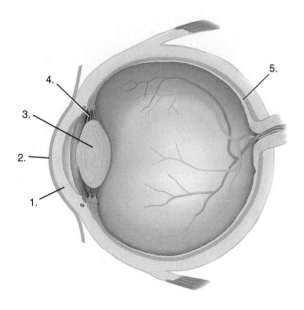
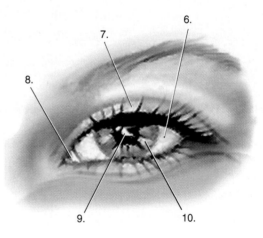

REVIEW ACTIVITIES

ABBREVIATION MATCHING

Match the following abbreviations with their definition.

_____ 1. COT   a. otorhinolaryngologist

_____ 2. TIA   b. both eyes

_____ 3. OU   c. living and well

_____ 4. TSH   d. extraocular (muscles) movement intact

_____ 5. PERRLA   e. light and accommodation

_____ 6. ENT   f. thyroid-stimulating hormone

_____ 7. OB   g. right eye

_____ 8. OD   h. certified occupational therapy assistant

_____ 9. EOMI   i. doctor of optometry

_____10. OAG   j. fasting sugar

         k. left ear

         l. open-angle glaucoma

         m. obstetrician

         n. certified ophthalmic technician

         o. follicle-stimulating hormone

         p. pupils equal, round, reactive to light and accommodation

         q. acute glaucoma

         r. transient ischemic attack

ABBREVIATION FILL-INS

Fill in the blanks with the correct abbreviation.

11. American Optometric Association _____

12. emergency medical technician _____

13. follicle-stimulating hormone _____

14. thyroid function tests _____

15. right eye _____

16. light and accommodation _____

CASE STUDIES

Write the term next to its meaning given on page 549. Then draw slashes to analyze the word parts. Note the use of medical abbreviations. Look these up in your dictionary or find them in Appendix B. If you have any questions about the answers, refer to your medical dictionary or check with your instructor for the answers in Appendix A.

REVIEW ACTIVITIES

CASE STUDY 15-1

Phacoemulsification

Surgeon: P.H. Ernest, M.D.

Preoperative and postoperative diagnoses

1. **cataract OD**, with low **corneal** endothelial cell count.

2. **myopia OD**

Operation performed: **Phacoemulsification** of right eye with insertion of foldable **intraocular** lens of 22 power.

Summary: 2% Xylocaine and Wydase administered by peribulbar injection. A Honan balloon was placed on the eye for 20 minutes at 5-minute intervals. Betadine drops were instilled into the cul-de-sac and cornea. A temporal approach was made. A **paracentesis** incision was made and Viscoelastic was used to replace the aqueous. At the limbus, a temporally approached 3.2-mm incision and then dissection into the cornea was made with crescent blade. A 2.3-mm **keratome** was used to make an internal corneal cut through Descemet's membrane creating a square wound. Under Viscoelastic, multiple sphincterotomies were performed. A 360-degree **capsulorrhexis** was performed. Hydrocortical cleavage and hydrodelineation was performed. Using phacoemulsification, the nucleus was sculpted into perpendicular grooves. Using an Ernest nuclear cracker, the nucleus was cracked into four quadrants. The **epinucleus** and any residual cortex was removed using pulsed phaco, irrigation, and aspiration. Under Viscoelastic, a foldable intraocular lens was inserted and positioned within the capsular bag. All Viscoelastic was removed both anterior and posterior from the intraocular lens using irrigation and aspiration. 500-cc balanced salt, 20-mg Vancomycin and 10-mg Tobramicin was instilled. The wound was tested to ensure no wound leaks. Maxitrol ointment and a shield was applied over the eye to ensure no inadvertent corneal **abrasion**. The patient was sent to the recovery room in good condition.

1. breakup of the lens _____

2. scrape wound _____

3. rupture of the capsule _____

4. within the eye _____

5. instrument used to cut thin
   slices of the cornea _____

6. nearsightedness _____

7. cloudy lesion on the lens _____

8. upon the nucleus _____

9. pertaining to the cornea _____

10. puncture for the removal of fluid _____

11. abbreviation, right eye _____

REVIEW ACTIVITIES

CROSSWORD PUZZLE

Check your answers by going back through the frames or checking the solutions in Appendix C.

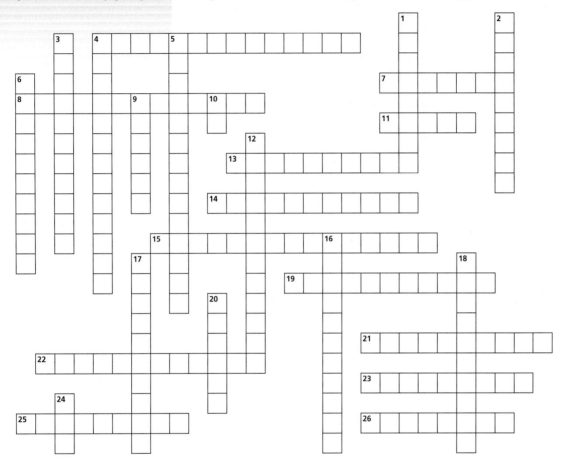

Across

4. instrument to look into the eye
7. measurement for lens prescription
8. study of hormones and glands
11. pertaining to vision
13. seeing red
14. synonym for dacryorrhea
15. hormone from the adrenal cortex
19. adrenal medulla hormone
21. tear duct stone
22. swollen eyelid
23. cross-eyed
25. bruise
26. wound with a flap

Down

1. synonym for diplopia
2. thyroid hormone
3. prolapsed iris
4. soft nails
5. slow thyroid
6. fix the retina
9. inflamed iris
10. optometrist (abbreviation)
12. hair eating
16. hair disease
17. pertaining to the eye
18. unequal pupils
20. white of the eye
24. otorhinolaryngologist (abbreviation)

REVIEW ACTIVITIES

GLOSSARY

abrasion	scrape
adrenocorticoid	hormone manufactured in the adrenal cortex
adrenolysis	destruction of the adrenal glands
adrenomegaly	enlarged adrenal glands
ambivalence	unable to decide, wavering on both sides
anisocoria	pupils of unequal size
blepharedema	swelling of the eyelid
blepharoplasty	plastic surgery of the eyelid
blepharoptosis	prolapse of the upper eyelid (drooping)
blepharorrhaphy	suturing of the eyelid
blepharospasm	twitching eyelid
chloropia	seeing green
contusion	bruise
corectasia	dilation of the pupil
corectopia	displaced pupil
corelysis	destruction of the pupil
coreometer	instrument used to measure pupil size
coreoplasty	plastic surgery of the pupil
corneitis	inflammation of the cornea (keratitis)
corneoiritis	inflammation of the cornea and the iris
corneoscleral	pertaining to the cornea and the sclera
cyclokeratitis	inflammation of the ciliary body and the cornea

cycloplegia	paralysis of the ciliary body
cytophagy	destruction of other cells by phagocytes (cytophagia, phagocytosis)
dacryoadenalgia	pain in the tear gland
dacryocystitis	inflammation of the tear sac
dacryocystocele	herniation of a tear sac
dacryocystoptosis	prolapse of the tear sac
dacryocystotome	instrument for incision of a tear sac
dacryolith	calculus in the tear duct or sac
dacryoma	tumor of the lacrimal tissue
dacryopyorrhea	discharge of pus from the tear gland
diascope	a glass plate used to look through to examine the skin
diopter	measurement unit of refraction
diplopia	double vision (ambiopia)
endocrine	glands that secrete hormones
endocrinologist	specialist in the study and treatment of disorders of the endocrine system
endocrinology	the science studying the endocrine system
epinephrine	hormone produced by the adrenal medulla
erythropia	seeing red
esotropia	condition in which the eyes point inward (cross-eyed)
euphoria	feeling good
evulsion	a tearing away

REVIEW ACTIVITIES

exotropia	condition in which the eyes point outward
fracture	break
glaucoma	condition in which the intraocular aqueous humor pressure is high
hyperopia	farsightedness
hypertropia	condition in which the eyes point upward
hyperthyroidism	overactive thyroid condition
hypotropia	condition in which the eyes point downward
hypothyroidism	underactive thyroid condition
iridalgia	iris pain
iridectomy	excision of the iris
iridocele	herniation of the iris
iridomalacia	softening of the iris
iridoplegia	paralysis of the iris (iridoparalysis)
iridoptosis	prolapse of the iris
iridorrhexis	rupture of the iris
keratectasia	protrusion of a thin scarred cornea
keratorrhexis	rupture of the cornea
keratoscleritis	inflammation of the cornea and sclera
keratotomy	incision into the cornea
laceration	a cut (verb form lacerate)
lacrimation	tearing (dacryorrhea)
macrophage	large phagocyte
microphage	small phagocyte
myopia	nearsightedness

nasolacrimal	pertaining to the nasal passages and the tear ducts
onychocryptosis	ingrown nail
onychoid	resembling a nail
onychoma	nail tumor
onychomalacia	softening of the nails
onychomycosis	fungus infection of the nail
onychophagia	nail biting
ophthalmalgia	eye pain (ophthalmodynia)
ophthalmic	pertaining to the eye
ophthalmocele	herniation of the eye
ophthalmologist	physician specialist in treatment of eye disease
ophthalmometer	instrument used to measure the eye
ophthalmopathy	any eye disease
ophthalmoplasty	surgical repair of the eye
ophthalmoplegia	ocular muscle paralysis
ophthalmoscope	instrument used to examine the interior of the eye
ophthalmoscopy	process of using an ophthalmoscope
optic	pertaining to vision
optometrist	specialist in assessing and treating visual acuity problems and other eye diseases (limited license)
optometry	the measurement of vision and the practice performed by the optometrist
paronychia	condition of infection around a nail
phacocele	dislocation of the lens of the eye

REVIEW ACTIVITIES

phacoemulsification	procedure to disintegrate cataracts	sclerostomy	make an opening in the sclera
phagocyte	cell that eats cells (macrophage, leukocyte)	suprarenal	upon the kidney, refers to the adrenal glands
phorometer	instrument used to measure ocular muscle movement	testosterone	hormone produced in the testes (androgen)
phoropter	instrument used to measure prescription strength for lenses	thyroxine	thyroid hormone
presbyopia	old eye, loss of accommodation	traumatology	the study of wound treatment
puncture	to make a hole	trichoglossia	condition of hair growth on the tongue
retinal	pertaining to the retina	trichoid	resembling hair
retinitis	inflammation of the retina	trichopathy	any hair disease
retinopexy	fixation of a detached retina (retinoplasty)	trichophagia	condition in which the person bites on or eats hair
retinoscope	instrument used to look at the retina	trichophobia	fear of hair growth (i.e., facial hair on women) or touching hair
sclerectomy	excision of the sclera	xanthopia	see yellow

APPENDIX A

ANSWERS TO UNIT REVIEW ACTIVITIES AND CASE STUDIES

UNIT 1

Circle and Correct

1. d 2. a 3. d 4. c 5. a 6. d 7. a 8. c 9. c 10. a 11. c 12. d 13. a 14. c 15. c 16. b

Select and Construct

1. acromegaly
2. microscope
3. anemic
4. radiographer
5. acrodermatitis
6. hydrophobia
7. thermometer
8. microsurgery
9. gastroduodenoscopy
10. cytometer

Plural/Singular Forms

1. bursae
2. cocci
3. carcinomata
4. protozoa
5. crises
6. appendices
7. ova

Adjectival Forms

1. cyanotic
2. anemic
3. duodenal
4. mucous
5. arthritic

UNIT 2

Circle and Correct

1. b 2. d 3. b 4. c 5. c 6. d 7. b 8. a 9. b 10. c 11. a 12. d 13. d 14. c 15. b

Select and Construct

1. gastrectomy
2. gastroduodenostomy
3. cyanoderma
4. dermopathy (dermatopathy)
5. erythrocyte
6. melanoblast
7. thrombocytopenia
8. gastromegaly (megalogastria)
9. megalomania
10. electrocardiograph
11. duodenotomy
12. cardiac
13. echography (sonography)
14. echocardiogram
15. radiographer
16. leukocytosis
17. acromegaly
18. tomogram
19. xanthosis, xanthoderma
20. cytology

Abbreviation Matching

1. l 2. k 3. d 4. b 5. h 6. g 7. m 8. n 9. i 10. c

Abbreviation Fill-in

11. CBC 12. WBC, RBC 13. MRI, XR 14. RT(R) 15. DMS, ECHO 16. CCU, EKG, ECHO 17. CPK, LDH

Case Study

1. acute
2. coronary cardiac
3. echocardiogram
4. substernal
5. telemetry
6. arteriosclerosis
7. angiography
8. cardiopulmonary
9. ambulance
10. etiology
11. electrocardiogram
12. x-ray

UNIT 3

Circle and Correct

1. a 2. c 3. b 4. a 5. c 6. c 7. b 8. b 9. d 10. b 11. c 12. a 13. c 14. b 15. d 16. d

ANSWERS

Select and Construct

1. encephalocele
2. electroencephalograph
3. cranioplasty
4. cerebrospinal
5. adenocarcinoma
6. mucoid
7. lipoma
8. craniomalacia
9. cerebrotomy
10. meningitis
11. oncologist
12. sarcoma
13. lymphadenoma, lymphoma
14. hypertrophy
15. hypotension
16. histologist
17. neoplasms
18. antineoplastic
19. histoblast
20. neonatal

Art Labeling

6–myel/o
4–crani/o
5–mening/o

2,3–cerebr/o
2,3–encepha/o
1–cephal/o

Abbreviation Matching

1. d   2. l   3. g   4. c   5. n   6. k   7. h   8. i   9. m   10. b

Abbreviation Fill-in

11. MLT   12. BP, mmHg, HCVD   13. TIA, CVA   14. BCC

Case Study

1. D&C
2. endocervical
3. poikilocytotic
4. dysplasia
5. atypia
6. grav 4, para 4 or G4, P4
7. carcinoma
8. colposcopy
9. conization
10. gynecology
11. Pap (smear)
12. biopsies

UNIT 4

Circle and Correct

1. c   2. d   3. a   4. b   5. c   6. a   7. d   8. b   9. c   10. d   11. d   12. b   13. c   14. a   15. d

Select and Construct

1. osteomalacia
2. abduction
3. hydrocyst
4. hydrocephalic
5. suprapubic
6. intercostal
7. abdominocentesis
8. arthroscopy
9. aberrant
10. orthodontist
11. tendinitis (tendonitis)
12. pelvimeter
13. cephalopelvic
14. orthopedist
15. osteosarcoma
16. hypertrophy
17. dysplasia
18. chondrodysplasia
19. amniocentesis
20. thoracic, supralumbar

Label the Diagram

4	pelv/i/o	pelvis
1	crani/o	cranium, skull
2	thorac/o	chest, thoracic cavity, thorax
3	abdomin/o	abdomen, abdominal cavity
5	lumb/o	lumbar spine
6	oste/o	bone
7	arthr/o	joint

Abbreviation Matching

1. d   2. n   3. h   4. p   5. r   6. b   7. m   8. k   9. o   10. c

Abbreviation Fill-in

11. DTs   12. RUQ   13. OMT   14. DDS   15. ORTHO (ORTH)

ANSWERS

Case Study

1. inflammation
2. arthroscope
3. mediolateral
4. meniscectomy
5. chondromalacia
6. arthritis
7. arthroscopic
8. patella
9. orthopedic
10. medial
11. pyorrhea
12. incision
13. arthrotomy
14. arthroplasty

UNIT 5

Circle and Correct

1. b 2. a 3. d 4. b 5. b 6. a 7. d 8. c 9. d 10. a 11. b 12. d 13. b 14. a 15. c 16. c 17. c 18. a 19. d 20. b 21. b 22. a

Select and Construct

1. bradycardia
2. tachyphagia
3. staphylitis (uvulitis)
4. cholelithiasis
5. otodynia (otalgia)
6. audiometry
7. dyspepsia
8. pyogenic
9. rhinorrhea
10. tympanogram
11. tympanites
12. cholecystogram
13. apnea
14. diathermy
15. polydipsia
16. synergy (synergistic)
17. microcephalus
18. macrocyte
19. prodromal
20. hypothermia

Mix and Match

1. f 2. d 3. a 4. c 5. b 6. e 7. g 8. h

Abbreviation Matching

1. r 2. l 3. f 4. a 5. q 6. p 7. d 8. s 9. n 10. o 11. i 12. m

Case Study

1. ductal
2. edematous
3. gallbladder
4. cholelith
5. cholangiogram
6. cm
7. epigastric
8. RUQ
9. cholecystectomy
10. ultrasound
11. T, °F

UNIT 6

Circle and Correct

1. b 2. c 3. d 4. b 5. a 6. d 7. b 8. b 9. c 10. a 11. c 12. a 13. b 14. c 15. c 16. d 17. b 18. d

Select and Construct

1. pyelonephritis
2. ureterorrhaphy
3. cystoscopy
4. nephroptosis
5. renogram, renograph
6. cystopexy
7. urethrorrhagia
8. nephrolysis
9. cystostomy
10. endometritis
11. hysteroptosis (metroptosis)
12. cryptorchidism
13. prostatectomy
14. gynecologist
15. oogenesis
16. balanorrhea
17. colpalgia (colpodynia)
18. hysteroscope
19. urologist
20. hysterosalpingogram
21. orchidopexy (orchiopexy)
22. colposcopy
23. endocervical

Art Labeling

Male Reproductive System

6—rect/o, rectum
3—cyst/o, urinary bladder
10—urethr/o, urethra

Female Reproductive System

11—colp/o, vagina
5—hyster/o, uterus
7—oophor/o, ovary

ANSWERS

Male Reproductive System *(continued)*

1—balan/o, glans penis
7—prostat/o, prostate gland
4—vas/o, vas deferens (ductus deferens)
8—orchid/o, testis
2—pen/o, penis
5—ureter/o, ureter
9—scrot/o, scrotum

Female Reproductive System *(continued)*

14—metr/o, uterine tissue
6—salping/o, uterine tubes, fallopian tubes
10—cervic/o, cervix
9—rect/o, rectum
3—clitor/o, clitoris
1—labi/o, labium
2—urethr/o, urethra
13—an/o, anus
8—ureter/o, ureter
12—cystovagin/o, cystovaginal wall
4—cyst/o, urinary bladder

Abbreviation Matching

1. q   2. s   3. g   4. h   5. i   6. m   7. o   8. p   9. n   10. b   11. e   12. l   13. a   14. d

Abbreviation Fill-in

15. MD   16. PSA   17. KUB   18. AIH   19. ESRD   20. Pap (smear)

Case Study

1. mg qid
2. benign
3. pathology
4. hyperplasia
5. prostatitis
6. chronic
7. H&P
8. hydronephrosis
9. TUR
10. hematuria
11. afebrile
12. cystoclysis
13. catheter
14. postoperative
15. transurethral

UNIT 7

Circle and Correct

1. d   2. c   3. b   4. b   5. c   6. d   7. a   8. b   9. c   10. d   11. d   12. c

Select and Construct

1. stomatomycosis
2. sublingual (hypoglossal, subglossal)
3. cheiloplasty
4. gingivitis
5. enterorrhagia
6. esophagogastroduodenoscopy
7. enteroptosis
8. rectoclysis
9. proctoplegia
10. pancreatolith
11. splenomegaly
12. gastrectasia
13. sigmoidoscope
14. hepatitis
15. rectocele
16. esophagogastric (gastroesophageal)
17. cholangiopancreatography
18. colorectal

Art Labeling

12—hepat/o, liver
4—gastr/o, stomach
6—col/o, colon
3—esophag/o, esophagus
1—stomat/o, mouth
5—pancreat/o, pancreas
7—sigmoid/o, sigmoid colon
2—pharyng/o, pharynx
11—cholecyst/o, gallbladder
8—rect/o, rectum
10—duoden/o, duodenum
9—appendic/o, appendix

Abbreviation Matching

1. f   2. k   3. i   4. j   5. g   6. h   7. o   8. q   9. r   10. e   11. a

Suffix Matching

1. j   2. e   3. a   4. f   5. h   6. c

Case Study

1. anterior
2. vomiting
3. hemorrhage
4. nasogastric
5. endoscope
6. mucosal
7. aspirate
8. isotonic
9. ulcer

ANSWERS

10. gastointestinal
11. melenic

12. hypotensive
13. duodenal

14. thrombi
15. EGD

UNIT 8

Circle and Correct

1. c   2. a   3. d   4. a   5. c   6. a   7. b   8. c   9. d   10. d   11. c   12. c   13. a   14. a

Select and Construct

1. arteriosclerosis
2. phlebectasia
3. enterorrhexis
4. angiogram (angiograph)
5. esthesiometer
6. anesthesiologist
7. analgesic
8. parahepatitis

9. neurosis, psychoneurosis
10. myograph
11. dyskinesia
12. pharmacist
13. psychotropic
14. paraplegia
15. fibromyoma
16. atherosclerosis

17. angioplasty
18. thrombosis
19. myospasm
20. fibroneuroma
21. thrombophlebitis
22. neurologist
23. cardiomyopathy
24. myocardial

Abbreviation Matching

1. k   2. t   3. l   4. j   5. g   6. e   7. p   8. f   9. d   10. r

Abbreviation Fill-in

11. HDL   12. MI   13. PT   14. CABG   15. IV   16. BK   17. MD   18. TENS   19. PND   20. OCD

Case Study

1. hypothyroidism
2. incontinence
3. psychiatric
4. obsessive compulsive disorder

5. UTI
6. EST
7. diarrhea
8. BP, P, R

9. Ua c̄ C+S
10. paranoia

UNIT 9

Circle and Correct

1. b   2. d   3. b   4. c   5. d   6. c   7. a   8. c   9. a   10. c   11. b   12. c   13. a   14. d   15. c   16. b

Select and Construct

1. gastroscopy
2. retroperitoneal
3. dialysis, hemodialysis
4. endoderm
5. ectopic
6. posteroanterior
7. procephalic
8. diagnosis
9. omphalitis

10. lateroanterior, anterolateral, ventrolateral, lateroventral
11. cephalocaudal
12. apepsia
13. pseudocyesis, pseudopregnancy
14. euphoria
15. euthanasia
16. dysmenorrhea
17. visceropleura, visceral pleura

18. hemostasis
19. aerobic
20. chromophilic
21. peritoneum, visceroperitoneum
22. omphalorrhea
23. syphilophobia
24. mediolateral
25. ectogenous

Diagram Labels

1. cephalic (cephalad)
2. superior (hyper, super, supra)
3. inferior (hypo, sub, infra)
4. anterior, ventral (pre, pro, ante)

5. circum
6. posterior, dorsal (retro, post)
7. abduct (lateral)
8. adduct (medial)

9. distal
10. proximal
11. sagittal

Abbreviation Matching

1. h   2. l   3. k   4. m   5. e   6. n   7. p   8. f   9. c   10. d

ANSWERS

Abbreviation Fill-in

11. LOA   12. STD   13. RPR (VDRL)   14. LAT   15. LMP   16. PA   17. OT   18. TB

Case Study

1. catheterization
2. apnea
3. IDDM
4. URI
5. narcolepsy
6. CPAP
7. hypoventilation
8. syndrome
9. symptoms
10. U
11. hypoglycemic
12. analgesic
13. cephalalgia
14. dyspnea
15. ventilatory

UNIT 10

Circle and Correct

1. b   2. d   3. a   4. b   5. d   6. c   7. b   8. b   9. c   10. d

Count with Prefixes

1. nulli, nulligravida
2. primi, primipara
3. mono, monocyte
4. bi, bifurcate, birfurcation
5. tri, trilateral
6. quad, quadriplegia
7. quint, quintuplets
8. sexti, sextigravida
9. septi, septipara
10. octo, octogenarian
11. noni, nonigravida
12. deca, decaliter
13. centi, centimeter
14. kilo, kilocalorie
15. multi, multiglandular

Prefix and Word

1. ab, abduct
2. de, descending
3. ex, excise
4. iso, isotonic
5. aniso, anisocytosis
6. dia, diathermy
7. per, percussion
8. peri, pericardium
9. circum, circumduction
10. sub, sublingual, subglossal (hypo, hypoglossal)

Select and Construct Part I

1. laparoscope
2. pyrosis
3. hyperhidrosis (hidrosis, hidrorrhea)
4. glycolysis
5. paracystitis
6. hypoglycemia
7. glucolipid (glycolipid)
8. decagram
9. millimeter
10. retromammary

Select and Construct Part II

1. excretion
2. abort
3. narcolepsy
4. mastocarcinoma
5. abrade
6. parahepatitis
7. narcotic
8. decalcification
9. isotonic
10. circumcision
11. ablation
12. percussion
13. anisocytosis
14. ablactation
15. dehydration
16. perfusion
17. circumduction
18. exhale, expiration
19. abrasion, abrade
20. pericardium

Abbreviation Matching

1. d   2. g   3. f   4. b   5. a   6. h   7. o   8. t   9. q   10. r   11. p   12. s   13. j

Abbreviations—Weights and Measures

1. kg
2. mg
3. cc
4. dL
5. mm
6. mcg, μg

Abbreviation Matching

1. g   2. h   3. m   4. i   5. f   6. j   7. c   8. b

Abbreviation Fill-in

9. q4h   10. D/W   11. NS   12. qid   13. †

ANSWERS

Case Study

1. subcuticular
2. anesthesia
3. multifocal
4. carcinoma in situ
5. dissected
6. axillary
7. hemostasis
8. mastectomy
9. mammogram
10. sterile
11. retraction
12. microcalcifications
13. biopsy

UNIT 11

Circle and Correct

1. c   2. d   3. a   4. d   5. a   6. b   7. c   8. a   9. d   10. b

Select and Construct

1. antibiotic (antiseptic)
2. contraceptive
3. homosexual
4. anisocytosis
5. sympodia
6. substernal (infrasternal)
7. mammography
8. ultrasonographer (sonographer)
9. epidural
10. extracystic
11. trilateral
12. metastasis

Prefix and Word

1. homo, homosexual
2. hetero, heterogeneous
3. sym, sympodia
4. super, superficial
5. supra, suprarenal
6. a/an, amenorrhea
7. a/an, anesthesia
8. epi, epigastric
9. extra, extracellular
10. infra, infrasternal
11. meta, metacarpals
12. ultra, ultrasound (ultrasonic)
13. bi, bilateral
14. anti, antiarthritic
15. contra, contraindicated
16. trans, transurethral

Abbreviation Matching

1. g   2. f   3. i   4. h   5. a   6. j   7. l   8. c

Abbreviation Fill-in

9. AAMA   10. s̄   11. inf   12. XM   13. subcu, subq, s.c.   14. FTM   15. TURP

Case Study

1. subdural
2. anesthesiologist
3. incision
4. hemostasis
5. subcutaneous
6. pericranium
7. retracted
8. perforator
9. dura mater
10. transferred
11. hemiparesis
12. temporoparietal

UNIT 12

Circle and Correct

1. c   2. d   3. b   4. d   5. c   6. d   7. c   8. a

Prefix and Word

1. ex, exhale
2. in, incise
3. in, incompetent
4. mal, malnutrition
5. tri, trigeminal
6. bi, bifocal
7. uni, unilateral
8. semi, semiconscious
9. hemi, hemiatrophy
10. con, congenital
11. dis, disinfectant
12. post, postmastectomy
13. pre, presurgical
14. pre, prefrontal
15. retro, retroesophageal
16. ante, antefebrile
17. intra, intradermal
18. inter, intercellular
19. sub, subcutaneous

ANSWERS

Select and Construct

1. antenatal (prenatal)
2. postpartum
3. hemicardia
4. semicomatose
5. unicellular
6. uninuclear
7. precancerous
8. inject
9. incontinent
10. insane
11. malformation
12. malaria
13. postcoital
14. antefebrile, prefebrile
15. postcibal
16. precancerous

Abbreviation Matching

1. g   2. f   3. i   4. c   5. h   6. k   7. l   8. b

Abbreviation Fill-in

9. exc   10. AIH   11. ID   12. iii   13. am   14. inf   15. prn

Case Study

1. bilateral
2. endometriomata
3. incised
4. transversely
5. visceroperitoneum
6. preoperative
7. dissect
8. posterior
9. intracystic
10. appendectomy
11. salpingo-oophorectomy
12. adhesions
13. postoperative
14. dissecting

UNIT 13

Circle and Correct

1. c   2. c   3. a   4. d   5. a   6. b   7. c   8. a   9. d   10. a   11. d   12. d

Art Labeling

1. e   2. d   3. c   4. h   5. g   6. a   7. f

Select and Construct

1. pulmonary (pulmonic)
2. pneumonomelanosis
3. dermatomycosis (mycodermatitis)
4. embolus (embolism)
5. mycology
6. nasomental
7. pharyngoscope
8. pleurocentesis
9. dextropedal
10. sinistromanual
11. pediatrician
12. histolysis
13. bronchitis
14. laryngalgia (laryngodynia)
15. phrenoplegia
16. bronchiectasis (bronchodilation)
17. psychiatrist
18. tracheostomy
19. chiropractor

Abbreviation Matching

1. f   2. n   3. a   4. l   5. m   6. k   7. h   8. j   9. c   10. p

Abbreviation Fill-in

11. PE   12. PFT   13. CO_2 14. R   15. COPD   16. RHIA

Matching

1. e   2. d   3. a   4. f   5. c   6. b   7. g

Case Study

1. bronchitis
2. pulse
3. tachypnea
4. intravenous
5. oximetry
6. O_2
7. %
8. respiratory
9. asthmaticus
10. viral
11. oxygen
12. IV
13. symptoms
14. syndrome

ANSWERS

UNIT 14

Circle and Correct

1. c 2. d 3. b 4. a 5. d 6. c 7. b 8. c 9. d 10. b 11. c 12. a

Select and Construct

1. sternalgia (sternodynia)
2. brachiocephalic
3. mycostasis (fungistasis)
4. ischiopubic
5. condylectomy
6. rachischisis
7. palatoschisis (uranoschisis)
8. xiphocostal
9. metacarpals
10. schizophasia
11. somnabulism (noctambulism)
12. nyctalopia
13. nycturia (nocturia)
14. ankylodactylia
15. iliac
16. pubic
17. femoral
18. patellar
19. fibular
20. tarsals
21. metatarsals
22. calcaneus, calcaneum
23. cost/o, costal
24. chondral

Skeletal Combining Forms and Adjectival Forms

1. cranio, cranial
2. cervico, cervical
3. cleido, clavicular
4. scapulo, scapular
5. acromio, acromial
6. humero, humeral
7. sterno, sternal
8. xipho, xiphoid
9. ulno, ulnar
10. radio, radial
11. carpo, carpal
12. metacarpo, metacarpal
13. phalango, phalangeal
14. ischio, ischial
15. ilio, iliac
16. pubo, pubic
17. femoro, femoral
18. patello, patellar
19. tibio, tibial
20. fibulo, fibular
21. tarso, tarsal
22. metatarso, metatarsal
23. calcaneo, calcaneal
24. costo, costal
25. chondro, chondral

Art Labeling

15—xiph/o, xiphoid
20—condyle/o, condyle
5—femor/o, femur
12—cleid/o, clavicle
6—phalang/o, phalanx
7—carp/o, carpus
9—radi/o, radius
10—humer/o, humerus
16—cost/o, rib
11—scapul/o, scapula
8—uln/o, ulna
1—metatars/o, metatarsal
2—tibi/o, tibia
3—fibul/o, fibula
17—vertebr/o, vertebra
14—stern/o, sternum
13—crani/o, cranium
18—ili/o, ilium
19—ischi/o, ischium
4—patell/o, patella

Abbreviation Matching

1. l 2. f 3. e 4. g 5. k 6. h 7. c 8. m

Abbreviation Fill-in

9. C_3 10. FxBB 11. OT(R), OTR 12. AOTA 13. R, rt 14. y/o (yr) 15. ORIF

Case Study

1. inspection
2. manually
3. lateral
4. incision
5. sterile
6. subcutaneous
7. anatomic
8. internal
9. fracture
10. pneumatic
11. anesthetized
12. reduction
13. fixation
14. epicondyle
15. humerus
16. M
17. y/o
18. right
19. par

ANSWERS

UNIT 15

Circle and Correct

1. d   2. c   3. b   4. a   5. d   6. b   7. a   8. d   9. a   10. d   11. b   12. b   13. c   14. a

Select and Construct

1. optometry
2. cycloplegia
3. onychomalacia
4. iritis
5. dacryorrhea
6. phacoemulsification
7. adrenalin (epinephrine)
8. hyperopia
9. retinoscope
10. traumatology
11. ophthalmoplasty
12. corectasis (corectasia)
13. blepharoptosis
14. keratotomy
15. thyromegaly
16. anisocoria
17. esotropia
18. presbyopia
19. onychocryptosis
20. retinoplasty

Art Labeling

1—corne/o, kerat/o cornea
5—retin/o, retina
8—lacrim/o, lacrimal
4—cycl/o, ciliary body
9—core/o, pupil
3—phac/o, lens
10—irid/o, iris
7—blephar/o, eyelid
2—conjunctiv/o, conjunction
6—scler/o, sclera

Abbreviation Matching

1. n   2. r   3. g   4. f   5. p   6. a   7. m   8. i   9. d   10. l

Abbreviation Fill-in

11. AOA   12. EMT   13. FSH   14. T3, T4   15. OD   16. L&A

Case Study

1. phacoemulsification
2. abrasion
3. capsulorrhexis
4. intraocular
5. keratome
6. myopia
7. cataract
8. epinucleus
9. corneal
10. paracentesis
11. OD

The following lists of abbreviations are grouped by topic. To assist you in learning, they are arranged in columns. Column 1 lists the abbreviation, column 2 the meaning, and column 3 is left blank as a work space. Study the abbreviation and its meaning. Then cover the abbreviation and read the meaning. Write the abbreviation correctly in the blank. You may use the same method to learn the meanings by covering the meaning and reading the abbreviation. Write the meaning correctly on a separate piece of paper. Abbreviations that correspond to word parts presented in the frames are also listed at the end of each unit.

Weights and Measures

Metric:

kg	kilogram(s) (1000 g)	_____
hg	hectogram (100 g)	_____
dag	decagram (10 g)	_____
gm or g	gram	_____
dg	decigram (0.1 g)	_____
cg	centigram (0.01 g)	_____
mg	milligram (0.001 g)	_____
mcg, μg	microgram (0.001 mg)	_____

Standard:

lb, #	pound	_____
oz, ℥	ounce	_____
dr, ʒ	dram	_____
gr	grain	_____

Volume:

cu mm	cubic millimeter (mm^3)	_____
cc	cubic centimeter (cm^3)	_____
cu m	cubic meter (m^3)	_____
cu in	cubic inch (in^3)	_____
cu ft	cubic foot (ft^3)	_____
cu yd	cubic yard (yd^3)	_____

Apothecary:

ī, īī, īīī	one, two, three	_____
īv, v̄, etc.	four, five, etc.	_____
īss	one and one half	_____

Lengths:

in, "	inch (2.54 cm)	_____
ft, '	foot (12 in)	_____
yd	yard (36 in)	_____
μm	micrometer (0.000001 m)	_____
mm	millimeter (0.001 m)	_____
cm	centimeter (0.01 m)	_____
m	meter	_____
km	kilometer (1000 m)	_____

Liquid Volume:

t, tsp	teaspoon	_____
T, Tbsp	tablespoon	_____
c	cup	_____
m, min	minim	_____

ABBREVIATIONS

ml	milliliter (0.001 L)
cc	cubic centimeter (1 ml)
cl	centiliter (0.01 L)
dl	deciliter (0.1 L)
L	liter (1000 ml)
dal	decaliter (10 L)
hl	hectoliter (100 L)
fl dr, fl ʒ	fluid dram (60 min)
fl oz, fl ʒ	fluid ounce (8 fl dr)
pt	pint (16 oz)
qt	quart (32 oz)
gal, °	gallon (4 qt)
gt	drop (1 min)
gtt	drops

Miscellaneous:

at wt	atomic weight
C, kcal	calorie
c, Ci	curie
ht	height
mA	milliampere
mEq	milliequivalent
MHz	megahertz
mg%	milligram percent
mw	molecular weight
IU	international units
U	units
°C	degrees Celsius
°F	degrees Fahrenheit

Chemical Symbols

Ag	silver (argentum—Latin)
$AgNO_3$	silver nitrate
Al	aluminum
Ar	argon
As	arsenic
Au	gold
B	boron
Ba	barium
Br	bromine
C	carbon
$C_6H_{12}O_6$	glucose
Ca	calcium (Ca^{++} ion)
Cd	cadmium
Cl	chlorine (Cl^- ion)
Co	cobalt
CO_2	carbon dioxide
Cr	chromium
Cu	copper (Cu^{++} ion)
F	fluorine
Fe	iron (ferrum—Latin)
H	hydrogen

ABBREVIATIONS

H_2O	water
HCl	hydrochloric acid
He	helium
Hg	mercury (hydrargyrum—Latin)
I	iodine (I^{131} radioactive)
K	potassium (kalium—Latin, K^+ ion)
Kr	krypton
Li	lithium
Mg	magnesium
Mn	manganese
N	nitrogen
Na	sodium (natrium—Latin Na^+ ion)
NaCl	sodium chloride (table salt)
Ne	neon
O	oxygen (O_2 molecule)
P	phosphorus
Pb	lead (plumbum—Latin)
pCO_2	partial pressure carbon dioxide
pO_2	partial pressure oxygen
Ra	radium
S	sulfur
Se	selenium
Si	silicon
U	uranium
Zn	zinc

Diagnoses

AB 1, 2, 3 . . .	abortion one, two, three . . .
ABE	acute bacterial endocarditis
ACVD	acute cardiovascular disease
AF (Afib)	atrial fibrillation
AI	aortic insufficiency
AID	acute infectious disease
	artificial insemination donor
AIDS	acquired immunodeficiency syndrome
AIH	artificial insemination husband
ALL	acute lymphocytic leukemia
ALS	amyotrophic lateral sclerosis
AMI	acute myocardial infarction
AML	acute myelocytic leukemia
AOD	arterial occlusive disease
ARC	AIDS-related complex (conditions)
ARD	acute respiratory disease
ARF	acute respiratory failure
	acute renal failure
	acute rheumatic fever
ARV	AIDS-related virus
AS	aortic stenosis
	arteriosclerosis
	left ear (auris sinistra)
ASCVD	arteriosclerotic cardiovascular disease

ABBREVIATIONS

ASHD	arteriosclerotic heart disease	_____
AV, A-V	arteriovenous, atrioventricular	_____
BCC	basal cell carcinoma	_____
BO	body odor	_____
BPH	benign prostatic hyperplasia (hypertrophy)	_____
CA	cancer	_____
CAD	coronary artery disease	_____
CD	childhood disease	_____
CE	cardiac enlargement	_____
CF	cystic fibrosis	_____
CHD	congestive heart disease	_____
	congenital hip dislocation	_____
	congenital or coronary heart disease	_____
CHF	congestive heart failure	_____
CIS	carcinoma in situ	_____
CLD	chronic liver disease	_____
	chronic lung disease	_____
COLD	chronic obstructive lung disease	_____
COPD	chronic obstructive pulmonary disease	_____
CP	cerebral palsy	_____
	cor pulmonale	_____
CPD	cephalopelvic disproportion	_____
CRF	chronic renal failure	_____
CT	carpal tunnel (syndrome)	_____
	coronary thrombosis	_____
CVA	cerebrovascular accident (stroke)	_____
CVD	cardiovascular disease	_____
DNR	do not resuscitate	_____
DOA	dead on arrival	_____
DRG	diagnostic-related group	_____
DTs	delirium tremens	_____
Dx	diagnosis	_____
EOMI	extraocular movement intact (muscles)	_____
ESRD	end stage renal disease (failure)	_____
FAS	fetal alcohol syndrome	_____
FB	foreign body	_____
FOD	free of disease	_____
FTND	full-term norm delivery	_____
FTT	failure to thrive	_____
FUO	fever of unknown origin	_____
Fx	fracture	_____
FxBB	fracture both bones	_____
GERD	gastroesophageal reflux disease	_____
GNID	gram-negative intracellular diplococci	_____
G, Grav 1 2, 3 . . ., G1, G2	pregnancy one, two, three . . .	_____
HA	headache	_____
	hearing aid	_____
	hemolytic anemia	_____
	hepatitis A	_____
HAA	hepatitis-associated antigen	_____

ABBREVIATIONS

HBV	hepatitis B virus	_____
HC	Huntington's chorea	_____
HCVD	hypertensive cardiovascular disease	_____
HD	Hodgkin's disease	_____
HDN	hemolytic disease of newborn	_____
HF	heart failure	_____
HH	hiatal hernia	_____
	hard of hearing	_____
HAV	hepatitis A virus	_____
HCV	hepatitis C virus	_____
HIV	human immunodeficiency virus	_____
HLV	herpes-like virus	_____
HPV	human papilloma virus	_____
HSV	herpes simplex virus	_____
HTLV/III	human T-cell lymphotropic virus/three	_____
HTN	hypertension	_____
Hx	history	_____
IDDM	insulin-dependent diabetes mellitus	_____
IHD	ischemic heart disease	_____
IM	infectious mononucleosis	_____
LAV	lymphadenopathy-associated virus	_____
LE	lupus erythematosus	_____
LGB	Landry-Guillain-Barré syndrome	_____
LOA	left occiput anterior	_____
MBD	minimal brain dysfunction	_____
MD	manic depression	_____
	muscular dystrophy	_____
	myocardial disease	_____
met., metas., mets.	metastasis, metastases	_____
MI	myocardial infarction	_____
mono	mononucleosis	_____
MP	metacarpophalangeal (joint)	_____
MS	mitral stenosis	_____
	multiple sclerosis	_____
MVP	mitral valve prolapse	_____
NMT	nebulizing mist treatment	_____
OA	osteoarthritis	_____
OAG	open-angle glaucoma	_____
OCD	obsessive-compulsive disorder	_____
OM	otitis media	_____
P (1, 2, 3 . . .)	preterm parity 1, 2, 3	_____
PAC	premature atrial contraction	_____
PAR	perennial allergic rhinitis	_____
	postanesthesia recovery	_____
para	paraplegic	_____
para 1, 2, 3 . . .	live births (one, two, three . . .)	_____
PAT	paroxysmal atrial tachycardia	_____
PCD	polycystic disease	_____
PD	Parkinson's disease	_____
	pulmonary disease	_____

ABBREVIATIONS

PE	pulmonary edema	_____
	pulmonary embolism	_____
PERRLA	pupils equal, round, reactive to light and accommodation	_____
PID	pelvic inflammatory disease	_____
PKU	phenylketonuria	_____
PMS	premenstrual syndrome	_____
PND	paroxysmal nocturnal dyspnea	_____
	postnasal drip	_____
preg	pregnant	_____
PVC	premature ventricular contraction	_____
Px	prognosis	_____
RA	rheumatoid arthritis	_____
ROP	right occiput posterior	_____
S-C disease	sickle cell hemoglobin-c disease	_____
schiz	schizophrenia	_____
SIDS	sudden infant death syndrome	_____
staph	staphylococcus	_____
STD	sexually transmitted disease	_____
STI	sexually transmitted infection	_____
strep	streptococcus	_____
T (1, 2, 3)	Term parity 1, 2, 3	_____
Tb	tubercle bacillus	_____
Top	termination of pregnancy	_____
type 1	diabetes (insulin dependent)	_____
type 2	diabetes (noninsulin, adult)	_____
TB	tuberculosis	_____
TCS	transcavital sonography	_____
thal	thalassemia	_____
TEE	transesophageal echocardiography	_____
TIA	transient ischemic attack	_____
TSD	Tay-Sachs disease	_____
TVS	transvaginal sonography	_____
URI	upper respiratory infection	_____
UTI	urinary tract infection	_____
VD	venereal disease (old, use. STD)	_____

Procedures

A, B, O, AB	blood typing groups	_____
AB	abortion	_____
ABG	arterial blood gas	_____
ACT	activated clotting time—Lee-White	_____
ACTH	adrenocorticotropic hormone (test)	_____
AFB	acid-fast bacillus	_____
AID	artificial insemination donor	_____
AIH	artificial insemination husband	_____
ANA	antinuclear antibodies (RIA)	_____
A&P	auscultation and percussion	_____
BaEn, BE	barium enema	_____
BP	blood pressure	_____
BUN	blood urea nitrogen	_____

ABBREVIATIONS

Bx	biopsy
C-section	cesarean section
CABG	coronary artery bypass graft
CAD	computer-aided design
CAPD	continuous ambulatory peritoneal dialysis
CAT, CAT scan	computerized axial tomography (scan)
cath	catheter
CBC	complete blood count
CH, chol	cholesterol
CPAP	continuous positive airway pressure
CPK	creatine phosphokinase
CPR	cardiopulmonary resuscitation
CSF	cerebrospinal fluid
CT	computerized tomography (scan)
CXR	chest x-ray
cysto	cystoscopy
C&S	culture and sensitivity
del	delivery
DHT	dihydrotestosterone
DNA	deoxyribonucleic acid
DPT DTP, DTaP	diphtheria-pertussis-tetanus (vaccine)
D&C	dilation and curettage
ECG, EKG	electrocardiogram
ECHO	echocardiogram
ECT	electroconvulsive therapy
EEG	electroencephalogram
EGD	esophagogastroduodenoscopy
EMG	electromyogram
ENG	electrony stagmography
EP	evoked potential
ERCP	endoscopic retrograde cholangiopancreatography
ERG	electroretinogram
ESR	erythrocyte sedimentation rate (sed. rate)
ESWL	extracorporeal shockwave lithotripsy
exam	examination
exc	excision
FBS	fasting blood sugar
FME	full mouth extraction
FSH	follicle-stimulating hormone
GA	gastric analysis
GTT	glucose tolerance test
GxT	graded exercise test
HA	hearing aid
HAA	hepatitis-associated antigen (test)
HAI	hemagglutination inhibition—rubella test
Hb, Hgb	hemoglobin
HBV	hepatitis B virus
HCG (hcg)	human chorionic gonadotropin

ABBREVIATIONS

Hct	hematocrit
HDL	high-density lipoprotein
HepB	hepatitis B vaccine
HGH	human growth hormone
Hib	*Hemophilus influenzae* vaccine
HSG	hysterosalpingogram
Hx	history
H&P	history and physical
IABP	intra-aortic balloon pump
ICAT	indirect Coomb's test
ICSH	interstitial cell-stimulating hormone
ID	intradermal (injection), identification
Ig	immunoglobulin, gamma (A, E, D, G, or M)
IM	intramuscular (injection)
inf	infusion
instill	instillation (drops)
IPPB	intermittent positive pressure breathing
IPV	inactivated polio virus vaccine (injectable)
IUD	intrauterine device
IV	intravenous (injection)
IVC	intravenous catheter
	intravenous cholangiogram
IVP	intravenous pyelogram
I&D	incision and drainage
I&O	intake and output
KUB	kidney-ureter-bladder (x-ray)
lab	laboratory
LASER	light amplification by stimulated emission of radiation
LAVH	laparoscopically assisted vaginal hysterectomy
LDH	lactose dehydrogenase
LDL	low-density lipoprotein
LH	luteinizing hormone
LP	lumbar puncture
MASER	microwave amplification by stimulated emission of radiation
MFT	muscle function test
MMRV	measles, mumps, rubella vaccine
MRI	magnetic resonance imaging
NCS	nerve conduction studies
OC	office call
OMT	osteopathic manipulative therapy
OPG	oculoplethysmography
OPV	oral polio vaccine
OREF	open reduction external fixation
ORIF	open reduction internal fixation
O&P	ova and parasites test
P+V	pyloroplasty and vagotomy

ABBREVIATIONS

Pap	Papanicolaou test (smear)
Pap	pulmonary artery pressure
PBI	protein bound iodine
PCTA	percutaneous transluminal angioplasty
PCV	packed cell volume, pneumococcal vaccine
PE	physical examination
PET	positron emission tomography
PFT	pulmonary function test
pH	hydrogen ion concentration, acid/base
PO, postop	postoperative
pro time, pt	prothrombin time
PSA	prostate specific antigen
PSG	polysomnogram
PTCA	percutaneous transluminal coronary angioplasty
PTT	partial thromboplastin time
2hr pc	two-hour postcibal blood glucose
2hr pg	two-hour postglucose blood glucose
2hr pp	two-hour postprandial blood glucose
P&A	percussion and auscultation
RATx	radiation therapy
RBC	red blood cell (count)
RIA	radioimmunoassay
RPG	retrograde pyelogram
RPR	syphilis test (also: DRT, VDRL, STS)
Rx	take, prescribe
S/A, S&A	sugar and acetone
SALT (old SGPT)	serum alanine aminotransferase
SAST (old SGOT)	serum aspartate aminotransferase
Sc, subcu, subq, sq	subcutaneous (injection)
SOP	standard operating procedure
sp gr, SpG	specific gravity (urine)
T, temp	temperature
T3	thyroid test (triiodothyronine)
T4	thyroid test (tetraiodothyronine)
tab	tablet(s)
TAH	total abdominal hysterectomy
Td	tetanus
TENS	transcutaneous electrical nerve stimulation
TSE	testicular self-exam
TSH	thyroid-stimulating hormone
TUR (TURP)	transurethral resection (of the prostate)
Tx	treatment, traction, transplant
UA	urinalysis
UV	ultraviolet (light)
V, Y, W, Z, -plasty	various types of plastic surgery
Var	vanan chickenpox vaccine (Varicella coster)
VCG	vectorcardiogram

ABBREVIATIONS

VDRL	Venereal Disease Research Laboratory (syphilis test)
WBC	white blood cell (count)
XM	crossmatch for blood (type and crossmatch)
XR	x-ray
YAG	yttrium-aluminum-garnet (laser)

Health Professions and Groups

AA	Alcoholics Anonymous
AAFP	American Academy of Family Physicians
AAMA	American Association of Medical Assistants
AAMT	American Association of Medical Transcriptionists
AANA	American Association of Nurse Anesthetists
AAP	American Academy of Pediatrics
AAPA	American Academy of Physician Assistants
AART	American Association of Rehabilitation Therapy
ACOA	Adult Children of Alcoholics
ACPMR	American Congress of Physical Medicine and Rehabilitation
ACS	American Cancer Society
	American College of Surgeons
ADA	American Dental Association
	American Diabetes Association
	American Dietetic Association
AHA	American Heart Association
AHIMA	American Health Information Management Association
AL-Anon, Alateen	Families of Alcoholics Groups
AMA	American Medical Association
ANA	American Nurses Association
	American Neurologic Association
AOA	American Optometric Association
	American Osteopathic Association
APA	American Psychiatric Association
APTA	American Physical Therapy Association
ARDMS	American Registry of Diagnostic Medical Sonographers
ARRT	American Registry of Radiologic Technologists
ART	Accredited Records Technician
ASCP	American Society of Clinical Pathologists
ASRT	American Society of Radiologic Technologists
BSN	Bachelors of Science in Nursing
CDC	Centers for Disease Control
CENA, CNA	Certified Nursing Assistant, Competency Eligible Nursing Assistant

ABBREVIATIONS

CHUC	Certified Health Unit Coordinator (Clerk)
CLA	Certified Laboratory Assistant
CMA	Certified Medical Assistant
CMT	Certified Medical Transcriptionist
COMA	Certified Ophthalmic Medical Assistant
COMT	Certified Ophthalmic Medical Technician
COTA	Certified Occupational Therapy Assistant
CRNA	Certified Registered Nurse Anesthetist
CRTT	Certified Respiratory Therapy Technician
CST	Certified Surgical Technologist
CT (ASCP)	Cyto technologist (American Society of Clinical Pathology)
DC	Doctor of Chiropractic
DDS	Doctor of Dental Surgery
DO	Doctor of Osteopathy
DPM	Doctor of Podiatric Medicine
EENT	Eye, Ear, Nose, and Throat specialist
EMT	Emergency Medical Technician
EMT-P	Emergency Medical Technician Paramedic
ENT	Ear, Nose, and Throat specialist
FACP	Fellow of the American College of Physicians
FACS	Fellow of the American College of Surgeons
GYN	Gynecologist
HMO	health maintenance organization
ICU	intensive care unit
LPN	Licensed Practical Nurse
LVN	Licensed Vocational Nurse
MD	Doctor of Medicine
MLT	Medical Laboratory Technician
MSN	Masters of Science in Nursing
MT (ASCP)	Medical Technologist (American Society of Clinical Pathologists)
NAHUC	National Association of Health Unit Coordinators (Clerks)
NANDA	North American Nursing Diagnosis Association
NLN	National League for Nursing
NP	Nurse Practitioner
OA	Overeaters Anonymous
OB	Obstetrician
ORTH	Orthopedist
OSHA	Occupational Safety and Health Administration
OT	Occupational Therapy
OTR	Occupational Therapist Registered
PA	Physician's Assistant
Pharm D	Doctor of Pharmacy
PT	Physical Therapy (Therapist)
RD	Registered Dietician

ABBREVIATIONS

RDCS	Registered Diagnostic Cardiac Sonographer
RDMS	Registered Diagnostic Medical Sonographer
RN	Registered Nurse
R.Ph	Registered Pharmacist
RRA	Registered Records Administrator
RRT	Registered Respiratory Therapist
RT (R)	Radiologic Technologist (Registered)
RT (N)	Radiologic Technologist (Nuclear)
RVT	Registered Vascular Technologist
USP	United States Pharmacopeia

Charting Abbreviations

aa	of each
ac	before meals *(ante cibum)*
AD	right ear *(auris dextra)*
ADLs	activities of daily living
ad lib	as desired (at liberty)
adm	admission
AE	above the elbow
AJ	ankle jerk
AK	above the knee
am	before noon *(ante meridiem)*
AMA	against medical advice
AMB	ambulate
ant	anterior
ANS	autonomic nervous system
AP	anteroposterior
approx	approximately
ASAP	as soon as possible
AS or LE	left ear *(auris sinistra)*, arteriosclerosis
AU	both ears *(auris uterque)*
AV	atrioventricular
BE	below the elbow
bid	twice a day *(bis in die)*
bin	twice a night *(bis in nocte)*
BK	below the knee
BM	bowel movement
BMR	basal metabolic rate
BP	blood pressure
BRP	bathroom privileges
c̄	with (Latin: *cum*)
$C_1, C_2, C_3 \ldots C_7$	cervical vertebrae first, second, third . . . seventh
$C_1, C_2 \ldots C_8$	cervical spinal nerve pairs
C	centigrade, celsius, or large calorie (kilocalorie)
cap(s)	capsules
CBR	complete bed rest
CC	chief complaint
CCU	cardiac care unit (coronary care unit)

ABBREVIATIONS

c/o	complains of
cont	continue
D	diopter (ocular measurement)
dc	discontinue
DC	discharge from hospital
DNA	does not apply
DNR	do not resuscitate
DNS	did not show
Dr	doctor
D/W	dextrose in water
Dx	diagnosis
EOM	extraocular movement
ER	emergency room
Ex	examination
F	Fahrenheit
FHS	fetal heart sounds
FHT	fetal heart tones
GB	gallbladder
GI	gastrointestinal
GU	genitourinary
h, hr, °	hour
Hb, Hgb	hemoglobin
hpf	high power field
hs	hour of sleep, bedtime (*hora somni*)
hypo	hypodermic injection
ICU	intensive care unit
IM	intramuscular
I&O	intake and output
$\overline{\text{iss}}$	one and one half
IU	international units
IV	intravenous
L, lt	left
$L_1, L_2, L_3 \ldots L_5$	lumbar vertebrae first, second, third . . . fifth (spinal nerve pairs)
L&A	light and accommodation
LAT	lateral
L&W	living and well
LLQ	left lower quadrant
LMP	last menstrual period
LOA	left occipitoanterior
LPF	low power field (10x)
LUQ	left upper quadrant of abdomen
MTD	right ear drum (membrana tympani dexter)
MTS	left ear drum (membrana tympani sinister)
neg	negative
NG	nasogastric
NPO	nothing by mouth
NS	norm saline
OD	right eye (*oculus dexter*)

ABBREVIATIONS

OP	outpatient
OR	operating room
OS or OL	left eye *(oculus sinister, oculus laevus)*
OU	each eye *(oculus uterque)*
	both eyes *(oculi unitas)*
P	pulse
PA	posteroanterior
pc	after meals *(post cibum)*
PDR	Physicians' Desk Reference
PI	present illness
po	by mouth *(per os)*
PO	postoperative
pm	afternoon or evening (post meridiem)
PNS	peripheral nervous system
prn	as needed or desired *(pro re nata)*
q	every *(quaque)*
qd	every day *(quaque die)*
qh	every hour *(quaque hora)*
q2h, q4h	every two hours, every four hours
qid	four times a day *(quater in die)*
qm	every morning *(quaque mane)*
qn	every night *(quaque nocte)*
R, rt	right, respiration
RBC	red blood cell, erythrocyte count
Rh	blood factor, Rh+ or Rh−
RLQ	right lower quadrant (abdomen)
R/O	rule out
ROM	range of motion
RPO	right occiput oblique
RUQ	right upper quadrant (abdomen)
$S_1, S_2, \ldots S_5$	sacral spinal nerve pairs
	without (sine)
sc, subcu, sq, subq	subcutaneously (into fat layer)
sed rate	sedimentation rate (erythrocyte)
SOB	short of breath
SOS	if necessary *(si opus sit)*
$\bar{\text{ss}}$, ½, .5	half (Latin: *semis*)
staph	staphylococcus
stat	immediately (statim)
strep	streptococcus
Sx	symptoms
$T_1, T_2, T_3 \ldots T_{12}$	thoracic vertebrae: first, second, third . . . twelfth (thoracic spinal nerve pairs)
T, temp	temperature
tab(s)	tablets
TC&DB	turn, cough, and deep breathe
tid	three times a day *(ter in die)*
tinct	tincture
TPN	total parenteral nutrition
trans	transverse

ABBREVIATIONS

ULQ	upper left quadrant (abdomen)
ung	ointment (unguentum)
URQ	upper right quadrant (abdomen)
VS	vital signs
WBC	white blood cell, leukocyte count
wm, bm	white male, black male
wf, bf	white female, black female
x	times, power
y/o, yr	year(s) old, year(s)
−	negative
F, ♀	female
M, ♂	male
+/−	positive or negative
*	birth
†	death
p̄	after (post–Latin)
ā	before (ante–Latin)
#	pound, number
↑	increase
↓	decrease
>	greater than
<	less than

APPENDIX C

PUZZLE SOLUTIONS

UNIT 1

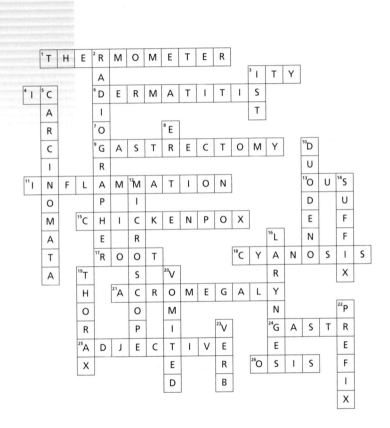

PUZZLE SOLUTIONS

UNIT 2

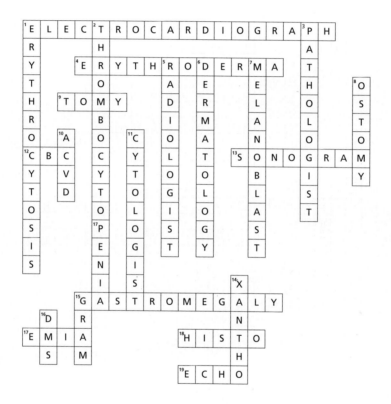

PUZZLE SOLUTIONS

UNIT 3

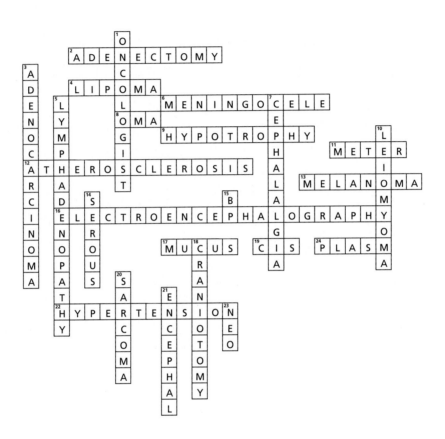

PUZZLE SOLUTIONS

UNIT 4

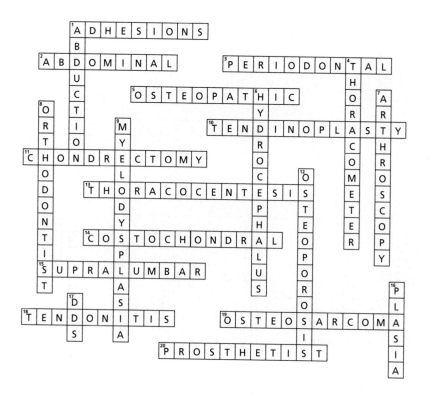

PUZZLE SOLUTIONS

UNIT 5

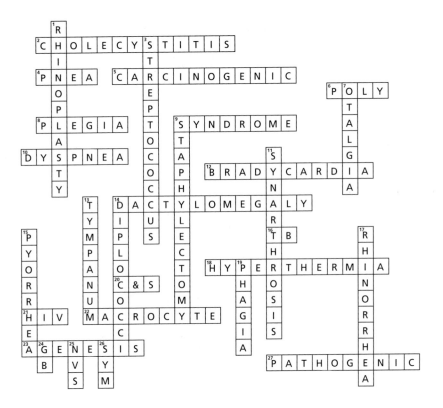

PUZZLE SOLUTIONS

UNIT 6

Across

1. CYSTORRHAPHY
3. PENILE
5. NEPHROPYELITIS
8. ENDOMETRIOSIS
12. BALANORRHEA
13. OLIGURIA
21. ORCHIOPEXY
23. URETEROLITH
25. TESTICULAR

Down

2. PROSTATECTOMY
4. TUP
6. HYSTEROSALPINGOGRAM
7. NEPHROPTOSIS
9. ORCHIDOPLASTY
10. UTERINE
11. RENAL
14. METROPA
15. MENORRHAGIA
16. HYSTEROCELE
17. OOPRITIS
18. POLYOTIA
19. CLPALGIA
20. HMATURIA
22. CRYPTO
24. PD

PUZZLE SOLUTIONS

UNIT 7

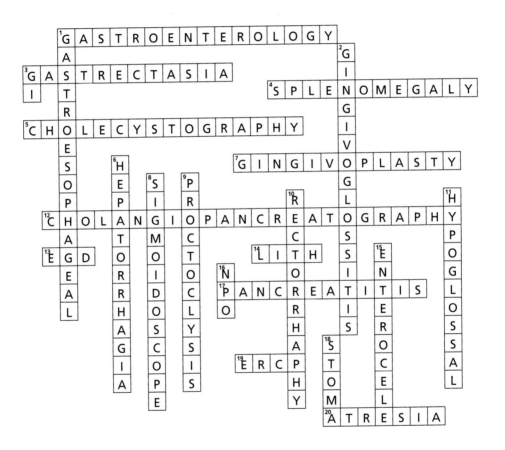

PUZZLE SOLUTIONS

UNIT 8

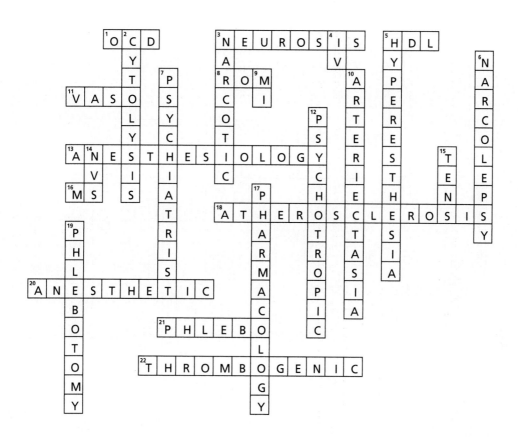

PUZZLE SOLUTIONS

UNIT 9

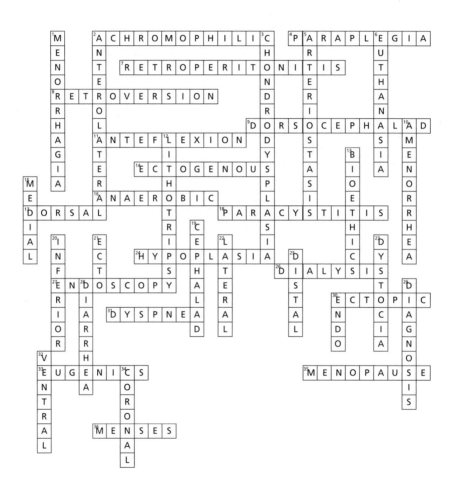

PUZZLE SOLUTIONS

UNIT 10a

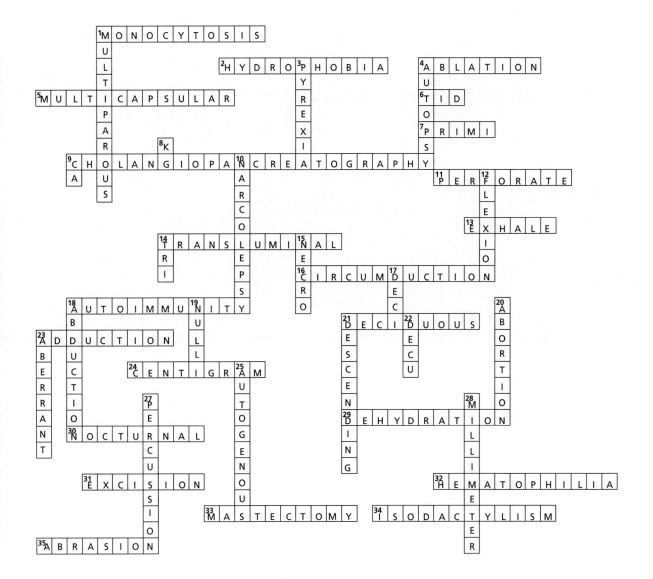

PUZZLE SOLUTIONS

UNIT 10b

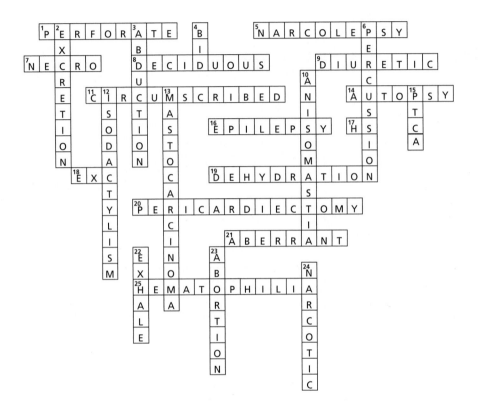

PUZZLE SOLUTIONS

UNIT 11

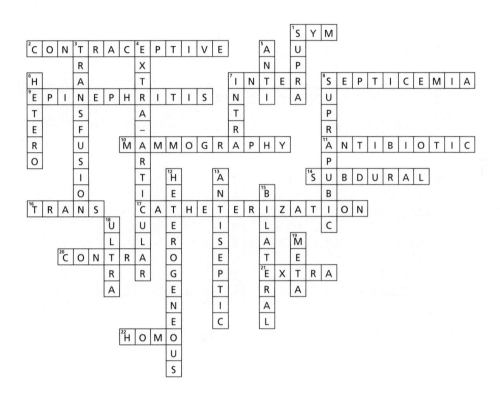

PUZZLE SOLUTIONS

UNIT 12

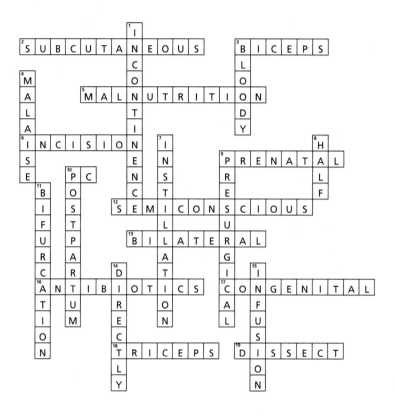

PUZZLE SOLUTIONS

UNIT 13

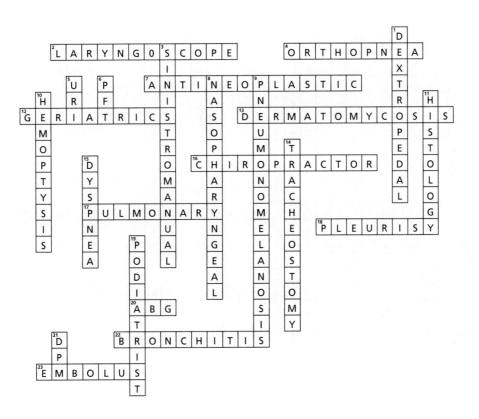

PUZZLE SOLUTIONS

UNIT 14

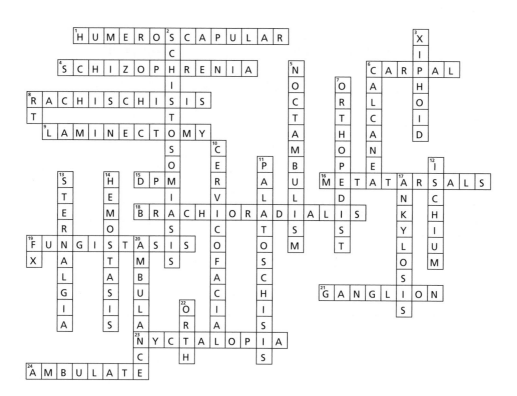

PUZZLE SOLUTIONS

UNIT 15

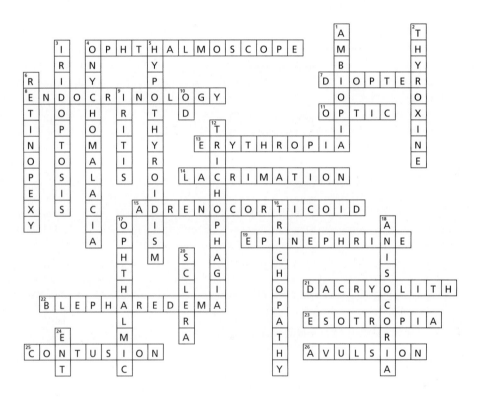

APPENDIX D

ADDITIONAL WORD PARTS

Following are word parts in addition to those presented in your study of the frames. Use these lists, your knowledge of word building, and your medical dictionary to enrich your medical vocabulary.

1. Pick a word part from the alphabetic list that interests you.
2. Look for it in your medical dictionary.
3. Find words that begin or end with this part and make a list.
4. Write the meanings of the new words you discovered.
5. Use the key in your dictionary to decipher the correct pronunciation, and practice saying the new words.

Word Part	Meaning	Example
acid/o	acid	acid/osis
acne	point	acne vulgaris
actin/o	ray (radiation)	actin/o/dermat/itis
acu	needle	acu/puncture
adenoid	resembling a gland	aden/oid/ectomy
adnex/al	adjacent, accessory	adnex/ectomy
albin/o	white	albin/ism
alkal/o	base	alkal/osis
all/o	other, different	all/o/pathy, all/ergy
ambly/o	dim, dull	ambly/opia
amyl/o	starch	amyl/ase
andr/o	man	andr/o/gen
aneurysm	abnormal dilation	aneurysm/o/rrhaphy
aort/o	aorta	aort/o/graphy
atel/o	imperfect, collapsed	atel/ectasis
bar/o	weight, heavy	bar/iatrics
bil/i	bile	bil/i/rubin
cac/o	bad, diseased	cac/hexia
cat/a	down, downward	cat/a/tonic
celi/o	abdominal region	celi/ac artery
cerumin	wax	cerumin/o/lysis
chalas/ia	relaxation	a/chalas/ia
chem/o	chemical, drug	chem/o/therapy
chron/o	time	chronological, chronic
chym/o	juice	ec/chym/o/sis
cirrhos	orange-yellow	cirrh/o/sis
clasia	breaking down	arthr/o/clasia
cleisis	closure, occlusion	colp/o/cleis/is
coll/o	glutinous, jellylike	coll/agen
cry/o	freezing	cry/o/surgery
decub/o	lying down	decubit/us ulcer
eczem/o	boil out	eczem/a
effer	to bring out	effer/ent
effus	to pour out	effus/ion
fec/a	feces	fec/a/lith
glomerul/o	glomerulus	glomerul/o/nephr/itis
gonad/o	ovaries, testes	gonad/o/tropin
halit/o	breath	halit/o/sis
kal/i	potassium	hyper/kal/emia
kary/o	nucleus	kary/o/type

Word Part	Meaning	Example
ket/o	ketones	ket/o/sis
klept/o	stealing	klept/o/mania
kyph/o	humped	kyph/o/sis
lord/o	bending	lord/o/sis
mediastin/o	mediastinum	mediastin/al
morph/o	form	meso/morph/ic
muscul/o	muscle	muscul/o/skelet/al
natr/i	sodium	hyper/natr/emia
orexis	appetite	an/orex/ia
pach/y	thick	pach/y/dermat/ous
-poiesis	produce, form	hemat/o/poies/is
poikil/o	irregular shape	poikil/o/cyt/o/sis
prax/ia	action	a/prax/ia
prur/i	itch	prur/itis
pteryg/o	wing	pteryg/o/mandibul/ar
ptyal/o	saliva	ptyal/in
radicul/o	root	radicul/o/neur/itis
roentgen/o	x-ray	roentgen/o/graphy
scoli/o	lateral curve	scoli/o/sis
scot/o	darkness	scot/oma
seb/o	fatty, sebum	seb/o/rrhea
sial/o	saliva	sial/aden/itis
somat/o	body	psych/o/somat/ic
sphygm/o	pulse	sphygm/o/man/o/meter
sphyxis	pulse (related to O_2)	a/sphyxia
stere/o	solid, three-dimensional	stere/o/metry
steth/o	chest	steth/o/scope
sthenia	strength	my/e/sthen/ia
stigma	point	a/stigmat/ism
stigmat/o	mark, point	a/stigmat/ism
taxia	muscle coordination	a/tax/ia
tel/e	distant, far	tel/e/metry
terat/o	monster, wonder	terat/o/genic
tetra	four	tetra/cycline
thel/o	nipple	thel/o/rrhagia
tresia	perforation, closure	a/tres/ia
vagin/o	vagina	vagin/itis
varic/o	twisted vein	varic/o/sity
vulv/o	vulva	vulv/o/vagin/itis
xen/o	strange, foreign	xen/o/phob/ia
xer/o	dry	xer/o/derma

APPENDIX E

GLOSSARY OF PROPER NAMES OF DISEASES AND PROCEDURES

Addison's disease	deficiency in adrenocortical hormones caused by a progressive destruction of the adrenal glands
Bartholin cyst	cyst of the gland located in the cleft between the labia minora and the hymenal ring that secretes mucous lubricant
Bell's palsy	idiopathic facial palsy of CN VII resulting in asymmetry of the palpebral fissures, nasolabial folds, mouth, and facial expression on the affected side
Biot's respirations	irregular respiratory pattern caused by damage to the medulla
Bouchard's node	bony enlargement of the proximal interphalangeal joint of the finger
Braxton Hicks contractions	uterine contractions that are irregular and painless; also known as false labor
Brushfield's spots	small, white flecks located around the perimeter of the iris and associated with Down syndrome
Cesarean section	delivery of the fetus by abdominal surgery (hysterotomy)
Chadwick's sign	blue soft cervix occurring normally during pregnancy
Chandelier's sign	cervix motion tenderness on palpation
Cheyne-Stokes respirations	crescendo/decrescendo respiratory pattern interspersed between periods of apnea
Cooley's anemia	thalasemia major
Coomb's test	postnatal blood test of cord blood for antibodies against fetal blood type (Rh neg mother, Rh pos fetus)
Cullen's sign	bluish color encircling the umbilicus and indicative of blood in the peritoneal cavity
Cushing's syndrome	hypersecretion of the adrenal cortex causing excessive production of glucocorticoids; may be caused by a tumor
Down syndrome	extra chromosome (trisomy) of 21 or 22, variety of signs and symptoms including retardation, sloping forehead, flat nose or absent bridge, and generally dwarfed physique
Electra complex	girls' sexual attraction toward their fathers and rivalry with their mothers
Fallopian tubes	uterine tubes
Giardia	genus of protozoan flagellate causing dysentery
Glasgow Coma Scale	international scale used in grading neurologic response
Graafian follicle	mature vesicular follicle of the ovary, matures ovum and secretes estrogen and progesterone
Grave's disease	disease characterized by hyperthyroidism, exophthalmic goiter, and thyromegaly, and dermopathy
Guillain-Barre syndrome	autoimmune inflammation causing destruction to the myelin sheath
Harlequin color change	one half of the newborn's body is red or ruddy and the other half appears pale
Heberden's node	enlargement of the distal interphalangeal joint of the finger
HELLP syndrome	pregnancy-induced hypertension, hemolysis, elevated liver enzymes and low platelets
Hirsutism	excessive body hair
Hodgkin's disease	cancerous lymphoreticular tumor
Homan's sign	pain in the calf when the foot is dorsiflexed

Horner's syndrome	paralysis of the cervical sympathetic nerve causing contracted pupil and blepharoptosis
Korotkoff's sounds	sounds generated when the flow of blood through an artery is altered by the inflation of a blood pressure cuff around the extremity
Korsakoff's syndrome	polyneuritic psychosis caused by chronic alcoholism
Kussmaul's respirations	respirations characterized by extreme increased rate and depth, as in diabetic ketoacidosis
Lou Gehrig's disease	amyotrophic lateral sclerosis
Mantoux test	test for tuberculosis
McBurney's point	anatomic location that is approximately at the normal location of the appendix in the RLQ; point of increased tenderness in appendicitis
Mongolian spots	various irregularly sized areas of deep bluish pigmentation on the upper back, shoulders, buttocks, and lumbosacral area of newborns of African, Latino, and Asian descent
Mongolism	obsolete term for Down syndrome
Montgomery's tubercles	sebaceous and milk glands present on the areola that produce secretions during breastfeeding
Murphy's sign	abnormal finding elicited during abdominal palpation in the RUQ and revealing gallbladder inflammation, patient will abruptly stop inspiration and complain of a sharp pain
Nabothian cysts	small, round, yellow lesions on the cervical surface
Non-Hodgkin's lymphoma	lymphoma that arises directly from the thymus gland
Oedipus complex	boys' sexual attraction to their mothers and feelings of rivalry toward their fathers

Paget's disease	1. malignant neoplasm of the mammary ducts 2. osteitis deformans
Papanicolaou test	Pap smear, tissue slide examination to detect cervical cancer
Parkinson's disease	chronic degenerative nerve disease characterized by palsy, muscle stiffness and weakness, tremor, and fatigue and malaise
Persian Gulf syndrome	variety of symptoms experienced by veterans of the Persian Gulf War including respiratory, gastrointestinal, joint, and muscle discomforts, fatigue, and memory loss
Rosving's sign	technique to elicit referred pain indicative of peritoneal inflammation
Skene's glands	paraurethral glands
Snellen chart	chart used for testing distance vision using standardized numbers and letters of various sizes
Stensen's ducts	openings from the parotids glands
Tay-Sachs disease	autosomal recessive trait inherited causing lack of hexosaminase A; disease is characterized by mental and physical retardation, blindness, convulsions, cephalomegaly, and death by age 4
Tourette's syndrome	symptoms include lack of muscle coordination, spasms, tics, grunts, barks, involuntary swearing, and coprolalia
Weber's test	tuning fork used to measure hearing loss and determine if it is conductive or sensoneural
Wharton's ducts	openings to the submaxillary glands

Reference: Estes, *Health Assessment & Physical Examination.* Delmar 1997, and *Tabor's Cyclopedic Medical Dictionary,* 18th Ed. F. A. Davis 1993.

INDEX OF TERMS

INDEX OF WORD PARTS LEARNED

License Agreement for Delmar Learning, a division of Thomson Learning

Educational Software/Data

You the customer, and Delmar Learning, a division of Thomson Learning, Inc. incur certain benefits, rights, and obligations to each other when you open this package and use the software/data it contains. BE SURE YOU READ THE LICENSE AGREEMENT CAREFULLY, SINCE BY USING THE SOFTWARE/DATA YOU INDICATE YOU HAVE READ, UNDERSTOOD, AND ACCEPTED THE TERMS OF THIS AGREEMENT.

Your rights:

1. You enjoy a non-exclusive license to use the software/data on a single microcomputer in consideration for payment of the required license fee, (which may be included in the purchase price of an accompanying print component), or receipt of this software/data, and your acceptance of the terms and conditions of this agreement.
2. You acknowledge that you do not own the aforesaid software/data. You also acknowledge that the software/data is furnished "as is," and contains copyrighted and/or proprietary and confidential information of Delmar Learning, a division of Thomson Learning, Inc. or its licensors.

There are limitations on your rights:

1. You may not copy or print the software/data for any reason whatsoever, except to install it on a hard drive on a single microcomputer and to make one archival copy, unless copying or printing is expressly permitted in writing or statements recorded on the diskette(s).
2. You may not revise, translate, convert, disassemble or otherwise reverse engineer the software/data except that you may add to or rearrange any data recorded on the media as part of the normal use of the software/data.
3. You may not sell, license, lease, rent, loan, or otherwise distribute or network the software/data except that you may give the software/data to a student or an instructor for use at school or, temporarily at home.

Should you fail to abide by the Copyright Law of the United States as it applies to this software/data your license to use it will become invalid. You agree to erase or otherwise destroy the software/data immediately after receiving note of Delmar Learning, a division of Thomson Learning, Inc. termination of this agreement for violation of its provisions.

Delmar Learning, a division of Thomson Learning, Inc. gives you a LIMITED WARRANTY covering the enclosed software/data. The LIMITED WARRANTY follows this License.

This license is the entire agreement between you and Delmar Learning, a division of Thomson Learning, Inc. interpreted and enforced under New York law.

This warranty does not extend to the software or information recorded on the media. The software and information are provided "AS IS." Any statements made about the utility of the software or information are not to be considered as express or implied warranties. Delmar Learning, a division of Thomson Learning, Inc. will not be liable for incidental or consequential damages of any kind incurred by you, the consumer, or any other user.

Some states do not allow the exclusion or limitation of incidental or consequential damages, or limitations on the duration of implied warranties, so the above limitation or exclusion may not apply to you.

This warranty gives you specific legal rights, and you may also have other rights which vary from state to state. Address all correspondence to: Delmar Learning, a division of Thomson Learning, Inc. Executive Woods, 5 Maxwell Drive, Clifton Park, New York 12065-2919. Attention: Technology Department

Limited Warranty

Delmar Learning, a division of Thomson Learning, Inc. warrants to the original licensee/purchaser of this copy of microcomputer software/data and the media on which it is recorded that the media will be free from defects in material and workmanship for ninety (90) days from the date of original purchase. All implied warranties are limited in duration to this ninety (90) day period. THEREAFTER, ANY IMPLIED WARRANTIES, INCLUDING IMPLIED WARRANTIES OF MERCHANTABILITY AND FITNESS FOR A PARTICULAR PURPOSE, ARE EXCLUDED. THIS WARRANTY IS IN LIEU OF ALL OTHER WARRANTIES, WHETHER ORAL OR WRITTEN, EXPRESS OR IMPLIED.

If you believe the media is defective please return it during the ninety day period to the address shown below. Defective media will be replaced without charge provided that it has not been subjected to misuse or damage.

This warranty does not extend to the software or information recorded on the media. The software and information are provided "AS IS." Any statements made about the utility of the software or information are not to be considered as express or implied warranties.

Limitation of liability: Our liability to you for any losses shall be limited to direct damages, and shall not exceed the amount you paid for the software. In no event will we be liable to you for any indirect, special, incidental, or consequential damages (including loss of profits) even if we have been advised of the possibility of such damages.

Some states do not allow the exclusion or limitation of incidental or consequential damages, or limitations on the duration of implied warranties, so the above limitation or exclusion may not apply to you. This warranty gives you specific legal rights, and you may also have other rights which vary from state to state. Address all correspondence to: Delmar Learning, a division of Thomson Learning, Inc. Executive Woods, 5 Maxwell Drive, Clifton Park, New York 12065-2919. Attention: Technology Department

Setup Instructions for Activity CD-ROM to accompany Medical Terminology: A Programmed Systems Approach, Ninth Edition

1. Double click My Computer.
2. Double click the Control Panel icon.
3. Double click Add/Remove Programs.
4. Click the Install button and follow the on-screen prompts from there.

System Requirements:

- Operating System: Microsoft® Windows® 95 or better
- Processor: Pentium or faster
- Memory: 24 MB or more
- Hard-disk space: 10 MB or more
- CD-ROM drive: 2x